Dilemmas in Clinical Cardiology

Books Available in Cardiovascular Clinics Series

Dilemmas in Clinical Cardiology

Melvin D. Cheitlin, M.D. / Editor

Professor of Medicine
University of California, San Francisco
Associate Chief of Cardiology
San Francisco General Hospital
San Francisco, California

CARDIOVASCULAR CLINICS
Albert N. Brest, M.D. / Editor-in-Chief

James C. Wilson Professor of Medicine
Director, Division of Cardiology
Jefferson Medical College
Philadelphia, Pennsylvania

 F. A. DAVIS COMPANY ● Philadelphia

Printed in the United States of America

Last digit indicates print number: 10 9 8 7 6 5 4 3 2 1

Printed on acid-free paper effective with Volume 17, Number 1.

NOTE: As new scientific information becomes available through basic and clinical research, recommended treatments and drug therapies undergo changes. The author(s) and publisher have done everything possible to make this book accurate, up-to-date, and in accord with accepted standards at the time of publication. However, the reader is advised always to check product information (package inserts) for changes and new information regarding dose and contraindications before administering any drug. Caution is especially urged when using new or infrequently ordered drugs.

Library of Congress Cataloging in Publication Data

Cardiovascular clinics. 21/1
    Philadelphia, F. A. Davis, 1969–
        v.   ill.   27 cm.
    Editor: v. 1-   A. N. Brest
    Key title: Cardiovascular clinics, ISSN 0069-0384.
    1. Cardiovascular system—Diseases—Collected works.   I.
Brest, Albert N., ed.
    [DNLM: W1 CA77N]
RC681.A1C27   616.1   70-6558
ISBN 0-8036-1712-7   MARC-S

Editor's Commentary

Dilemmas abound in clinical cardiology. Should all patients have cardiac catheterization after myocardial infarction? Is multivessel angioplasty preferable to coronary bypass surgery? Is valve surgery indicated in asymptomatic patients with severe valvular regurgitation? Should all patients with atrial fibrillation be anticoagulated prior to cardioversion? The contributors to this book discuss these controversial issues, as well as many other important dilemmas faced regularly by clinical practitioners. I am extremely grateful to Melvin D. Cheitlin for his guidance in the formulation of this issue, and we are both indebted to the individual authors for their thoughtful contributions.

Albert N. Brest, M.D.
Editor-in-Chief

Contributors

Mark W. Anderson, M.D
Professor of Radiology
University of California, San Francisco Medical Center
San Francisco, California

Michael A. Azrin, M.D.
Cardiology Division
Yale University School of Medicine
New Haven, Connecticut

Kanu Chatterjee, M.B., F.R.C.P.
Lucie Stern Professor of Medicine
Associate Chief, Division of Cardiology
University of California, San Francisco
San Francisco, California

Melvin D. Cheitlin, M.D.
Professor of Medicine
University of California, San Francisco
Associate Chief of Cardiology
San Francisco General Hospital
San Francisco, California

Richard B. Devereux, M.D.
Associate Professor of Medicine
Cornell University Medical College
Director, Echocardiography Laboratory
The New York Hospital
New York, New York

Laurence M. Epstein, M.D.
Clinical Cardiac Electrophysiology and Cardiovascular Research
University of California, San Francisco
San Francisco, California

Annmarie Errichetti, M.D.
Assistant Professor of Medicine
University of Massachusetts Medical School
Director of Cardiac Noninvasive Laboratory
The Medical Center of Central Massachusetts/Memorial
Worcester, Massachusetts

Michael D. Ezekowitz, M.D., Ph.D.
Associate Professor of Medicine (Cardiology)
Yale University School of Medicine
New Haven, Connecticut

Valentin Fuster, M.D.
Arthur M. and Hilda A. Master Professor of Medicine
Chief, Division of Cardiology
Mt. Sinai Medical Center
New York, New York

William H. Gaasch, M.D.
Professor of Medicine
University of Massachusetts Medical School
Chief, Cardiology Section
The Medical Center of Central Massachusetts/Memorial
Worcester, Massachusetts

Barry H. Greenberg, M.D.
Professor of Medicine
Division of Cardiology
Oregon Health Sciences University
Portland, Oregon

Joshua M. Greenberg, M.D.
Assistant Professor of Medicine
University of Massachusetts Medical School
Director, Cardiac Catheterization Laboratory
The Medical Center of Central Massachusetts/Memorial
Worcester, Massachusetts

Rolf M. Gunnar, M.D., F.A.C.P., F.R.C.P.
John W. Clarke Professor of Medicine
Chairman, Department of Medicine
Loyola University School of Medicine
Maywood, Illinois

Jonathan L. Halperin, M.D.
Associate Professor of Medicine
Division of Cardiology
Mount Sinai Medical Center
New York, New York

Charles B. Higgins, M.D.
Professor of Radiology
Chief, Magnetic Resonance Imaging
University of California, San Francisco Medical Center
San Francisco, California

Russell J. Ivanhoe, M.D.
Attending Cardiologist
Florida Hospital
Orlando, Florida

Spencer B. King III, M.D.
Professor of Medicine (Cardiology) and Radiology
Director, Andreas Gruentzig Cardiovascular Center
Emory University School of Medicine
Atlanta, Georgia

Paul Kligfield, M.D.
Associate Professor of Medicine
Director, Cardiac Graphics Laboratory
Cornell University Medical College
The New York Hospital
New York, New York

Daniel L. Kulick, M.D.
Assistant Professor of Medicine
Director, Cardiac Catheterization Laboratory
University of Southern California School of Medicine
Los Angeles, California

Herbert J. Levine, M.D.
Professor of Medicine
Cardiology Section
Tufts University School of Medicine
Senior Physician
New England Medical Center
Boston, Massachusetts

Howard S. Lewis, M.D.
Division of Cardiology
Oregon Health Sciences University
Portland, Oregon

Barry M. Massie, M.D.
Professor of Medicine
University of California, San Francisco
Director, Coronary Care Unit and Hypertension Unit
Veterans Administration Medical Center
San Francisco, California

Charles R. McKay, M.D.
Associate Professor of Medicine
Department of Internal Medicine
Division of Cardiovascular Disease
University of Iowa College of Medicine
Iowa City, Iowa

Khether E. Raby, M.D.
Department of Medicine
Cardiovascular Division
Brigham and Women's Hospital
Boston, Massachusetts

Shahbudin H. Rahimtoola, M.B., F.R.C.P.
George C. Griffith Professor of Cardiology
Professor of Medicine
Chief, Section of Cardiology
University of Southern California School of Medicine
Los Angeles, California

Stuart Rich, M.D.
Associate Professor of Medicine
Chief, Division of Cardiology
University of Illinois at Chicago
Chicago, Illinois

Melvin M. Scheinman, M.D.
Professor of Medicine
Chairman, Clinical Cardiac Electrophysiology Section
University of California, San Francisco
San Francisco, California

Andrew P. Selwyn, M.D.
Associate Professor of Medicine
Harvard Medical School
Director, Cardiac Catheterization Laboratory
Brigham and Women's Hospital
Boston, Massachusetts

James P. Srebro, M.D.
Assistant Professor of Medicine
Division of Cardiology
University of California, San Francisco
San Francisco, California

Peter Stecy, M.D.
Assistant Professor of Medicine
Loyola University School of Medicine
Maywood, Illinois

Bernardo Stein, M.D.
Division of Cardiology
Mount Sinai Medical Center
New York, New York

Eric J. Topol, M.D.
Associate Professor of Internal Medicine
Director, Cardiac Catheterization Laboratories
University of Michigan Medical Center
Ann Arbor, Michigan

Contents

PART 1

Coronary Heart Disease

CHAPTER 1

Is Noninvasive Risk Stratification Sufficient, or Should All Patients Undergo Cardiac Catheterization and Angiography after a Myocardial Infarction?

Daniel L. Kulick, M.D.
Shahbudin H. Rahimtoola, M.B., F.R.C.P.

DEFINITION OF THE PROBLEM

Approximately 500,000 to 900,000 patients are hospitalized yearly in the United States with acute myocardial infarction.[1-3] In 1986, 758,000 hospital admissions were recorded for this condition.[4] Of these patients, 80 percent or more will survive to hospital discharge.[2] Among these survivors of the early phase of myocardial infarction, the one-year mortality has ranged from 8 to 13 percent,[1-3,5-10] with a subsequent mortality of 3 to 5 percent per year thereafter.[1,2,5-7,11] Of the patients dying in the first year following hospital discharge, 50 to 75 percent of the deaths occur in the first three to six months.[3,8,10,12-16] Hospital survivors of acute myocardial infarction can be subdivided into a high-risk group with a mortality in the first year of up to 50 percent and into a low-risk group with a one-year mortality of 5 percent or less.[2,12,17,18] In recent years, there has been a major thrust to identify these two subgroups of patients early, preferably before hospital discharge, in order to apply appropriate therapeutic options in individual patients.

In the hospital phase of acute myocardial infarction, subgroups of patients at high risk of adverse events in the months following hospital discharge can be identified by four general criteria: (1) Spontaneous myocardial ischemia occurring more than 24 to 48 hours after hospital admission has been reported in up to 18 percent of patients[19-21] and identifies a group of patients with an increased rate of early reinfarction[22,23] and mortality.[7,10,19,23] These patients also have an increased incidence of multivessel coronary artery disease.[19,21,24] (2) Clinical congestive heart failure and/or left ventricular systolic dysfunction is a powerful predictor of increased

3

mortality after myocardial infarction.[2,10,12,17,18,25,26] In fact, the postinfarction left ventricular ejection fraction may be the single most important predictor of survival.[3,27,28] (3) The presence of complex and/or frequent ventricular arrhythmias in the late hospital phase of myocardial infarction is associated with an increased mortality in the year following hospital discharge.[10,17,29-32] (4) A history of prior myocardial infarction confers an increased mortality risk.[2,8,10,25,33] Overall, the reported incidence of myocardial infarction complicated by one or more of the above variables has been reported to range from 15 to 48 percent.[21,34-37]

Whereas patients with myocardial infarction with the above complications are clearly at an increased risk of subsequent mortality, what is the outcome of the majority of survivors of myocardial infarction who do not fall into any of the above high-risk subgroups? We have learned that within this large group of patients, there are those who will have a relatively poor prognosis in the year following infarction (moderate risk) and others in whom the one-year mortality is truly small (low risk). *The clinical challenge is to identify the patients at moderate risk, as well as those few patients in the low-risk group who are at risk of death.*

With the demonstration of the safety of predischarge submaximal exercise testing following an uncomplicated myocardial infarction,[38-44] numerous studies have demonstrated the efficacy of noninvasive testing in identifying patients at increased risk following myocardial infarction.[34,35,37-39,41,43-47] Based on these findings, many have advocated a noninvasive risk stratification approach to the management of patients following myocardial infarction, reserving cardiac catheterization and angiography for those patients who fall into high-risk subgroups based on clinical parameters and results of noninvasive testing, including some form of exercise test and measure of left ventricular function.[3,12,18,48,49]

This is a reasonable strategy that is generally accepted and with which we concur in principle. However, an alternative strategy is to consider early cardiac catheterization and angiography in all or most patients with acute myocardial infarction. At present, there is little debate over the approach to the patient with a complicated myocardial infarction; as already noted, the poor prognosis associated with recurrent myocardial ischemia, left ventricular dysfunction, or complex ventricular arrhythmias following myocardial infarction mandates an intensive approach to these patients. The issue lies with the patient with an uncomplicated first myocardial infarction, in whom both moderate- and low-risk subsets clearly exist. In light of the important diagnostic, therapeutic, and prognostic information that can be gained from cardiac catheterization and angiography, as well as certain limitations inherent in noninvasive testing, a strong case can be made for performing cardiac catheterization in all these patients. The balance of this discussion will defend this position.

INFORMATION LEARNED FROM CARDIAC CATHETERIZATION AND ANGIOGRAPHY

Following acute myocardial infarction, cardiac catheterization with left ventricular and coronary angiography as a single test yields important information regarding cardiac hemodynamics, left ventricular function, and the extent and severity of coronary artery disease (Table 1–1). Furthermore, the angiographic severity of a given coronary artery stenosis may reveal direct information about the physiologic significance of the obstruction.[50] From an integrated analysis of left

Table 1–1. Information Learned from
Cardiac Catheterization and
Angiography

Cardiac hemodynamics
Left ventricular function
Extent and severity of coronary artery disease
Physiologic significance of coronary artery disease
Estimation of amount of jeopardized myocardium
Clues to presence of hibernating or stunned myocardium

ventricular wall motion and coronary artery stenoses, one might estimate the amount of still viable, but *jeopardized* or *vulnerable myocardium*.[33,51] Moreover, it may provide important clues to the presence of hibernating, and possibly stunned, myocardium (Figs. 1–1 and 1–2).[52,54] All of this information provides important prognostic and therapeutic data *(vide infra)* in the patient following a myocardial infarction.

Cardiac catheterization and angiography carries a mortality risk of less than or equal to 0.1 to 0.3 percent[55–58] and has been demonstrated to be safe in acutely ill patients in general[59] and in patients following acute myocardial infarction specifically.[21,25,27,35,60–64] For the experienced and skilled operator functioning in a quality laboratory, therefore, the risk of cardiac catheterization should not be a significant factor in the decision-making process of whether or not to perform the procedure.

What, then, are the expected results of coronary angiography in a group of survivors of acute myocardial infarction? Numerous angiographic studies of such patients have demonstrated a high incidence of multivessel coronary artery disease, ranging from 30 to 88 percent, with the vast majority of such studies reporting an incidence of approximately 50 to 75 percent (Table 1–2).[21,24,25,27,33,35,36,60–62,65–86] Furthermore, the incidence of three-vessel coronary artery disease in these patients has been reported to range from 25 to 50 percent,[21,27,33,60,65,68,69,74] and the incidence of left main coronary artery disease from 1 to 12 percent.[21,24,27,33,35,60,61,66,69,74] Thus a large proportion, if not the majority, of patients surviving an acute myocardial infarction have coronary artery disease of such severity and magnitude that many would be offered coronary revascularization on the basis of coronary artery anatomy alone by most physicians.[52,87,88]

Cardiac catheterization and angiography offer powerful prognostic information for survivors of acute myocardial infarction. Numerous studies have demonstrated that the survival of patients with coronary artery disease is directly related to the number of diseased vessels,[26,89–95] and this relationship is specifically true for patients following myocardial infarction. Schulman and associates[33] have demonstrated an event-free survival (freedom from death, nonfatal recurrent myocardial infarction, need for coronary artery bypass surgery) of only 38 percent at five years in patients with three-vessel coronary artery disease documented after acute myocardial infarction; other investigators have similarly demonstrated that the presence of multivessel coronary artery disease following myocardial infarction is a potent predictor of increased mortality.[25,72,76] Furthermore, four independent series have shown the presence of multivessel coronary artery disease to be the best predictor of long-term mortality following myocardial infarction, having more predictive power than either clinical variables or noninvasive testing.[24,27,35,96]

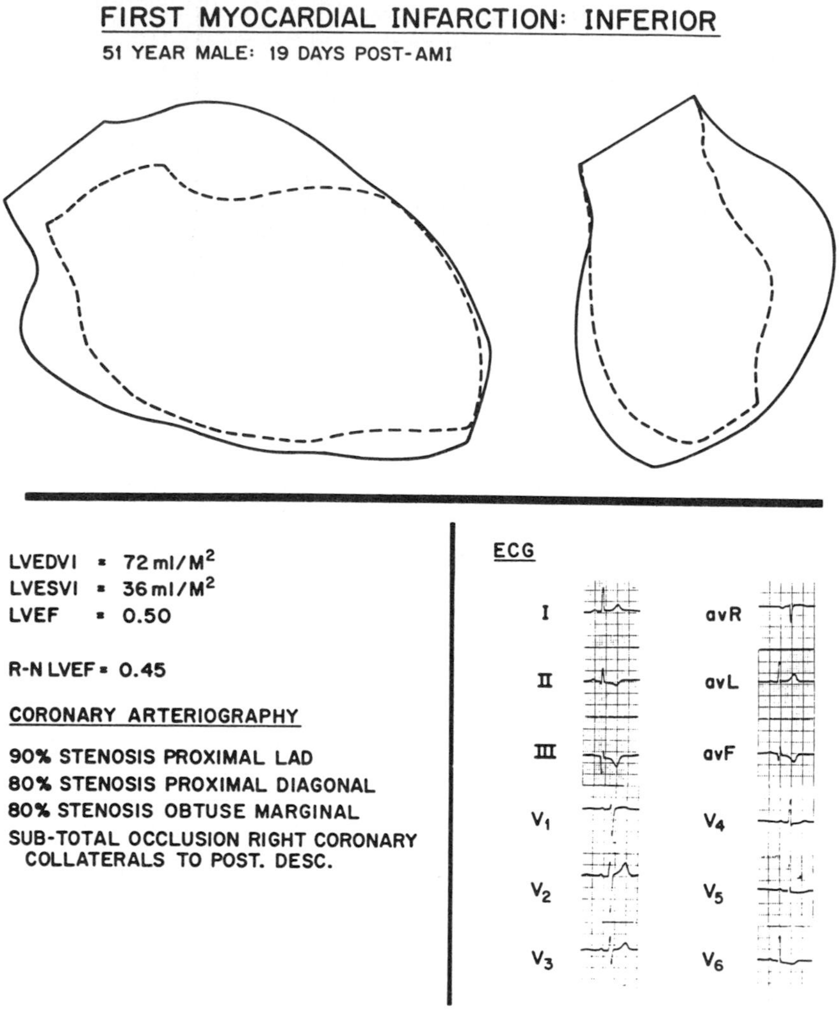

FIRST MYOCARDIAL INFARCTION: INFERIOR
51 YEAR MALE: 19 DAYS POST-AMI

LVEDVI = 72 ml/M^2
LVESVI = 36 ml/M^2
LVEF = 0.50

R-N LVEF = 0.45

CORONARY ARTERIOGRAPHY

90% STENOSIS PROXIMAL LAD
80% STENOSIS PROXIMAL DIAGONAL
80% STENOSIS OBTUSE MARGINAL
SUB-TOTAL OCCLUSION RIGHT CORONARY
  COLLATERALS TO POST. DESC.

ECG

I   aVR
II aVL
III aVF
V$_1$ V$_4$
V$_2$ V$_5$
V$_3$ V$_6$

Figure 1–1. Asymptomatic patient prior to sudden onset of acute inferior myocardial infarction. Borderline impaired LVEF at rest. Hypokinetic/akinetic inferior wall with Q waves in leads II, III, and aVF. Anterior wall is akinetic, but in leads V$_1$–V$_6$, I, and aVL, there are no pathologic Q waves and the R waves are normal. There are severe proximal coronary artery lesions. The anterior wall is hibernating and the inferior wall is stunned; however, because blood flow may not have been fully restored to the posterior descending artery, the inferior wall could have been hibernating as well. (From Rahimtoola,[54] with permission.)

In addition to multivessel coronary artery disease, the presence of disease in the proximal segment of the left anterior descending (LAD) coronary artery is an independent "high-risk" lesion.[33,91,97] Schuster and coworkers[98] have demonstrated that the majority of patients dying from acute myocardial infarction have proximal LAD thrombosis, and Vlodaver and Edwards[99] found a 78 percent incidence of proximal LAD disease in a large autopsy series. In two large prospective series, Taylor[25] and DeFeyter[24] and their colleagues found that 85 percent and 82 percent, respectively, of all mortality in patients following myocardial infarction occurred in the subgroup with proximal LAD disease.

In addition to the extent of coronary artery disease, the degree of left ven-

FIRST MYOCARDIAL INFARCTION: INFERIOR

51 YEAR MALE: 20 DAYS POST-AMI, CBS:

    LIMA TO LAD
    SVG's TO DIAGONAL, OBTUSE MARGINAL
        AND POST. DESCENDING

---

7 MONTHS POST-OP:

RN-LVEF = 0.63
NORMAL WALL MOTION
(infero-apical slightly reduced motion?)

TREADMILL: 11 MINUTES BRUCE PROTOCOL

HR: 101% AGE-PREDICTED MAXIMUM
BP: NORMAL
ECG: NORMAL
THALLIUM-201: UPTAKE - NORMAL AND UNIFORM
                WASHOUT - NORMAL AND UNIFORM
INFERO-POST: SMALL AREA OF THINNING

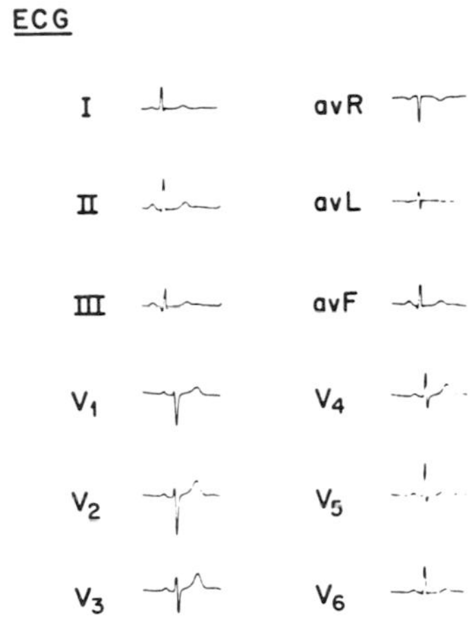

ECG

I   avR
II   avL
III   avF
V1   V4
V2   V5
V3   V6

Figure 1-2. Same patient as depicted in Figure 1-1. Patient had four coronary bypass grafts and is asymptomatic. Seven months after surgery, left ventricular ejection fraction at rest is normal. ECG, regional wall motion, and treadmill with thallium 201 are all virtually normal. LIMA = left internal mammary artery graft; LAD = left anterior descending coronary artery; SVG = saphenous vein grafts. (From Rahimtoola,[54] with permission.)

tricular dysfunction, as reflected by the left ventricular ejection fraction, is a potent independent predictor of prognosis following myocardial infarction.[2,3,12,17,18,24,25,27,33,100] In a detailed prospective analysis of angiographic and exercise variables, Norris and coworkers[28] found the left ventricular ejection fraction to be the single best predictor of survival following myocardial infarction. Schulman and associates[33] recently demonstrated that the identification of risk segments on the postmyocardial infarction left ventricular angiogram, defined as segments of myocardium still contracting but supplied by high-grade coronary artery stenoses, provided important long-term prognostic information following myocardial infarction. It is clear, therefore, that a single cardiac catheterization provides important prognostic data derived from both coronary artery anatomy and left ventricular function, as well as an integrated analysis of the two.

Although the valuable prognostic data learned from cardiac catheterization and angiography are well documented, another question is whether one can offer therapy that may alter the prognosis favorably in patients identified to be at high risk following myocardial infarction. Whereas this issue was unsettled 10 years ago,[101] it is now clear that many of these high-risk patients can benefit from revascularization therapy. The data from three large, multicenter randomized trials and two nonrandomized studies of coronary artery bypass surgery in patients with coronary artery disease clearly demonstrate a survival benefit with revascularization in

Table 1–2. Coronary Arteriography after Myocardial Infarction

Authors	Cited Ref. No.	MVD	3V CAD	LMCAD
Turner, et al	21	67%	35%	8.5%
DeFeyter, et al	24	55%		1%
Taylor, et al	25	74%		
Sanz, et al	27	59%	26%	1%
Schulman, et al	33	73%	50%	8%
Gibson, et al	35	61%		2%
Schwartz, et al	36	71%		
Betriu, et al	60	59%	25%	1%
Roubin, et al	61	35%	9%	1%
Bertrand, et al	62	75%		
Griffith, et al	65	68%	45%	
Veenbrink, et al	67	25%		
Akhras, et al	68	73%	49%	
Starling, et al	69	72%	40%	2%
Williams, et al	70	65%		
Wasserman, et al	71	69%		
Abraham, et al	72	43%		
Weiner, et al	73	59%		
Morris, et al	74	88%	47%	12%
Abraham, et al	75	30%		
Nicod, et al	76	62%		
Patterson, et al	77	63%		
Schulze, et al	78	63%		
Tubau, et al	79	64%		
Turner, et al	80	78%		
Castellanet, et al	81	78%		
Paine, et al	82	66%		
Savran, et al	83	45%		
Pichard, et al	84	70%		
Rigo, et al	85	63%		
Van Der Wall, et al	86	44%		
Average		62%	36%	4%

MVD = multivessel coronary artery disease; 3V CAD = 3-vessel coronary artery disease; LMCAD = left main coronary artery disease

patients with left main coronary artery disease, three-vessel coronary artery disease with or without abnormal left ventricular function, and two-vessel coronary artery disease that includes the proximal segment of the left anterior descending artery (especially in the presence of significant myocardial ischemia); the benefit may be greater in patients with depressed left ventricular function.[52,88,102–108] In patients with unstable angina following myocardial infarction, the excellent long-term survival following coronary bypass surgery is most impressive.[109,110] In a retrospective, nonrandomized analysis of patients surviving myocardial infarction with three-vessel coronary artery disease, Akhras and colleagues[68] demonstrated only a 2 percent mortality at 37 months in the group receiving coronary bypass surgery, as opposed to a 38 percent mortality in the group receiving medical therapy. Rogers and associates[51] have shown that coronary bypass surgery markedly enhances three-year survival in patients following myocardial infarction who have multiple *jeopardized* segments (identical to "risk" segments, defined above) on left ventricular angiography. One may conclude from the above data that the identification of high-risk patients at cardiac catheterization following myocardial infarction allows for the implementation of therapy that may substantially improve the prognosis for these patients.

LIMITATIONS OF NONINVASIVE TESTING FOLLOWING MYOCARDIAL INFARCTION

Since initial reports demonstrating the safety and efficacy of predischarge exercise testing in defining high- and low-risk subgroups of patients with myocardial infarction not complicated by recurrent ischemia, heart failure, or complex ventricular arrhythmias, it has become commonplace to stratify such patients according to risk as determined by clinical criteria and noninvasive tests prior to hospital discharge, reserving cardiac catheterization and angiography for patients demonstrating abnormalities on noninvasive testing.[3,12,18,48] All noninvasive risk stratification strategies employ some form of exercise testing, as well as an independent measure of left ventricular function (radionuclide angiography or echocardiography). If one elects to follow such an approach, it is necessary to be aware of certain limitations inherent in noninvasive testing following myocardial infarction.

First and foremost, studies that have evaluated the prognostic role of exercise testing following uncomplicated myocardial infarction have not considered three key subgroups: (1) the "elderly" (patients aged 65 to 70 years and older), (2) patients unable to perform the exercise test, and (3) patients who have received thrombolytic treatment. As will be discussed in detail later, "elderly" patients and those receiving thrombolytic treatment may represent subsets with a unique risk, and inasmuch as they have been excluded from clinical studies of exercise testing following myocardial infarction, there are no published data to support noninvasive risk stratification in these patients. For a variety of reasons, exercise testing cannot be performed in all patients following myocardial infarction; these include obvious high-risk cardiac conditions, such as heart failure, conduction disturbances, arrhythmias, and severe myocardial ischemia, as well as noncardiac conditions including peripheral vascular disease, noncardiac medical illness, and musculoskeletal disorders. Available data indicate that 10 to 22 percent of patients will be unable to perform an exercise test following an uncomplicated myocardial infarction (Table 1–3).[34,35,37,42,111–114] Those patients unable to exercise have been

Table 1–3. Patients Unable to Exercise Following Uncomplicated Myocardial Infarction, and Their Mortality

Authors	Cited Ref. No.	% Unable to Exercise	Mortality
Deckers, et al	34	16%	10% (1 yr)
Gibson, et al	35	15%	
Fuller, et al	37	10%	
Ibsen, et al	42	15%	
Gibson, et al	111	12%	13% (22 mo)
Chaitman, et al	112	15%	
Gibson, et al	113	19%	
Krone, et al	114	22%	14% (1 yr)
Average		15%	12%

demonstrated to be at significantly increased risk of mortality and cardiac morbidity in the year following myocardial infarction,[10,34,111,114] suggesting that simple inability to perform an exercise test represents a high-risk subgroup that may benefit from early invasive testing.

To interpret clinical trials of exercise testing following myocardial infarction, one must be clear as to which exercise variable carries the most prognostic value; the available data on this question are conflicting. Early studies by Theroux[38] and DeBusk[39] and their colleagues suggested that although ST segment depression on the exercise electrocardiogram was predictive of increased mortality, chest pain during exercise testing was not. Conversely, Schwartz and coworkers[36] found ST segment depression not to be predictive of increased mortality, whereas exercise-induced angina was prognostically useful. Starling and associates[69] found that a combination of ST segment depression and chest pain during exercise testing was more predictive of multivessel coronary artery disease than was either variable alone, although the most sensitive variable was an inadequate blood pressure response during exercise. Other studies have found maximal exercise workload attained[34] or exercise duration[41] to be the best predictors of survival, with ST segment depression to be of much less prognostic value. Further complicating test interpretation, Handler and Sowton[115] have demonstrated marked day-to-day variability in patients undergoing consecutive predischarge submaximal exercise tests following myocardial infarction.

In an attempt to provide improved and more specific prognostic data, many investigators have advocated additional tests for the noninvasive assessment of patients following myocardial infarction. The addition of immediate and delayed imaging with thallium-201 to standard exercise testing has been demonstrated to be superior to simple exercise testing for the prediction of mortality, cardiac events, and multivessel coronary artery disease in many studies;[35,77,80,85,96] however, other studies have reported no increased benefit with thallium imaging.[72,86] The response of left ventricular ejection fraction during exercise, as measured by radionuclide angiography, has been reported to be of prognostic value following myocardial infarction,[71,76,116,117] although two series have found no additional prognostic benefit of exercise-induced changes in left ventricular function to that gained from resting studies alone.[118,119] Preliminary data are also available on the use of exercise two-dimensional echocardiography in the assessment of patients following myocardial infarction.[120,121] The addition of more complex tests to simple exercise testing following myocardial infarction raises several key issues. These tests may not be widely available, and they require complex equipment and expert interpretation to provide the high-quality results reported in the literature. *Importantly, the addition of multiple and sometimes repetitive tests can markedly increase the cost of a noninvasive approach to risk stratification following myocardial infarction.*

Another limitation of predischarge submaximal exercise testing is that many of the so-called negative tests are in fact inconclusive, because patients do not attain a sufficiently high workload to exclude myocardial ischemia reliably. From 25 to 35 percent of patients with a "negative" predischarge submaximal exercise test have been found to demonstrate ischemia on a standard full Bruce protocol test 6 to 12 weeks later.[37,47] This finding underscores the need for a second, more rigorous exercise test in patients discharged as being at "low risk" following myocardial infarction. Inasmuch as the majority of the mortality in the first year following myocardial infarction occurs in the first three to six months,[9,10,14] there is a small but finite

Table 1–4. Cardiac Mortality in Patients with Abnormal and Negative Predischarge Exercise Test Results after Uncomplicated Myocardial Infarction (% of all Cardiac Deaths Occurring in Group)

Authors	Cited Ref. No.	Abnormal Exercise Test	Negative Exercise Test
Theroux, et al	38	85%	15%
DeBusk, et al	39	40%	60%
Weld, et al	41	33%	67%
Sami, et al	123	43%	57%
Handler	124	81%	19%
Average		56%	44%

risk of a "low-risk" patient dying before a second, more definitive exercise test is performed; in one recent series, this sequence occurred in 2 percent of patients waiting for a second test.[122]

Although predischarge exercise testing may be able to separate large groups of survivors of myocardial infarction into high- and low-risk subsets, there will yet remain a number of patients classified as being at low risk by noninvasive testing who will nonetheless experience cardiac mortality in the year following myocardial infarction. In dealing with individual patients, if this number of noninvasive "false-negatives" is substantial, the clinician is faced with a difficult dilemma. If one carefully analyzes the available data, it becomes apparent that this is a significant issue. DeBusk and coworkers[39] reported a six-month cardiac mortality of 7 percent (2 of 31 patients) in patients with an abnormal exercise test 21 days following an uncomplicated myocardial infarction, as opposed to only a 1 percent (3 of 307 patients) cardiac mortality in those with a negative test. In this series, however, over 90 percent of the patients had a negative test, so, in fact, 60 percent of all cardiac deaths (3 of 5 deaths) occurring over a six-month period occurred in the "low-risk" group. Other investigators have similarly reported that 15 to 67 percent of all cardiac deaths will occur in patients without ischemic changes on exercise testing (Table 1–4).[38,41,123,124]

Given the powerful adverse prognostic implications of multivessel coronary artery disease associated with acute myocardial infarction, could the large percentage of cardiac deaths occurring in patients with negative exercise tests be related to poor sensitivity of this test for the detection of multivessel disease? In an analysis of 14 reported series in which patients underwent early exercise testing and coronary angiography following myocardial infarction, from 9 to 57 percent of patients with multivessel coronary artery disease had negative exercise tests, giving the test a sensitivity of 43 to 91 percent for the detection of multivessel disease (Table 1–5);[36,37,69,72–74,77,79–81,85,86,112,125] in 12 of these 14 studies, the sensitivity of exercise testing for the detection of multivessel disease was less than 80 percent. The addition of thallium imaging to the exercise test does not appear to improve on this finding, inasmuch as the reported sensitivity of exercise thallium testing for the detection of multivessel coronary artery disease following myocardial infarction ranges from only 51 to 71 percent.[72,77,80,85,86,113] Similarly, the predictive value of a negative predischarge exercise test for the absence of multivessel coronary artery disease is only

Table 1–5. Value of Exercise Test for Detection of Multivessel Coronary Artery Disease after Myocardial Infarction

	Cited Ref. No.	Sensitivity of ETT for MVD	Sensitivity of Ex-Tl 201 for MVD	Predictive Value of Negative ETT for Absence of MVD
Schwartz, et al	36	56%		44%
Fuller, et al	37	65%		72%
Griffith, et al	65			43%
Starling, et al	69	88%		69%
Abraham, et al	72	64%	64%	
Weiner, et al	73	91%		
Morris, et al	74	43%		
Patterson, et al	77	71%	65%	
Tubau, et al	79	72%		57%
Turner, et al	80	48%	68%	
Castellanet, et al	81	69%		
Rigo, et al	85	49%	51%	
Van Der Wall, et al	86	77%	66%	
Chaitman, et al	112	67%		
Gibson, et al	113		71%	
DeFeyter, et al	125	67%		
Average		66%	64%	57%

ETT = exercise treadmill test; Ex-Tl 201 = exercise test with immediate and delayed thallium 201 imaging; MVD = multivessel coronary artery disease

43 to 72 percent, suggesting that 28 to 57 percent of patients with negative tests will have multivessel disease.[36,37,65,69,79]

In summary, the limitations of noninvasive risk assessment following uncomplicated myocardial infarction are significant (Table 1–6).

EXPECTATIONS OF NONINVASIVE RISK STRATIFICATION

Keeping the aforementioned limitations of postmyocardial infarction exercise testing in mind, what are the expectations of a noninvasive risk stratification approach when applied to a large group of patients (Fig. 1–3). If one starts with 100 patients surviving a myocardial infarction uncomplicated by recurrent ischemia, heart failure, or complex ventricular arrhythmias, and excluding patients over the

Table 1–6. Limitations of Noninvasive Risk Assessment Following Myocardial Infarction

1. Only limited data are available in many subgroups
2. Exercise testing cannot be performed in all patients
3. High-quality, "state-of-the-art" testing may not be available in most centers
4. Of the patients who experience late cardiac mortality, about half of the deaths occur in the group with "negative" tests
5. Suboptimal sensitivity of exercise testing for the detection of multivessel coronary artery disease
6. Submaximal exercise testing may not achieve a sufficient workload to confidently exclude myocardial ischemia
7. Not an inexpensive approach, if one considers the frequent use of additive, repetitive tests

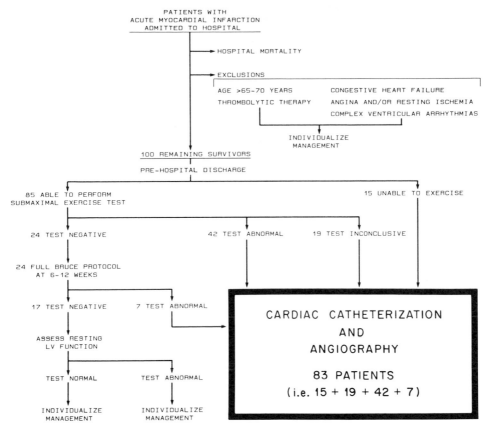

Figure 1–3. Expected results of a noninvasive risk-stratification approach to 100 hospital survivors of an uncomplicated acute myocardial infarction.

age of 65 to 70 years or those who have received thrombolytic treatment, the following analysis may be applied. From 10 to 22 percent of these patients will be unable to perform an exercise test;[34,35,37,42,111–114] this number can be approximated to 15 percent. Given the high risk in patients unable to perform an exercise test following myocardial infarction,[10,34,111,114] these 15 patients should undergo cardiac catheterization and angiography. Of the remaining 85 patients, from 9 to 72 percent will have an abnormal submaximal exercise test;[35–39,47,65,69,82,124,126,127] the average of these 12 series results in a 49 percent rate of positive exercise tests. Employing this average rate of exercise test positivity, 49 percent of 85 patients will yield an additional 42 patients requiring cardiac catheterization and angiography. Furthermore, from 16 to 29 percent of patients will have an "inconclusive" exercise test;[67,82] such patients have been demonstrated to have a high prevalence of multivessel coronary artery disease.[82] If one assumes an average of 22 percent of tests to be inconclusive, an additional 19 patients would warrant cardiac catheterization, bringing the total to 76 patients. Of the remaining 24 patients, 25 to 35 percent will have an abnormal full Bruce protocol stress test six to 12 weeks later;[37,47] assuming an average of 30 percent, an additional 7 patients will require cardiac catheterization. Overall, therefore, of 100 hospital survivors of an uncomplicated myocardial infarction who are less than or equal to 65 to 70 years of age and did not receive thrombolytic treatment, 83 will ultimately require cardiac catheterization and angiography following a risk stratification scheme using exercise testing alone. In addition, if one employs an independent noninvasive test of left ventricular function, some percentage of the remaining 17 patients will have occult left ventricular dysfunction and may ultimately require cardiac catheterization.

If one adds thallium imaging to the initial submaximal exercise test, 15 of 100 patients will still be unable to exercise; and of the remaining 85 patients, 65 percent (55 patients) will have an abnormal thallium study suggesting reversible ischemia.[35] Using this approach, therefore, at least 70 of 100 patients will still require cardiac catheterization and angiography. It is clear, therefore, that if one employs a noninvasive approach to risk assessment in patients following an uncomplicated myocardial infarction, then a significant majority will still require cardiac catheterization and angiography.

SPECIAL CONSIDERATIONS

Certain subsets of hospital survivors of acute myocardial infarction may possess unique risks and are discussed below.

Non-Q Wave Myocardial Infarction

Approximately 25 percent of all myocardial infarctions are of the non-Q wave variety.[5,128] This incidence may be increasing, and it will likely increase further with more widespread use of interventions to limit myocardial infarct size. Although the mortality in the first weeks following myocardial infarction is lower in these patients than in those with Q-wave myocardial infarction, their mortality at the end of 1 to 3 years is equal to that of patients with Q-wave infarction,[128–131] demonstrating that the late mortality in patients with non-Q wave myocardial infarction is in fact increased. In addition to having a high late mortality, patients with non-Q wave myocardial infarction have an increased reinfarction rate, ranging from 18 to 21 percent,[22,111,131,132] and a high rate of need for revascularization procedures.[111] Although one study found an increased incidence of multivessel coronary artery disease in patients with non-Q wave myocardial infarction,[133] the majority of studies have found no difference in the incidence of multivessel disease between patients with Q wave and non-Q wave myocardial infarction.[21,75,111,128,134] The primary explanation for the increased late mortality and morbidity in patients with non-Q wave myocardial infarction appears to be the high incidence of ischemia these patients exhibit following infarction; the incidence of recurrent ischemia in these patients has been reported to range from 30 to 64 percent.[20,128,132,135,136] Gibson and associates[111] demonstrated that 75 percent of their patients with non-Q wave myocardial infarction exhibited redistribution defects on exercise thallium testing. Inasmuch as this high incidence of late ischemia has been correlated with the increased morbid event rate observed in these patients,[22,111] a case can be made for performing early cardiac catheterization and angiography in most survivors of a non-Q wave myocardial infarction.

"Young" Patients

Recommendations exist in the literature for cardiac catheterization and angiography of all hospital survivors of acute myocardial infarction below a certain age,[5,49] although the precise age is somewhat arbitrary. Studies limiting coronary angiography to relatively "young" survivors of myocardial infarction (generally below the age of 60) have found a 25 to 59 percent incidence of multivessel coronary artery disease.[27,60,61,67,72,75,83] Given the earlier stated incidence of "false-negative" exercise tests in patients with multivessel disease, and the anticipated longer life expectancy (and longer "at-risk" period) of the younger patient, the recommendation to perform early cardiac catheterization in "young" patients (below age 50?) may not be unreasonable.

"Older" Patients

As stated earlier, nearly every reported clinical study on noninvasive risk stratification following myocardial infarction has excluded patients older than 65 to 70 years of age. For this reason, there are no data on the applicability of noninvasive risk assessment in this group of patients. In view of the increasing proportion of older patients in this country, and inasmuch as over three fourths of all deaths due to coronary artery disease in the United States occur in patients above the age of 65,[137] this issue is highly pertinent. Numerous studies have demonstrated up to a threefold increase in late mortality following myocardial infarction in patients over the ages of 60 to 70 years as opposed to those younger.[13,100,129,138-140] Patients in this "older" age group have been similarly demonstrated to have an increased incidence of high-risk multivessel coronary artery disease following myocardial infarction.[74,140] In the only reported study of risk assessment following myocardial infarction not excluding older patients, Morris and colleagues[74] found an 88 percent incidence of multivessel disease in a group of patients ranging in age to 83 years; most importantly, in those with multivessel disease, 57 percent had a negative exercise test. Appropriate "older" patients have been demonstrated to do as well following coronary artery bypass surgery as younger patients,[141] and they are also potential candidates for percutaneous transluminal coronary angioplasty. For this reason, early cardiac catheterization and angiography may be appropriate for most older (above ages 65 to 70 years?) survivors of acute myocardial infarction, if they are in otherwise good medical condition.

Patients Receiving Thrombolytic Treatment

Patients receiving thrombolytic treatment have not been included in reported clinical studies of noninvasive risk stratification following myocardial infarction; such patients represent an increasing proportion of all myocardial infarction patients. Thrombolytic treatment has been demonstrated to alter the natural history of acute myocardial infarction favorably by decreasing both early and late mortality;[142-144] the proper approach to early management of these patients is thus important to define. Thrombolytic treatment will be unsuccessful in establishing arterial patency in at least 25 percent of patients,[142,145,146] and from 12 to 29 percent of patients will have reocclusion of a successfully recanalized artery.[142,147,148] Califf and associates[149] recently demonstrated coronary angiography to be the only reliable means of assessing successful thrombolysis.

Following successful reperfusion, a significant residual stenosis often remains in the infarct-related artery, and this may impair recovery of left ventricular function.[150] Data exist suggesting that further reduction of the residual high-grade stenosis with percutaneous transluminal coronary angioplasty may enhance recovery of left ventricular function.[151-153] Stack and coworkers[154] recently demonstrated a combined approach of thrombolytic treatment and percutaneous transluminal coronary angioplasty to result in only a 2 percent one-year mortality in hospital survivors of acute myocardial infarction. For the assessment of successful reperfusion and possible need for further revascularization therapy, early cardiac catheterization and angiography may be appropriate in all patients following thrombolytic treatment; this approach has been suggested by some authors.[49,155] Large-scale randomized trials are presently ongoing to address this issue specifically.

Inferior Myocardial Infarction

Many studies have found an increased incidence of multivessel coronary artery disease in survivors of an uncomplicated inferior myocardial infarction.[24,62,70,72,79,112,156] Importantly, 31 to 38 percent of these patients will have severe disease in the proximal segment of the left anterior descending artery or left main coronary artery.[21,112,156] The presence of anterior ST-segment depression[157] or right ventricular infarction[158] in these patients is not reliably predictive of multivessel disease. For these reasons, cardiac catheterization and angiography may be appropriate in survivors of an inferior myocardial infarction.

Hibernating and Stunned Myocardium

Following myocardial infarction, areas of partially infarcted but reperfused and still viable myocardium may be "stunned," with delayed recovery of function. Furthermore, in patients with multivessel coronary artery disease, areas of noninfarcted but chronically hypoperfused myocardium may be hypocontractile, or *hibernating.*[52-54] Inasmuch as this dysfunction is reversible following successful coronary revascularization (Figs. 1–1 and 1–2),[54,159] cardiac catheterization and angiography would identify patients with reversible resting left ventricular dysfunction.

COST ANALYSIS

Concern exists regarding a perceived increased cost of performing cardiac catheterization and angiography in all survivors of myocardial infarction. As will be outlined below, the cost differential may not be substantial, particularly if one considers the frequent use of repetitive, additive noninvasive tests following myocardial infarction. As stated earlier, a single cardiac catheterization will yield important information on both the extent and the severity of coronary artery disease and left ventricular dysfunction, as well as an index of the amount of *jeopardized* myocardium present. Of course, following cardiac catheterization, some patients will require exercise testing to assess ischemic risk of moderate coronary artery disease, in order to assess the need for revascularization therapy.[35,76] *It is difficult to obtain precise costs of various procedures;* however, a reasonable comparative cost analysis can be estimated. All costs are expressed in multiples of a standard exercise test, which is assigned an arbitrary cost of one dollar:

Exercise treadmill test . . . . $ 1
Exercise test with thallium imaging 4
Radionuclide ventriculogram 3
Two-dimensional echocardiogram 3
Cardiac catheterization with left ventricular and
        coronary angiography 15

Table 1–7. Cost Analysis of Noninvasive Versus Invasive Risk Assessment Following Uncomplicated Myocardial Infarction*

100 Patients with Uncomplicated First Myocardial Infarction		
A. Noninvasive I	$100 \times \$4$	$ 400
100 exercise tests with thallium imaging		
70 positive/inconclusive test results = 70 catheterizations/ angiographies	$70 \times \$15$	$1050
30 negative test results = assess resting LV function with two-dimensional echocardiography or radionuclide angiography	$30 \times \$3$	$ 90 $1540
B. Noninvasive II	$100 \times \$1$	$ 100
100 standard exercise tests		
76 abnormal, inconclusive, unable to perform → catheterization and angiography	$76 \times \$15$	$1140
24 negative → 2nd test at 6–12 weeks	$24 \times \$1$	$ 24
7 positive → catheterization and angiography	$7 \times \$15$	$105
17 negative → assess resting LV function with two-dimensional echocardiography or radionuclide angiography	$17 \times \$3$	$ 51 $1420
C. Invasive		
100 catheterization and angiography	$100 \times \$15$	$1500
50 secondary exercise tests to assess physiologic significance of coronary artery disease	$50 \times \$1$	$ 50 $1550

From the foregoing cost estimates, a relative cost analysis of invasive and non-invasive approaches to risk assessment following myocardial infarction can be derived (Table 1–7). If one employs a noninvasive approach utilizing radionuclide imaging in 100 patients surviving an uncomplicated myocardial infarction, 100 exercise tests with thallium imaging will cost $400. Assuming 70 patients will have positive or inconclusive test results,[35] cardiac catheterization and angiography in these patients will cost an additional $1050. Of the 30 patients with negative exercise thallium tests, independent assessment of left ventricular function by radionuclide angiography or echocardiography will cost an additional $90. The net cost of this noninvasive approach to risk assessment in these 100 patients will thus be $1540.

If one uses a noninvasive approach employing standard exercise testing initially, 100 tests will cost $100. If 76 of these test results are abnormal, inconclusive, or if they cannot be performed,[34–39,42,47,65,67,69,82,111–114,124,126,127] cardiac catheterization and angiography in these patients will cost an additional $1140. In the 24 patients with negative test results, a second, more rigorous test 6–12 weeks later will cost an additional $24, and cardiac catheterization in the 7 patients with positive test results[37,47] will cost $105. Noninvasive assessment of left ventricular function in the remaining 17 patients will cost $51, making the net cost of this approach $1420.

If one follows an initial invasive approach to these same 100 patients, the cost for 100 cardiac catheterization and angiography procedures will be $1500. If approximately half of these patients require physiologic assessment of moderate coronary artery disease, the cost of 50 exercise tests will be $50. The net cost of this approach will be $1550. It is clear, therefore, that the performance of early cardiac catheterization and angiography in all survivors of uncomplicated myocardial infarction need not be significantly more expensive than a noninvasive risk stratification approach, if all tests are employed judiciously.

SUMMARY

From the foregoing discussion, it becomes apparent that although noninvasive risk stratification is a reasonable approach to assessment of patients following an uncomplicated myocardial infarction, the performance of early cardiac catheterization and angiography on nearly all such patients is not unreasonable and may in fact be the most practical approach. The basis for this rationalization may be summarized as follows:

1. Many subgroups will need early catheterization anyway
   a. Myocardial infarction complicated by recurrent ischemia, heart failure, or complex ventricular arrhythmias
   b. Patients receiving thrombolytic treatment
   c. "Young" patients (less than 50 years old?)
   d. "Older" patients (over ages 65 to 70?) in otherwise good medical condition
   e. Patients unable to exercise
   f. Patients with abnormal or inconclusive noninvasive test results (approximately 70 percent of patients)
2. Cardiac catheterization and angiography as a single test provides the two most powerful prognostic variables following myocardial infarction, namely, the extent of coronary artery disease and residual left ventricular function. This knowledge is reassuring to both physician and patient and allows for planning of optimal long-term management.
3. Certain limitations exist in noninvasive risk assessment strategies (Table 1–6).
4. This approach need not be significantly more costly, if all tests are used wisely.

The *major risk* inherent in the definition of the extent of coronary artery disease in all survivors of acute myocardial infarction might be the performance of unnecessary revascularization procedures (percutaneous transluminal coronary angioplasty or coronary bypass surgery).[101,160] The burden rests with the individual clinician to (1) collect all useful and necessary data; (2) assess reliability and accuracy of various tests available at one's own institution; (3) avoid performing unnecessary and repetitive tests; (4) interpret the data in the proper context; and (5) counsel patients appropriately, correctly, and judiciously about their prognosis and therapeutic options. In this manner, all patients who might benefit *appropriately* from revascularization can be discovered early and offered this therapeutic option. Other patients can also be managed more appropriately; for example, those who are truly at very low risk (normal left ventricular function and either normal coronary arteries or "mild" coronary artery disease). However, it is most important to avoid unnecessary revascularization procedures.

Although this discussion has focused on noninvasive and invasive testing following myocardial infarction, it is necessary to emphasize that comprehensive management of coronary artery disease and its complications should not be neglected in these patients;[161] for example, control or amelioration of risk factors for coronary artery disease is mandatory in all these patients, and in their families as well.

REFERENCES

1. Dwyer, EM: After the myocardial infarction: A review and approach to risk stratification. Cardiology Clinics 6(1):153, 1988.
2. Moss, AJ: Prognosis after myocardial infarction. Am J Cardiol 52:667, 1983.
3. Beller, GA and Gibson, RS: Risk stratification after myocardial infarction. Mod Concepts Cardiovasc Dis 55:5, 1986.
4. The TIMI Research Group: Immediate vs. delayed catheterization and angioplasty following thrombolytic therapy for acute myocardial infarction: TIMI II-A Results. JAMA 260:2849, 1988.
5. Kelly, DT: Clinical decisions in patients following myocardial infarction. Curr Probl Cardiol 10(1):1, 1985.
6. Gomez-Marin, O, Folsom, AR, Kottke, TE, et al: Improvement in long-term survival among patients hospitalized with acute myocardial infarction, 1970–1980. N Engl J Med 316.1353, 1987.
7. Waters, DD, Bosch, X, Bouchard, A, et al: Comparison of clinical variables and variables derived from a limited predischarge exercise test as predictors of early and late mortality after myocardial infarction. J Am Coll Cardiol 5:1, 1985.
8. Madsen, EB, Gilpin, E, Henning, H, et al: Prediction of late mortality after myocardial infarction from variables measured at different times during hospitalization. Am J Cardiol 53:47, 1984.
9. Gilpin, EA, Koziol, JA, Madsen, EB, et al: Periods of differing mortality distribution during the first year after acute myocardial infarction. Am J Cardiol 52:240, 1983.
10. Dwyer, EM, McMaster, P, Greenberg, H, et al: Nonfatal cardiac events and recurrent infarction in the year after acute myocardial infarction. J Am Coll Cardiol 4:695, 1984.
11. Kannel, WB, Sorlie, P, and McNamara, PM: Prognosis after initial myocardial infarction: The Framingham study. Am J Cardiol 44:53, 1979.
12. Epstein, SE, Palmeri, ST, and Patterson, RE: Evaluation of patients after myocardial infarction: Indications for cardiac catheterization and surgical intervention. N Engl J Med 307:1487, 1982.
13. Davis, HT, DeCamilla, J, Bayer, LW, et al: Survivorship patterns in the post-hospital phase of myocardial infarction. Circulation 60:1252, 1979.
14. Moss, AJ, DeCamilla, JJ, and Davis H: Cardiac death in the first six months after myocardial infarction: Potential for mortality reduction in the early post-hospital period. Am J Cardiol 39:816, 1977.
15. Mulcahy, R, Hickey, N, Graham, I, et al: Factors influencing long-term prognosis in male patients surviving a first coronary attack. Br Heart J 37:158, 1975.
16. Dalen, JE, Gore, JM, Braunwald, E, et al: Six- and twelve-month follow-up of the Phase I Thrombolysis in Myocardial Infarction (TIMI) trial. Am J Cardiol 62:179, 1988.
17. The Multicenter Post-Infarction Research Group: Risk stratification and survival after myocardial infarction. N Engl J Med 309:331, 1983.
18. O'Rourke, RA: Clinical decisions for post-myocardial infarction patients. Mod Concepts Cardiovasc Dis 55:55, 1986.
19. Schuster, EH and Bulkley, BH: Early post-infarction angina: Ischemia at a distance and ischemia in the infarct zone. N Engl J Med 305:1101, 1981.
20. Bosch, X, Theroux, P, Waters, DD, et al: Early post-infarction ischemia: Clinical, angiographic, and prognostic significance. Circulation 75:988, 1987.
21. Turner, JD, Rogers, WJ, Mantle, JA, et al: Coronary angiography soon after myocardial infarction. Chest 77:58, 1980.
22. Marmor, A, Geltman, EM, Schechtman, K, et al: Recurrent myocardial infarction: Clinical predictors and prognostic implications. Circulation 66:415, 1982.
23. Figueras, J, Cinca, J, Valle, V, et al: Prognostic implications of early spontaneous angina after acute transmural myocardial infarction. Int J Cardiol 4:261, 1983.
24. DeFeyter, PJ, Van Eenice, MJ, Dighton, DH, et al: Prognostic value of exercise testing, coronary angiography, and left ventriculography six to eight weeks after myocardial infarction. Circulation 66:527, 1982.

25. Taylor, GJ, Humphries, JO, Mellits, ED, et al: Predictors of clinical course, coronary anatomy, and left ventricular function after recovery from acute myocardial infarction. Circulation 62:960, 1980.

26. Mock, MB, Ringqvist, I, Fisher, LD, et al: Survival of medically treated patients in the Coronary Artery Surgery Study (CASS) registry. Circulation 66:562, 1982.

27. Sanz, G, Castaner, A, Betriu, A, et al: Determinants of prognosis in survivors of myocardial infarction: A prospective clinical angiographic study. N Engl J Med 306:1065, 1982.

28. Norris, RM, Barnaby, PF, Brandt, PWT, et al: Prognosis after recovery from first acute myocardial infarction: Determinants of reinfarction and sudden death. Am J Cardiol 53:408, 1984.

29. Rapaport, E and Remedios, P: The high risk patient after recovery from myocardial infarction: Recognition and management. J Am Coll Cardiol 1:391, 1983.

30. Moss, AJ, DeCamilla, J, Engstrom, F, et al: The post-hospital phase of myocardial infarction: Identification of patients with increased mortality risk. Circulation 49:460, 1974.

31. Moss, AJ, DeCamilla, JJ, Davis, HT, et al: Clinical significance of ventricular ectopic beats in the early post-hospital phase of myocardial infarction. Am J Cardiol 39:635, 1977.

32. Bigger, JT, Fleiss, JL, Kleiger, R, et al: The relationships among ventricular arrhythmias, left ventricular dysfunction, and mortality in the two years after myocardial infarction. Circulation 69:250, 1984.

33. Schulman, SP, Achuff, SC, Griffith, LSC, et al: Prognostic cardiac catheterization variables in survivors of acute myocardial infarction: A five year prospective study. J Am Coll Cardiol 11:1164, 1988.

34. Deckers, JW, Fioretti, P, Brower, RW, et al: Prediction of one year outcome after complicated and uncomplicated myocardial infarction: Bayesian analysis of predischarge exercise test results in 300 patients. Am Heart J 113:90, 1987.

35. Gibson, RS, Watson, DD, Craddock, GB, et al: Prediction of cardiac events after uncomplicated myocardial infarction: A prospective study comparing predischarge exercise thallium-201 scintigraphy and coronary angiography. Circulation 68:321, 1983.

36. Schwartz, KM, Turner, JD, Sheffield, LT, et al: Limited exercise testing soon after myocardial infarction: Correlation with early coronary and left ventricular angiography. Ann Intern Med 94:727, 1981.

37. Fuller, CM, Raizner, AE, Verani, MS, et al: Early post-myocardial infarction treadmill stress testing: An accurate predictor of multivessel coronary disease and subsequent cardiac events. Ann Int Med 94:734, 1981.

38. Theroux, P, Waters, DD, Halphen, C, et al: Prognostic value of exercise testing soon after myocardial infarction. N Engl J Med 301:341, 1979.

39. DeBusk, RF, Kraemer, HC, and Nash, E: Stepwise risk stratification soon after myocardial infarction. Am J Cardiol 52:1161, 1983.

40. Markiewicz, W, Houston, N, and DeBusk, RF: Exercise testing soon after myocardial infarction. Circulation 56:26, 1977.

41. Weld, FM, Cho, KL, Bigger, JT, et al: Risk stratification with low-level exercise testing two weeks after acute myocardial infarction. Circulation 64:306, 1981.

42. Ibsen, H, Kjoller, E, Styperek, J, et al: Routine exercise ECG three weeks after acute myocardial infarction. Acta Med Scand 198:463, 1975.

43. Miller, DH and Borer, JS: Exercise testing early after myocardial infarction: Risks and benefits. Am J Med 72:427, 1982.

44. Baron, DB, Licht, JR, and Ellestad, MH: Status of exercise stress testing after myocardial infarction. Arch Intern Med 144:595, 1984.

45. Theroux, P, Marpole, DGF, and Bourassa, MG: Exercise stress testing in the post-myocardial infarction patient. Am J Cardiol 52:664, 1983.

46. Cohn, PF: The role of noninvasive cardiac testing after an uncomplicated myocardial infarction. N Engl J Med 309:90, 1983.

47. Starling, MR, Crawford, MH, Kennedy, GT, et al: Treadmill exercise tests predischarge and six weeks post-myocardial infarction to detect abnormalities of known prognostic value. Ann Intern Med 94:721, 1981.

48. Froelicher, VF, Perdue, ST, Atwood, JE, et al: Exercise testing of patients recovering from myocardial infarction. Curr Probl Cardiol 11(7):369, 1986.

49. Crawford, MH and O'Rourke, RA: The role of cardiac catheterization in patients after myocardial infarction. Cardiology Clinics 2(1):105, 1984.

50. Gould, KL, Lipscomb, K, and Hamilton, GW: Physiologic basis for assessing critical coronary stenosis: Instantaneous flow response and regional distribution during coronary hyperemia as measures of coronary flow reserve. Am J Cardiol 33:87, 1974.

51. Rogers, WJ, Smith, LR, Oberman, A, et al: Surgical vs. nonsurgical management of patients after myocardial infarction. Circulation 62(Suppl I):I67, 1980.

52. Rahimtoola, SH: A perspective on the three large multicenter randomized clinical trials of coronary bypass surgery for chronic stable angina. Circulation 72(Suppl V):V123, 1985.

53. Braunwald, E and Rutherford, JD: Reversible ischemic left ventricular dysfunction: Evidence for the hibernating myocardium. J Am Coll Cardiol 8:1467, 1986.

54. Rahimtoola, SH: The hibernating myocardium. Am Heart J 117:211, 1989.

55. Braunwald, E: Deaths related to cardiac catheterization: Circulation 37(Suppl III):III17, 1968.

56. Davis, K, Kennedy, JW, Kemp, HG, et al: Complications of coronary arteriography from the Collaborative Study of Coronary Artery Surgery (CASS). Circulation 59:1105, 1979.

57. Bourassa, MG and Noble, J: Complication rate of coronary arteriography: A review of 5250 cases studied by a percutaneous femoral technique. Circulation 53:106, 1976.

58. Wyman, RM, Safian, RD, Portway, V, et al: Current complications of diagnostic and therapeutic cardiac catheterization. J Am Coll Cardiol 12:1400, 1988.

59. Trenouth, RS, Rosch, J, Antonovic, R, et al: Ventriculography and coronary arteriography in the acute ill patient: Complications, extent of coronary artery disease, and abnormalities of left ventricular function. Chest 69:647, 1976.

60. Betriu, A, Castaner, A, Sanz, GA, et al: Angiographic findings one month after myocardial infarction: A prospective study of 259 survivors. Circulation 65:1099, 1982.

61. Roubin, GS, Harris, PJ, Bernstein, L, et al: Coronary anatomy and prognosis after myocardial infarction in patients 60 years of age and younger. Circulation 67:743, 1983.

62. Bertrand, ME, Lefebvre, JM, Laisne, CL, et al: Coronary arteriography in acute transmural myocardial infarction. Am Heart J 97:61, 1979.

63. DeWood, MA, Stifter, WF, Simpson, CS, et al: Coronary arteriographic findings soon after non-Q wave myocardial infarction. N Engl J Med 315:417, 1986.

64. DeWood, MA, Spores, J, Notske, R, et al: Prevalence of total coronary occlusion during the early hours of transmural myocardial infarction. N Engl J Med 303:897, 1980.

65. Griffith, LSC, Varnauskas, E, Wallin, J, et al: Correlation of coronary arteriography after acute myocardial infarction with predischarge limited exercise test response. Am J Cardiol 61:201, 1988.

66. DeFeyter, PJ, Van Den Brand, M, Serruys, PW, et al: Early angiography after myocardial infarction: What have we learned? Am Heart J 109:194, 1985.

67. Veenbrink, TWG, Van Der Werf, T, Westerhof, PW, et al: Is there an indication for coronary angiography in patients under 60 years of age with no or minimal angina pectoris after a first myocardial infarction? Br Heart J 53:30, 1985.

68. Akhras, F, Upward, J, Keates, J, et al: Early exercise testing and elective coronary artery bypass surgery after uncomplicated myocardial infarction: Effect on morbidity and mortality. Br Heart J 52:413, 1984.

69. Starling, MR, Crawford, MH, Richards, KL, et al: Predictive value of early post-myocardial infarction modified treadmill exercise testing in multivessel coronary artery disease detection. Am Heart J 102:169, 1981.

70. Williams, RA, Cohn, PF, Vokonas, PS, et al: Electrocardiographic, arteriographic, and ventriculographic correlations in transmural myocardial infarction. Am J Cardiol 31:595, 1973.

71. Wasserman, AG, Katz, RJ, Cleary, P, et al: Noninvasive detection of multivessel disease after myocardial infarction by exercise radionuclide ventriculography. Am J Cardiol 50:1242, 1982.

72. Abraham, RD, Freedman, SB, Dunn, RF, et al: Prediction of multivessel coronary artery disease and prognosis early after acute myocardial infarction by exercise electrocardiography and thallium-201 myocardial perfusion scintigraphy. Am J Cardiol 58:423, 1986.

73. Weiner, DA, McCabe, C, Klein, MD, et al: ST segment changes post-infarction: Predictive value for multivessel coronary disease and left ventricular aneurysm. Circulation 58:887, 1978.

74. Morris, DD, Rozanski, A, Berman, DS, et al: Noninvasive prediction of the angiographic extent of coronary artery disease after myocardial infarction: Comparison of clinical, bicycle exercise electrocardiographic, and ventriculographic parameters. Circulation 70:192, 1984.

75. Abraham, RD, Roubin, GS, Harris, PJ, et al: Coronary and left ventricular angiographic anatomy and prognosis of survivors of first acute myocardial infarction. Am J Cardiol 52:257, 1983.

76. Nicod, P, Corbett, JR, Firth, BG, et al: Prognostic value of resting and submaximal exercise radio-

nuclide ventriculography after acute myocardial infarction in high-risk patients with single and multivessel disease. Am J Cardiol 52:30, 1983.

77. Patterson, RE, Horowitz, SF, Eng, C, et al: Can noninvasive exercise test criteria identify patients with left main or three vessel coronary artery disease after a first myocardial infarction? Am J Cardiol 51:361, 1983.

78. Schulze, RA, Humphries, JO, Griffith, LSC, et al: Left ventricular and coronary angiographic anatomy: Relationship to ventricular irritability in the late hospital phase of acute myocardial infarction. Circulation 55:839, 1977.

79. Tubau, JF, Chaitman, BR, Bourassa, MG, et al: Detection of multivessel coronary disease after myocardial infarction using exercise stress testing and multiple ECG lead systems. Circulation 61:44, 1980.

80. Turner, JD, Schwartz, KM, Logic, JR, et al: Detection of residual jeopardized myocardium three weeks after myocardial infarction by exercise testing with thallium-201. Circulation 61:729, 1980.

81. Castellanet, MJ, Greenberg, PS, and Ellestad, MH: Comparison of ST segment changes on exercise testing with angiographic findings in patients with prior myocardial infarction. Am J Cardiol 42:29, 1978.

82. Paine, TD, Dye, LE, Roitman, DI, et al: Relation of graded exercise test findings after myocardial infarction to extent of coronary artery disease and left ventricular dysfunction. Am J Cardiol 42:716, 1978.

83. Savran, SV, Bryson, AL, Welch, TG, et al: Clinical correlates of coronary cineangiography in young males with myocardial infarction. Am Heart J 91:551, 1976.

84. Pichard, AD, Ziff, C, Holt, J, et al: Angiographic study of the infarct-related coronary artery in the chronic stage of acute myocardial infarction. Am Heart J 106:687, 1983.

85. Rigo, P, Bailey, IK, Griffith, LSC, et al: Stress thallium-201 myocardial scintigraphy for the detection of individual coronary arterial lesions in patients with and without previous myocardial infarction. Am J Cardiol 48:209, 1981.

86. Van Der Wall, EE, Eenige Van, MJ, Visser, FC, et al: Thallium-201 exercise testing in patients 6–8 weeks after myocardial infarction: Limited value for the detection of multivessel disease. Eur Heart J 6:29, 1985.

87. Rahimtoola, SH: Coronary bypass surgery for chronic angina—1981. Circulation 65:225, 1982.

88. Deumite, NJ, Chaitman, BR, Davis, KB, et al: Asymptomatic left main coronary artery disease (CASS) (abstr). J Am Coll Cardiol 5:518, 1985.

89. Friesinger, GC, Page, EE, and Ross, RS: Prognostic significance of coronary arteriography. Trans Assoc Am Physicians 83:78, 1970.

90. Humphries, JO, Kuller, L, Ross, RS, et al: Natural history of ischemic heart disease in relation to arteriographic findings. Circulation 49:489, 1974.

91. Platia, EV, Grunwald, L, Mellits, ED, et al: Clinical and arteriographic variables predictive of survival in coronary artery disease. Am J Cardiol 46:543, 1980.

92. Bruschke, AVG, Proudfit, WL, and Sones, FM: Progress study of 590 consecutive nonsurgical cases of coronary disease followed 5–9 years: Arteriographic correlations. Circulation 47:1147, 1973.

93. Reeves, TJ, Oberman, A, Jones, WB, et al: Natural history of angina pectoris. Am J Cardiol 33:423, 1974.

94. Burggraf, GW and Parker, JO: Progress in coronary artery disease: Angiographic, hemodynamic, and clinical factors. Circulation 51:146, 1975.

95. Harris, PJ, Harrell, FE, Lee, KL, et al: Survival in medically treated coronary artery disease. Circulation 60:1259, 1979.

96. Kaul, S, Lilly, DR, Gascho, JA, et al: Prognostic utility of the exercise thallium-201 test in ambulatory patients with chest pain: Comparison with cardiac catheterization. Circulation 77:745, 1988.

97. Rahimtoola, SH: Left main equivalence is still an unproved hypothesis but proximal left anterior descending coronary artery disease is a "high risk" lesion. Am J Cardiol 53:1719, 1984.

98. Schuster, EH, Griffith, LS, and Bulkley, BH: Preponderance of acute proximal left anterior descending coronary arterial lesions in fatal myocardial infarction: A clinicopathologic study. Am J Cardiol 47:1189, 1981.

99. Vlodaver, Z and Edwards, JE: Pathology of coronary atherosclerosis. Prog Cardiovasc Dis 14:256, 1971.

100. Ahnve, S, Gilpin, E, Dittrich, H, et al: First myocardial infarction: Age and ejection fraction identify a low-risk group. Am Heart J 116:925, 1988.

101. Rahimtoola, SH: Coronary arteriography in asymptomatic patients after myocardial infarction: The need to distinguish between clinical investigation and clinical care. Chest 77:53, 1980.

102. Chaitman, BR, Fisher, LD, Bourassa, MG, et al: Effect of coronary bypass surgery on survival patterns in subsets of patients with left main coronary artery disease: Report of the Collaborative Study in Coronary Artery Surgery (CASS). Am J Cardiol 48:765, 1981.

103. Detre, KM, Takoro, T, Hultgren, H, et al: Long-term mortality and morbidity results of the Veterans Administration randomized trial of coronary artery bypass surgery. Circulation 72(Suppl V):V84, 1985.

104. Varnauskas, E and the European Coronary Surgery Study Group: Survival, myocardial infarction, and employment status in a prospective randomized study of coronary bypass surgery. Circulation 72(Suppl V):V90, 1985.

105. Passamani, E, Davis, KB, Gillespie, MJ, et al: A randomized trial of coronary artery bypass surgery: Survival of patients with a low ejection fraction. N Engl J Med 312:1665, 1985.

106. Bounous, EP, Mark, DB, Pollock, BG, et al: Surgical survival benefits for coronary disease patients with left ventricular dysfunction. Circulation 78(Suppl I):I151, 1988.

107. Alderman, EL, Fisher, LD, Litwin, P, et al: Result of coronary artery surgery in patients with poor left ventricular function (CASS). Circulation 68:785, 1983.

108. Pigott, JD, Kouchoukos, NT, Oberman, A, et al: Late results of surgical and medical therapy for patients with coronary artery disease and depressed left ventricular function. J Am Coll Cardiol 5:1036, 1985.

109. Rahimtoola, SH: Coronary bypass surgery for unstable angina. Circulation 69:842, 1984.

110. Rahimtoola, SH, Nunley, D, Grunkemeier, G, et al: Ten-year survival after coronary bypass surgery for unstable angina. N Engl J Med 308:676, 1983.

111. Gibson, RS, Beller, GA, Gheorghiade, M, et al: The prevalence and clinical significance of residual myocardial ischemia two weeks after uncomplicated non-Q wave infarction: A prospective natural history study. Circulation 73:1186, 1986.

112. Chaitman, BR, Waters, DD, Corbara, F, et al: Prediction of multivessel disease after inferior myocardial infarction. Circulation 57:1085, 1978.

113. Gibson, RS, Taylor, GT, Watson, DD, et al: Predicting the extent and location of coronary artery disease during the early post-infarction period by quantitative thallium-201 scintigraphy. Am J Cardiol 47:1010, 1981.

114. Krone, RJ, Gillespie, JA, Weld, FM, et al: Low-level exercise testing after myocardial infarction: Usefulness in enhancing clinical risk stratification. Circulation 71:80, 1985.

115. Handler, CE and Sowton, E: Diurnal variation and reproducibility of predischarge submaximal exercise testing after myocardial infarction. Br Heart J 52:299, 1984.

116. Hung, J, Goris, ML, Nash, E, et al: Comparative value of maximal treadmill testing, exercise thallium myocardial perfusion scintigraphy and exercise radionuclide ventriculography for distinguishing high- and low-risk patients soon after acute myocardial infarction. Am J Cardiol 53:1221, 1984.

117. Corbett, JR, Dehmer, GJ, Lewis, SE, et al: The prognostic value of submaximal exercise testing with radionuclide ventriculography before hospital discharge in patients with recent myocardial infarction. Circulation 64:535, 1981.

118. Morris, KG, Palmeri, ST, Califf, RM, et al: Value of radionuclide angiography for predicting specific cardiac events after myocardial infarction. Am J Cardiol 55:318, 1985.

119. Borer, JS, Rosing, DR, Miller, RH, et al: Natural history of left ventricular function during one year after acute myocardial infarction: Comparison with clinical, electrocardiographic, and biochemical determinations. Am J Cardiol 46:1, 1980.

120. Ryan, T, Armstrong, WF, O'Donnell, JA, et al: Risk stratification after acute myocardial infarction by means of exercise two dimensional echocardiography. Am Heart J 114:1305, 1987.

121. Armstrong, WF, O'Donnell, J, Ryan, T, et al: Effect of prior myocardial infarction and extent and location of coronary disease on accuracy of exercise echocardiography. J Am Coll Cardiol 10:531, 1987.

122. Senaratne, MPJ, Hsu, L, Rossall, RE, et al: Exercise testing after myocardial infarction: Relative values of the low level predischarge and the post-discharge exercise test. J Am Coll Cardiol 12:1416, 1988.

123. Sami, M, Kraemer, H, and DeBusk, RF: The prognostic significance of serial exercise testing after myocardial infarction. Circulation 60:1238, 1979.

124. Handler, CE: Submaximal predischarge exercise testing after myocardial infarction: Prognostic value and limitations. Eur Heart J 6:510, 1985.

125. DeFeyter, PJ, Van Eenige, MJ, Dighton, DH, et al: Exercise testing early after myocardial infarction: Detection of multivessel coronary artery disease and extent of left ventricular dysfunction six to eight weeks after infarction using a 12-lead exercise electrocardiogram. Chest 83:853, 1983.

126. Starling, MR, Crawford, MH, Kennedy, GT, et al: Exercise testing early after myocardial infarction: Predictive value for subsequent unstable angina and death. Am J Cardiol 46:909, 1980.

127. Saunamaki, KI and Andersen, JD: Clinical significance of the ST-segment response and other early exercise test variables in uncomplicated vs. complicated myocardial infarction. Eur Heart J 8:603, 1987.

128. Gibson, RS: Non-Q wave myocardial infarction: Diagnosis, prognosis, and management. Curr Probl Cardiol 13:1, 1988.

129. Krone, RJ, Friedman, E, Thanavaros, S, et al: Long-term prognosis after first Q-wave (transmural) or non-Q wave (non-transmural) myocardial infarction: Analysis of 593 patients. Am J Cardiol 52:234, 1983.

130. Connolly, DC and Elveback, LR: Coronary heart disease in residents of Rochester, Minnesota: VI. Hospital and post-hospital course of patients with transmural and subendocardial myocardial infarction. Mayo Clin Proc 60:375, 1985.

131. Hutter, AM, DeSanctis, RW, Flynn, T, et al: Nontransmural myocardial infarction: A comparison of hospital and late clinical course of patients with that of matched patients with transmural anterior and transmural inferior myocardial infarction. Am J Cardiol 48:595, 1981.

132. Madigan, NP, Rutherford, BD, and Frye, RL: The clinical course, early prognosis, and coronary anatomy of subendocardial infarction. Am J Med 60:634, 1976.

133. Ogawa, H, Hiramori, K, Haze, K, et al: Comparison of clinical features of non-Q wave and Q-wave myocardial infarction. Am Heart J 111:513, 1986.

134. Schulze, RA, Pitt, B, Griffith, LSC, et al: Coronary angiography and left ventriculography in survivors of transmural and nontransmural myocardial infarction. Am J Med 64:108, 1978.

135. Gibson, RS, Boden, WE, Theroux, P, et al: Diltiazem and reinfarction in patients with non-Q wave myocardial infarction: Results of a double-blind, randomized multicenter trial. N Engl J Med 315:423, 1986.

136. Nicholson, MR, Roubin, GS, Bernstein, L, et al: Prognosis after an initial non-Q wave myocardial infarction related to cornary anatomy. Am J Cardiol 52:462, 1983.

137. United States Department of Health and Human Services, Public Health Service, National Institutes of Health: Report of the Working Group on Arteriosclerosis of the National Heart, Lung and Blood Institute. NIH Publication No. 81-2034, p 39, June 1981.

138. Norris, RM, Caughey, DE, Mercer, CJ, et al: Prognosis after myocardial infarction: Six-year follow-up. Br Heart J 36:786, 1974.

139. Henning, H, Gilpin, EA, Covell, JW, et al: Prognosis after acute myocardial infarction: A multivariate analysis of mortality and survival. Circulation 59:1124, 1979.

140. Tofler, GH, Muller, JE, Stone, PH, et al: Factors leading to shorter survival after acute myocardial infarction in patients ages 65 to 75 years compared with younger patients. Am J Cardiol 62:860, 1988.

141. Rahimtoola, SH, Grunkemeir, GL, and Starr, A: Ten year survival after coronary artery bypass surgery for angina in patients aged 65 years and older. Circulation 74:509, 1986.

142. Mardor, VJ and Sherry, S: Thrombolytic therapy: Current status. N Engl J Med 318:1512, 1585, 1988.

143. Gruppo Italiano per lo Studio Della Streptochinasi Nell'Infarto Miocardico (GISSI): Effectiveness of intravenous thrombolytic treatment in acute myocardial infarction. Lancet 1:397, 1986.

144. Gruppo Italiano per lo Studio Della Streptochinasi Nell'Infarto Miocardico (GISSI): Long-term effects of intravenous thrombolysis in acute myocardial infarction: Final report of the GISSI study. Lancet 2:871, 1987.

145. Anderson, JL: Streptokinase and acylated streptokinase: Biochemical properties and clinical effects. In Topol, EJ (ed): Acute Coronary Intervention. Alan R. Liss, New York, 1988.

146. Collen, D and Topol, EJ: Tissue-type plasminogen activator. In Topol, EJ (ed): Acute Coronary Intervention. Alan R. Liss, New York, 1988.

147. Topol, EJ, Califf, RM, George, BS, et al: A randomized trial of immediate versus delayed elective angioplasty after intravenous tissue plasminogen activator in acute myocardial infarction. N Engl J Med 317:581, 1987.

148. Harrison, DG, Ferguson, DW, Collins, SM, et al: Rethrombosis after reperfusion with streptokinase: Importance of geometry of residual lesions. Circulation 69:991, 1984.

149. Califf, RM, O'Neill, W, Stack, RS, et al: Failure of simple clinical measurements to predict perfusion status after intravenous thrombolysis. Ann Intern Med 108:658, 1988.
150. Sheehan, FH, Mathey, DG, Schofer, J, et al: Factors that determine recovery of left ventricular function after thrombolysis in patients with acute myocardial infarction. Circulation 71:1121, 1985.
151. O'Neill, WO, Timmis, GC, Bourdillon, PD, et al: A prospective randomized clinical trial of intracoronary streptokinase versus coronary angioplasty for acute myocardial infarction. N Engl J Med 314:812, 1986.
152. Topol, EJ, Weiss, JL, Brinker, JA, et al: Regional wall motion improvement after coronary thrombolysis with recombinant tissue plasminogen activator: Importance of coronary angioplasty. J Am Coll Cardiol 6:426, 1985.
153. Guerci, AD, Gerstenblith, G, Brinker, JA, et al: A randomized trial of intravenous tissue plasminogen activator for acute myocardial infarction with subsequent randomization to elective coronary angioplasty. N Engl J Med 317:1613, 1987.
154. Stack, RS, Califf, RM, Hinohara, T, et al: Survival and cardiac event rates in the first year after emergency coronary angioplasty for acute myocardial infarction. J Am Coll Cardiol 11:1141, 1988.
155. Willerson, JT: Selection of patients for coronary arteriography. Circulation 72(Suppl V):V3, 1985.
156. Miller, RR, DeMaria, AN, Vismara, LA, et al: Chronic stable inferior myocardial infarction: Unsuspected harbinger of high-risk proximal left coronary arterial obstruction amenable to surgical revascularization. Am J Cardiol 39:954, 1977.
157. Gibson, RS, Crampton, RS, Watson, DD, et al: Precordial ST-segment depression during acute inferior myocardial infarction: Clinical, scintigraphic, and angiographic correlation. Circulation 66:732, 1982.
158. Haines, DE, Beller, GA, Watson, DD, et al: A prospective clinical, scintographic, angiographic, and functional evaluation of patients after inferior myocardial infarction with and without right ventricular dysfunction. J Am Coll Cardiol 6:995, 1985.
159. Cohen, M, Charney, R, Hershman, R, et al: Reversal of chronic ischemic myocardial dysfunction after transluminal coronary angioplasty. J Am Coll Cardiol 12:1193, 1988.
160. Rahimtoola, SH: Comments. In Gibson, RS: Non Q-wave myocardial infarction: Diagnosis, prognosis, and management. Curr Probl Cardiol 13(1):55, 1988.
161. Rahimtoola, SH: A brief overview of the treatment of patients with angina: A clinical cardiologist's perspective. In Weiner, D and Frishman, W (eds): Therapy of Angina Pectoris. Marcel Dekker, New York, 1986.

Commentary

By Melvin D. Cheitlin, M.D.

Kulick and Rahimtoola have crafted a well-thought-out and provocative argument for a radical approach to patients who have suffered a myocardial infarction. Their thesis that coronary arteriography and left ventriculography is the preferred risk stratification tool for "nearly everyone" after a myocardial infarction rests on their conclusion that "nearly everyone" after myocardial infarction is either already a proved high-risk patient with a complicated infarction or with angina at minimal activity; is unable to exercise; will have evidence of ischemia on noninvasive evaluation; or will have a noninvasive test result that is uninterpretable. In all these cases, coronary arteriography is the only answer to risk stratification. They further argue that because coronary arteriography reveals areas of contracting myocardium supplied by diseased vessels as well as certain pathologic combinations such as left main disease and multivessel disease with decreased left ventricular function proved to benefit from revascularization, coronary arteriography is inherently better in risk stratification than noninvasive techniques. Finally, they argue that because some "low-risk patients" identified by noninvasive techniques still do have myocardial infarction and die, somehow coronary arteriography will identify these patients and prevent this outcome.

Although the arguments are, on the surface, compelling, in actuality each of these arguments has problems. First, in an effort to be fair, Kulick and Rahimtoola have averaged a number of studies to obtain figures that reflect the number of patients who are at high risk after myocardial infarction and thus will require coronary arteriography without further workup. The frequency of high-risk patients such as those with congestive heart failure, with angina at rest or on minimal activity, or with late ventricular fibrillation or tachycardia depends upon the patient population selected for the study. To select a single figure, only studies of consecutive patients should be included. In our experience—and we, like the authors, also practice at a county hospital with an older and sicker population than most community hospitals—only a minority of patients, possibly 25 percent, have one or more indications for cardiac catheterization without further evaluation. DeBusk and colleagues' report[1] of 702 consecutive patients surviving 3 weeks after myocardial infarction indicates that about 10 percent of patients have had prior myocardial infarction, congestive heart failure, or angina at low activity, and these patients had the highest risk of having reinfarction or death within 6 months (18 percent).

The statement that about half the patients after an uncomplicated myocardial infarction will have a stress test abnormality again depends on the population selected for the study (frequently differing from one study to the next) as well as on the definition of "stress test abnormality." Most studies use ST segment depression as an end point and do not specify at what stage of exercise or double product the ST segment depression occurs. As is well recognized, patients who can complete stage 3 of the Bruce protocol are at low risk of future complications, even if they develop 1 mm ST segment depression. DeFeyter and colleagues,[2] quoted by the authors, point out that death or recurrent myocardial infarction is an infrequent occurrence in their study. In 179 survivors of myocardial infarction, there were 11 cardiac deaths and 12 reinfarctions in a mean follow-up time of 28 months. Patients completing 10 minutes on the Bruce protocol are at extremely low risk, with only one having a recurrent myocardial infarction and none dying in over 2 years of follow-up.

Another issue is whether risk stratification should be done before discharge after an uncomplicated myocardial infarction or postponed until 3 to 6 weeks after discharge when a higher degree of exercise can be done, as it was in DeFeyter's[2] and DeBusk's[1] studies. DeBusk pointed out that the extremely low incidence of death and reinfarction between hospital discharge and 3 weeks after discharge in the low-risk patients suggests that the predischarge study can be eliminated in this group. If the object is to identify high-risk patients and not all areas of myocardium that will become ischemic at high double product, low-level stress tests should be sufficient. In the Multicenter Postmyocardial Infarction Study,[4] four clinical descriptors were independent predictors of future mortality: a history of symptoms before the myocardial infarction, PVCs greater than 10 per hour, the presence of other than basilar rales during the myocardial infarction, or an ejection fraction equal to or less than 40 percent. In this study, without description of the coronary arteries at all and without even an evaluation of persistent ischemic areas of muscle at risk, 72 percent of the patients had none or only one abnormality, and the mortality with none of the risk factors was 1.5 percent per year and with one risk factor was between 2 and 4 percent per year. Mortality increased markedly with two, three, and four abnormalities, but this was present in less than a third of the patients with three and four abnormalities in a very small percentage (7 percent for three and 2 percent for four factors). In the two thirds with one or no abnormalities, it is difficult to comprehend how even noninvasive testing, let alone coronary arteriography, could improve this low mortality.

The importance of morphology, revealing the presence of left main lesions or a combination of important lesions that place a large amount of myocardium at risk, hardly can be argued; however, these are the patients in whom exercise testing results are most likely to be positive. In a study done in 1974, we[5] looked at 120 patients who had both exercise tests and coronary arteriography. At that time we defined anatomically high-risk patients as those with a 50 percent or greater left main lesion, 75 percent or greater left anterior descending and left circumflex lesions before any branches, and 90 percent LAD lesions proximal to the first septal perforator. We classified these patients as having less than 1 mm, 1 to 1.9 mm, or 2 mm or more resting ST segment depression. All patients with left main lesions had at least 2 mm ST segment depression, and all but two patients with one or more of the high-risk lesions had at least 1 mm ST segment depression. In this latter group all but two of the high-risk patients, those with single-vessel 90 percent LAD lesions, would have had at least 1 mm ST segment depression. Other studies have supported these findings.

Most false-negative stress test results occur in patients with one-vessel disease, with a smaller number having two-vessel disease. Patients with three-vessel disease have an 80 to 90 percent incidence of ST segment depression with exercise. That patients with really high-risk lesions will be missed is unlikely, especially if other factors—such as inability to increase systolic blood pressure or heart rate or inability to exercise into stage 3 of the Bruce protocol—are used as indicators of high risk, as well as simply ST segment depression. When large areas of ischemia are present, especially those distant from the infarct, thallium 201 studies have been most useful in identifying location of the ischemia as well as the general amount of ischemic muscle.[7]

A fascinating question is whether the morphology of the lesion predicts propensity for future occlusive events. It has been suggested that ulcerated plaques are more likely to occlude than smooth obstructions. If this could be shown, then only coronary arteriography could reveal this propensity. To date, morphology of the lesions has not been proved to be predictive of future events. We should continue to try to identify such patients, although the low risk already demonstrated by noninvasive testing would suggest that increased benefit of coronary arteriography is small.

At present, all noninvasive and even coronary arteriographic assessments of risk depend on the presence of fixed, high-grade, coronary obstruction. Inasmuch as these noninvasive evaluations do indeed predict groups who are at high and low risk, the degree and extent of these coronary arterial obstructions must be important.

The development of a new event such as increased angina or recurrent myocardial infarction depends almost entirely upon a change in coronary blood flow due to a sudden increase in obstruction. Almost always, this increase in obstruction is due to rupture of a plaque or the development of a thrombus rather than simply increased vasomotor tone or spasm. The question has been raised as to whether it is possible to predict from coronary arteriography the lesion that will progress and be the site of a future occlusion. Little and colleagues[8] recently published a study of 42 consecutive patients who had undergone coronary arteriography before and up to 1 month after suffering an acute myocardial infarction. Twenty-nine patients had a newly occluded coronary artery, and 25 of these had at least one artery with greater than 50 percent stenosis on the initial angiogram. In 19 of 29 patients (66 percent), the artery that subsequently occluded had a lesion less than 50 percent on the first study, and in 28 of the 29 (97 percent) the stenosis was less than 70 percent. In only 10 of the 29 (34 percent) did the infarction occur due to occlusion of an artery that previously contained the most severe stenosis. In another study, by Moise and colleagues,[9] in 313 patients with coronary artery disease who had two coronary arteriograms, 116 had newly occluded coronary arteries. They found the presence of a greater than 80 percent stenosis, extent of coronary disease, male sex, and smoking to be the factors most predictive of development of a new coronary artery occlusion; however, 72 percent of the new occlusions in their studies occurred in coronary segments that previously contained less than a 75 percent stenosis. Apparently, in those patients judged at low risk by noninvasive techniques, the future occlusive events in the few who will have them probably will not be predicted by coronary arteriography anyway. In these patients the factors predicting the possible progression of disease and precipitation of new occlusive events may not be predictable by any of the presently available techniques, because they all depend upon finding myocardium at risk due to high-grade fixed obstruction. Inasmuch as these noninvasive techniques are predictive of future events, the presence and extent of high-grade obstructions must be important even if future occlusion may not occur at the site of most severe obstruction.

That patients after myocardial infarction or even all patients with coronary artery disease require more than a history to indicate the need for further study presents no conflict. It is also agreed that some patients without angina or with angina controlled on medical management are at high risk and need to be identified and offered revascularization. The major point of contention is the thesis that this risk stratification can be done in the majority of patients by clinical and noninvasive means and that coronary arteriography is not the only way—or even the best way—of doing this. Furthermore, it may not be possible to identify the few low-risk patients who will have future myocardial infarction or die even by coronary arteriography.

Probably the most serious problem besides the marked increase in expense that coronary arteriography in all postmyocardial infarction patients would incur would be the danger, already evident, of assuming that obstructions per se are dangerous and should be eliminated. The overuse of angioplasty in situations in which benefit has not yet been demonstrated is a real problem, but no amount of reminding physicians of their responsibility to use judgment can convince technically proficient cardiologists dedicated to the elimination of obstructions not to do angioplasty, even though by examination of a lesion one may not predict its physiologic importance. Until some unique contribution to prediction of coronary arteriography is shown, noninvasive evaluation of the patient after myocardial infarction should remain the risk stratification technique for most patients.

REFERENCES

1. DeBusk, RF, Kraemer, HC, Nash, E, et al: Stepwise risk stratification soon after acute myocardial infarction. Am J Cardiol 52:1161, 1983.
2. DeFeyter, PJ, Van Eenice, MJ, Dighton, DH, et al: Prognostic value of exercise testing, coronary angiography, and left ventriculography six to eight weeks after myocardial infarction. Circulation 66:527, 1982.
3. DeBusk, RF and Dennis, CA: "Submaximal" predischarge exercise testing after acute myocardial infarction: Who needs it? Am J Cardiol 55:499, 1985.
4. The Multicenter Post-Infarction Research Group: Risk stratification and survival after myocardial infarction. N Engl J Med 309:331, 1983.
5. Cheitlin, MD, Davia, JE, DeCastro, CM, et al: Correlation of "critical" left coronary lesions with positive submaximal exercise tests in patients with chest pain. Am Heart J 89:305, 1975.
6. Levites, R and Anderson, JJ: Detection of critical coronary artery lesions with treadmill exercise testing: Fact or fiction? Am J Cardiol 42:533, 1978.
7. Schulman, SP, Achuff, SC, Griffith, LSC, et al: Prognostic cardiac catheterization variables in survivors of acute myocardial infarction: A five year prospective study. J Am Coll Cardiol 11:1164, 1988.
8. Little, WC, Constantinescu, M, Applegate, RJ, et al: Can coronary angiography predict the site of a subsequent myocardial infarction in patients with mild-to-moderate coronary artery disease? Circulation 78:1157, 1988.
9. Moise, A, Lesperance, J, Theroux, P, et al: Clinical and angiographic predictors of new total coronary occlusion in coronary artery disease: Analysis of 313 nonoperated patients. Am J Cardiol 54:1176, 1984.

CHAPTER 2

Should the Asymptomatic Patient with a Significant Proximal LAD Stenosis Undergo PTCA?

Kanu Chatterjee, M.B., F.R.C.P.
James P. Srebro, M.D.

Since the introduction of the technique by Gruentzig and colleagues[1,2] in 1977, percutaneous transluminal coronary angioplasty (PTCA) has become an established method of improving blood flow to ischemic myocardium in patients with obstructive atherosclerotic coronary artery disease. It is of interest that the first PTCA performed on a human was on a young Swiss man with a tight proximal left anterior descending coronary artery stenosis, the subject of the present discussion. With increasing experience and technologic improvements, the indications for PTCA have expanded to include patients with multivessel disease; with stable, unstable, and postinfarction angina; and in patients with evolving acute myocardial infarction. With a higher and higher primary success rate, enthusiasm has grown, not unexpectedly, to perform PTCA based on anatomic considerations alone, often disregarding the physiologic implications of the stenosis. It should be emphasized that the purpose of revascularization therapy—whether by coronary artery bypass surgery, PTCA, or by any other technique—is to relieve myocardial ischemia and to avert its adverse consequences. Thus, the presence of myocardial ischemia should be an important consideration before any therapy is contemplated in patients with obstructive coronary artery lesions. Furthermore, when several therapeutic options are available, the relative merits of different options, including the potential to improve symptoms and prognosis, must be carefully evaluated. The recommendation to treat at all becomes difficult in asymptomatic or mildly symptomatic patients, because the benefit of such therapy may not be discernible immediately and potential complications of treatment can mask the potential benefits. Thus, the question of whether an asymptomatic patient with proximal left anterior descending (LAD) coronary artery stenosis should undergo PTCA cannot be answered without considering many related questions: (1) What is the risk that proximal LAD stenosis will decrease survival? (2) Is the prognosis different among

patients with silent or manifest ischemia resulting from proximal LAD stenosis? (3) Is the magnitude of myocardium at risk an important consideration for selection of therapy? (4) Is conservative therapy any worse than more aggressive therapy, such as PTCA? (5) Is coronary artery bypass graft surgery better than PTCA in such patients? (6) What is the cost effectiveness of PTCA compared with the other therapeutic modalities?

It is apparent that the general answers to these questions are not available at present and that specific recommendations have to be made with an individual patient in mind. In practice the decision about PTCA for proximal LAD stenosis remains largely empirical. In this discussion we outline an approach, which, admittedly, may not be universally applicable; it should be helpful, however, to the clinician faced with this therapeutic dilemma.

PROGNOSIS OF LEFT ANTERIOR DESCENDING CORONARY ARTERY (LAD) STENOSIS

The natural history of isolated LAD stenosis in asymptomatic individuals remains unknown. However, some general statements can be made from the information available regarding the influence of symptoms on the prognosis of patients with coronary artery disease. A large number of studies have been performed that relate prognosis to the extent, severity, and distribution of coronary artery disease. Several nonangiographic studies have assessed the relationship of clinical manifestations of coronary artery disease to long-term prognosis. In the Framingham Study,[3] a large sample population was followed for 10 years. Following the onset of angina, the annual mortality was 4 percent and increased to 5 percent following a nonfatal myocardial infarction. The population with neither of these manifestations of ischemic heart disease had an excellent prognosis. Unfortunately, the specific coronary anatomy was not known, so the impact of the severity and distribution of the coronary artery disease could not be identified. In the Helsinki coronary risk factor study,[4] 1711 men aged 40 to 59 years were followed for 15 years and compared with the population without manifestations of coronary artery disease. The total coronary mortality in the study population was 9.3 per 1000 person years. In patients with documented myocardial infarction based on electrocardiographic criteria, deaths per 1000 person years were 71.3. In the population with symptoms of angina or exercise stress test evidence of myocardial ischemia, the mortality was 18.5 per 1000 person years. In the absence of ischemia, the risk was fourfold less, only 4.7 per 1000 person years. Again, the severity of coronary artery disease and specific anatomy were not known, and the prognosis of isolated LAD stenosis could not be ascertained. Electrocardiographic evidence of myocardial ischemia at rest or during exercise irrespective of symptoms imparts a poorer prognosis compared with control groups.[5] An annual mortality of greater than 5 percent has been reported in patients who develop 1 mm or more ST segment depression during a final exercise stage of I or less. In contrast, an annual mortality of less than 1 percent was reported in patients who experience less than 1 mm ST depression at the completion of stage III of a Bruce protocol. It seems clear from these studies that myocardial ischemia is the primary factor contributing to prognosis.

With the advent of coronary angiography, the significance of the severity and distribution of coronary artery disease in relation to long-term prognosis has been determined in a number of retrospective studies. Analysis of pooled data from sev-

eral major centers indicates that if only one of the three major coronary arteries had significant obstructive lesions, the annual mortality was approximately 2 percent. If two major vessels were involved, the mortality was approximately 7 percent; and if all three were significantly obstructed, the rate was approximately 11 percent.[6] The Cleveland Clinic experience also suggests that the annual mortality of patients with one-vessel coronary artery disease is approximately 3 percent.[7] More recent studies, however, have indicated a more favorable prognosis in patients with single-vessel coronary artery disease. The Coronary Artery Surgery Study (CASS) found that the survival rate of patients with single-vessel coronary artery disease was decreased by only 5 percent over 4 years of observation compared with the control group without significant coronary artery disease.[8]

Califf and associates[9] studied the outcome of patients with single-vessel coronary artery disease. The overall annual mortality in the nonsurgically treated patients with single-vessel disease was less than 2 percent, not markedly worse than that of the control population. In this study, however, the prognosis of patients with LAD stenosis was worse than that of those with right coronary artery (RCA) stenosis. The 1-year and 5-year survival rates in patients with LAD stenoses were 96 percent and 92 percent, respectively, and those with RCA disease were 99 percent and 96 percent, respectively. Although other studies have indicated a poorer prognosis for patients with LAD stenosis,[10] a totally benign outcome of such patients has also been reported.[11] Kouchoukos and coworkers[11] reported no mortality of nonsurgically treated patients with LAD stenosis during an average follow-up period of 3.5 years.

Whether the location of the stenosis within the LAD influences the prognosis also has been evaluated in a number of studies.[9,12] Califf and colleagues[9] compared the survival rate of nonsurgically treated patients with stenoses of LAD before and after the first septal perforator. The group with lesions before the first septal perforator had a lower survival rate than the group with more distal lesions. At 5 years, the patients with distal lesions had a survival rate of 98 percent, compared with 90 percent in patients with lesions proximal to the first septal perforator. In this study the annual mortalities were found to be 2 percent in patients with proximal LAD stenosis and only 0.4 percent in those with distal LAD stenosis. Patients with proximal RCA or left circumflex lesions did not have higher mortality compared with those with distal lesions. Brooks and associates[12] reported that only patients with proximal LAD stenosis seemed to be at high risk of mortality over a mean follow-up period of 2 years. All these studies tend to support the hypothesis that significant proximal LAD stenosis is associated with a worse prognosis. It needs to be emphasized, however, that asymptomatic patients with LAD stenosis were not specifically evaluated, although some patients had only mild symptoms.

A few studies have suggested that patients with asymptomatic coronary artery disease have a better prognosis than those with angina. Cohn and colleagues[13] found a survival rate of 81 percent in asymptomatic patients (yearly mortality 2.7 percent) compared with 62 percent in the symptomatic group (yearly mortality 5.4 percent). The worst prognosis was found in asymptomatic patients with three-vessel disease who had a survival rate of 4.7 percent compared with 8.7 percent in symptomatic individuals. In this study the small number of patients with isolated LAD stenosis limits the ability to extrapolate the prognosis of asymptomatic LAD stenosis with confidence. Furthermore, the majority of asymptomatic patients with coronary artery disease in this study had ECG evidence of prior myocardial infarction. Thus, the prognosis of patients without any manifestations of coronary artery disease appears difficult to know with certainty.

Other studies suggest that the prognosis of patients with "manifest" ischemia is very similar to that of patients with "silent" ischemia. Silent myocardial ischemia in patients after myocardial infarction is associated with a poorer prognosis that is very similar to that of patients with postinfarction[14,15] and unstable angina.[16]

Falcone and associates[17] reported that the clinical course of patients with exercise-induced angina is similar to that of exercise-induced silent ischemia. No difference in survival was noted in either group during a follow-up period of four years. In the Coronary Artery Surgery Study, the severity of coronary artery disease and prognosis of patients with silent ischemia on treadmill test and patients with angina were compared. There was no significant difference in the extent of coronary artery disease found on angiography and in their seven-year survival rates.[18]

In patients without previous clinical manifestations of coronary artery disease, silent myocardial ischemia does not necessarily influence the prognosis unfavorably. In asymptomatic individuals who underwent treadmill testing, Erikssen and coworkers[20] identified the incidence of coronary artery disease by this method to be 2.5 percent. In follow-up, there was a 0.5 percent incidence of sudden death, which occurred only in patients with three-vessel disease. Thus, patients without known coronary artery disease who have asymptomatic myocardial ischemia enjoy a better prognosis than those with established coronary artery disease and silent ischemia.

Silent myocardial ischemia in patients with asymptomatic coronary artery disease appears to be associated with higher incidence of unfavorable cardiac events. Cohn[21] summarized data from three studies with a total of 141 patients with asymptomatic coronary artery disease and silent ischemia and reported an average incidence of cardiac events of 34 percent over a follow-up period of three to eight years. DeWood[22] compared the mortality and incidence of cardiac events in 26 patients with silent ischemia detected by ambulatory electrocardiograms to those of 32 patients who exhibited no electrocardiographic evidence of ischemia. The patients with silent ischemia had a higher cardiac event rate (46 percent) and mortality (9 percent) over a follow-up period of three years compared with an event rate of 23 percent and a mortality of 6 percent in the group without ischemia. Walters and associates[23] reported a worse prognosis in patients with an exercise-induced thallium defect without symptoms compared with those who developed angina.[23] These studies indicate that the presence of symptoms is not as important as the presence of ischemia. The relevance of this concept is that one should consider the identification of myocardial ischemia very carefully in asymptomatic patients with coronary artery disease because *it is ischemia that appears to determine the prognosis, regardless of whether it is associated with symptoms.* Thus, in the evaluation of asymptomatic patients with significant proximal LAD stenosis, the detection of ischemia becomes imperative.

THERAPY AND PROGNOSIS

The two major goals of therapy are (1) to ameliorate symptoms and to improve life-style and (2) to improve prognosis. In asymptomatic patients, it is difficult to improve life-style with any therapy. Indeed, the potential exists for deterioration in life-style resulting from the complications of therapy. Nitrates, beta-adrenergic blocking agents, and calcium entry blocking agents are the three classes of drugs employed to treat myocardial ischemia and its manifestations. Each class of drugs, when used alone or in combination, can produce significant undesirable side effects. Thus, asymptomatic patients may become symptomatic, and normal lifestyle may deteriorate because of therapeutic intervention. Morbidity associated with coronary artery bypass surgery also may alter the life-style of patients subjected to such therapy. Although PTCA has less morbidity than coronary artery bypass surgery, PTCA is not an entirely benign procedure. Additionally, anxiety from the fear of restenosis may alter life-style after PTCA.

As discussed earlier, the survival of medically treated symptomatic patients with single-vessel coronary artery disease is excellent, although the prognosis of patients with proximal LAD stenosis appears to be somewhat worse. The prognosis of patients with asymptomatic LAD stenosis is not known, but it is unlikely to be any worse than that of symptomatic patients. It appears from the presently available data that the prognosis of patients with coronary artery disease and myocardial ischemia is similar regardless of symptoms. Thus, it is reasonable to expect that the prognosis of asymptomatic patients with proximal LAD stenosis would be similar to those with symptoms. One would expect a very favorable prognosis in patients with isolated single-vessel disease compared with those with more extensive disease.

Is revascularization therapy any better than medical therapy in patients with proximal LAD stenosis? A number of prospective, randomized studies have reported no difference in survival between medically and surgically treated patients with single-vessel disease.[24] Some uncontrolled studies, however, have suggested that patients with proximal LAD stenosis, particularly in association with left ventricular dysfunction, may experience a marginally better prognosis with coronary artery bypass surgery compared with medical therapy.[9] In the Coronary Artery Surgery Study, it was also noted that patients with angina and reduced left ventricular ejection fraction had better survival following coronary artery bypass surgery than with continued medical therapy.[25] Ellis and associates[26] have compared the 3 to 5-year mortality and infarction rates after PTCA (627 patients) and medical therapy (865 patients) for one- or two-vessel disease including the left anterior descending coronary artery. There was no difference in overall survival (PTCA 95 percent and medical therapy 93 percent at five years). However, after correction of baseline differences, PTCA improved survival of patients with left ventricular ejection fraction less than 50 percent ($P < 0.02$). Results of these studies suggest that if left ventricular dysfunction results primarily from myocardial ischemia, improved perfusion to the ischemic myocardium may result in a better prognosis. Inasmuch as ischemia appears to be the predominant prognostic factor, the magnitude of myocardium at risk rather than the coronary anatomy should be considered. Patients with silent myocardial ischemia and left ventricular dysfunction also appear to benefit from coronary artery bypass surgery. In certain subsets of patients with proximal LAD stenosis, one can appreciate the appeal of catheter-based and surgical revascularization therapy.

However, one must also consider the advantages and disadvantages of each modality in making a decision. Coronary artery bypass surgery can be performed with a very low operative mortality (0 to 0.6 percent) in patients with single-vessel coronary artery disease.[9] Furthermore, the use of an internal mammary artery (IMA) as a conduit is associated with a higher late-graft patency rate and a better survival compared with saphenous vein conduits. Several studies have claimed patency rates of 85 to 96 percent for IMA grafts.[27,28] Loop and associates[27] reported a mean patency rate of 96 percent for IMA grafts compared with 81 percent for saphenous vein grafts at 10 years. Follow-up angiographic studies have frequently demonstrated progressive atherosclerosis and stenosis of saphenous vein grafts, especially in the fifth to twelfth postoperative years. The 10-year actuarial survival was 86.6 percent for patients receiving an IMA graft compared with 75.9 percent for patients receiving saphenous vein grafts.

Zeff and colleagues[29] compared the patency rates of IMA and saphenous vein grafts to the LAD in a prospective, randomized study. During a follow-up period of 10 years, the patency rate of IMA grafts was 94.6 percent, whereas that of saphenous vein grafts was 76.3 percent. Although some patients received vein grafts to other vessels as well, those who received an IMA graft to the LAD continued to have a better prognosis. Cardiac mortality in patients receiving IMA conduits at 10 years was 7.7 percent (annual mortality of 0.77 percent) compared with 12.8 percent in those who received saphenous vein grafts (annual mortality of 1.28 percent). These reports suggest that patency is much improved if an IMA is used for revascularization of the LAD. Long-term prognosis is also expected to be excellent following IMA bypass of the LAD.

How does PTCA compare with coronary artery bypass surgery? It is now well established that the primary success rate for effective dilatation of the stenotic coronary artery has increased considerably in recent years, presumably due to increasing experience and improved technology (Table 2–1).[30] In the most recent PTCA registry, 1802 patients were entered during 1985 to 1986. In 839 patients with single-vessel disease, the success rate (defined as a reduction of stenosis by 20 percent or more) was 89 percent. This primary success rate is considerably higher than that in the initial PTCA registry of 1977 to 1981.[30] In patients with single-vessel disease, the recent incidence of PTCA-related deaths, nonfatal myocardial infarction, and the need for emergent coronary artery bypass surgery was 0.2 percent, 3.5 percent, and 2.9 percent, respectively.[30] Thus, successful PTCA is expected in the vast majority of patients with single-vessel disease and should be performed with very low morbidity and mortality. However, it needs to be emphasized that one of the major limitations of PTCA is restenosis, which occurs in approximately 25 to 35 percent of subjects. In patients with moderate or severe angina and an ideal single-vessel lesion, PTCA may be the most desirable mode of treatment. However, such decisions are usually made empirically and based on experience rather than on the

Table 2–1. Comparison of Outcomes in the PTCA Registry: 1977–81 and 1985–86

Outcome	Group % of Patients	
	1977–81 (*n* = 1155)	1985–86 (*n* = 1802)
One or more lesions reduced ≥20%	67.5	90.7
All lesions attempted reduced ≥20% and no death, infarction, or coronary operation	61.0	78.3
Death	1.2	1.0
Nonfatal infarction	4.9	4.3
Coronary artery bypass grafting	26.5	5.6

Table 2–2. Complications of Angioplasty by Number of Diseased
Vessels in 1985–86 Cohort of PTCA Registry (1802 Patients)

Complication	Vessel Disease*								
	Single (n = 839)		Double (n = 559)		Triple (n = 367)		Left Main (n = 37)		
	Number of Patients	%	Number of Patients	%	Number of Patients	%	Number of Patients	%	P Value
Death	2	0.2	5	0.9	8	2.8	3	8.1	<0.001
Nonfatal MI	29	3.5	29	5.2	19	5.2	1	2.7	NS
Emergency CABG	24	2.9	22	3.9	16	4.4	1	2.7	NS
Death, MI, or emergency CABG	46	5.5	45	8.1	34	9.3	4	10.8	<0.05
Occlusion	33	3.9	25	4.5	29	7.9	1	2.7	<0.01
Prolonged angina	29	3.5	29	5.2	24	6.5	2	5.4	<0.05

*χ^2 tests for linear trend were used to compare the groups with single-, double-, and triple-vessel disease because of the small number of patients with left main coronary artery disease.

Abbreviations: CABG = coronary artery bypass grafting, MI = myocardial infarction, NS = not significant.

From Holmes, DR, Jr, Holubkov, R, Vlietstra, RE, et al: Comparison of complications during percutaneous transluminal coronary angioplasty from 1977–81 and from 1985–86: The National Heart, Lung, and Blood Institute Percutaneous Transluminal Coronary Angioplasty Registry. J Am Coll Cardiol 12:1149, 1988.

results of controlled studies. Even when single-vessel disease is present, certain characteristics of the lesion may be associated with a higher incidence of complications. The severity of the lesion, length, calcification, eccentricity, ostial involvement, and the presence of thrombus increase the potential for immediate and delayed complications.[31] It also has been reported that PTCA of very proximal LAD stenoses may be associated with a higher risk of complications.[32] Subacute progression of left main stenosis following LAD dilatation has been reported by Haraphorgse and Rossall.[33] Although rare, occlusion of the left main coronary artery following PTCA has been reported.[34,35] Percutaneous transluminal coronary angioplasty of a very proximal LAD lesion also may cause occlusion of adjacent major branches. Strategies such as dual wires and *kissing balloon* technique increase the complexity of the procedure,[36] but they may provide an extra margin of safety in certain situations. The potential complications (Table 2–2) always should be carefully considered in PTCA, particularly in asymptomatic patients.

The cost effectiveness of PTCA compared with medical or surgical therapy remains controversial. Although the immediate cost of PTCA is considerably less than coronary artery bypass surgery, repeat cardiac catheterization to evaluate restenosis is practiced in many centers, and repeat PTCA in patients with restenosis increases cost. Thus, the long-term cost related to PTCA may not be substantially less than that related to coronary artery bypass surgery, particularly when an IMA is used. However, one should not overlook many benefits of PTCA, such as minimal discomfort and morbidity, lack of prolonged hospitalization, and avoidance of sternotomy.

Table 2–3. Several Approaches to Proximal LAD Stenosis

Physiologic Test for Ischemia	LAD Stenosis Anatomy	Amount of Jeopardized Myocardium	Suggested Approach
Negative or mildly positive	Noncritical	Small	Medical therapy Modify risk factors Periodic screen for progression If patient cannot tolerate medical therapy, consider interventional approach
Positive	Favorable (discrete, concentric, not involving other vessels)	Large	PTCA, especially if EF is <40%
Positive	Unfavorable (elongated, complex, involving other branches)	Large	CABG with IMA, especially if EF <40%

It is apparent that a decision regarding PTCA of proximal LAD stenosis in an asymptomatic patient should be made with a number of factors in mind: (1) the general prognosis of medically treated patients with single-vessel disease, including those with lesions distal to the first septal perforator, is excellent and comparable with that of surgically treated patients and that of patients treated by PTCA; (2) revascularization may provide a better prognosis in patients with ischemia and left ventricular dysfunction; (3) the prognoses of patients with manifest and silent myocardial ischemias are similar, and the objective of therapy is to avert the consequences of myocardial ischemia; (4) the IMA graft to the LAD provides long-term conduit patency and improves survival; (5) abrupt reclosure and a 25 to 35 percent delayed restenosis rate are the major limitations of PTCA; and (6) PTCA is generally more attractive than coronary artery bypass surgery owing to lower morbidity, although immediate and late mortality following PTCA or coronary artery bypass surgery with an IMA conduit appears to be similar. It also needs to be emphasized that most of the information regarding relative advantages and disadvantages of PTCA and coronary artery bypass surgery in patients with LAD stenoses are circumstantial and derived from studies of symptomatic patients. Nevertheless, it is reasonable to extrapolate these data to formulate a therapeutic approach for the management of asymptomatic patients with proximal LAD stenosis (Table 2–3).

SUGGESTED MANAGEMENT APPROACH

Left anterior descending coronary artery stenosis is usually discovered in asymptomatic patients in the following clinical settings: (1) positive stress test performed to screen patients with risk factors for coronary artery disease, (2) during postinfarction risk stratification for adverse cardiac events and prognosis, and (3) following thrombolytic therapy to assess the severity of coronary artery disease.

In patients without previous myocardial infarction it is desirable to assess the magnitude of ischemia and myocardium at risk. This information is usually obtained by performing conventional exercise stress tests, exercise or dipyridamole thallium scintigraphy, or exercise radionuclide ventriculography. In the absence of significant ischemia or when left ventricular wall motion remains normal during exercise, no specific therapy is required except the modification of risk factors. These patients can be followed with exercise tests to assess the progression of disease. In postinfarction patients or in patients following thrombolytic therapy who have fixed perfusion defects or no reversible wall motion abnormalities, medical therapy such as the use of beta-adrenergic blocking drugs and aspirin may be all that is required.

Risk factors such as hypertension and hyperlipidemia should be aggressively treated. Weight reduction, smoking cessation, and graded exercise are also important and may contribute to stabilizing the atherosclerotic process and, in some cases, may lead to regression. After an appropriate period of time, a test for ischemia should be repeated. If the test result is negative or improved, one would be encouraged to follow the clinical course and repeat the tests at regular intervals of time.

In some patients, medical management will be especially problematic because side effects may be intolerable despite their salutary effect on ischemia. If the patient is asymptomatic, limitations of life-style, the inconvenience of taking medications, and the continuing financial cost without a perceptible benefit to the patient may affect compliance. These considerations may make an interventional approach more attractive.

In patients who have large reversible perfusion defects, markedly positive stress tests at low levels of exercise, or a large area of jeopardized myocardium, the clinical situation warrants a more aggressive approach. This is especially true with an extremely tight stenosis and with anatomy that is favorable for intervention. In the case of PTCA, this means a discrete, concentric focal stenosis that does not involve the left main or circumflex coronary arteries. Features such as eccentricity and calcification are only relative contraindications. The presence of intraluminal thrombus may increase the risk of further thrombosis or distal embolization.

In patients who are deemed to be at high risk for PTCA, there are several strategies that may improve perfusion to the watershed myocardium in the result of failure. These include coronary sinus retroperfusion (investigational), peripheral cardiopulmonary bypass, and intracoronary catheter-based perfusion systems. Each has theoretic advantages and limitations, and efficacy has not been documented in large trials. Nonetheless, these are potentially useful adjuncts in high-risk cases.

Patients who undergo percutaneous angioplasty probably should be treated with calcium entry blocking agents and aspirin for several months after the procedure, although there is no conclusive evidence that this reduces the restenosis rate. Follow-up usually involves repeat exercise studies, especially in the first year. If the patient continues to manifest ischemia, repeat cardiac catheterization is necessary. If restenosis occurs, it is generally acceptable to redilate the lesion. In our institution, we generally try a slightly larger balloon, higher inflation pressures, or longer inflation times. If the patient again experiences restenosis, referral for catheter-based atherectomy, laser-assisted angioplasty, or intravascular stent placement may be considered. These modalities are investigational at present. Alternatively, the patient may be considered for surgical revascularization.

Coronary artery bypass grafting is generally reserved for those patients with single-vessel disease who have intractable symptoms. This concept can be extended in patients considered to be high-risk as already discussed. The patient should have anatomy that is amenable to graft implantation with good distal runoff. The myocardium subserved by the vessel should be viable. Internal mammary arteries are much preferred in this situation because of their prolonged patency rates.

SUMMARY

The approach to a proximal LAD stenosis in an asymptomatic patient depends on a number of factors. Most important among these are the presence and extent of ischemia, anatomic considerations, and the functional status of the myocardium subserved by the vessel. In patients with functionally and hemodynamically insignificant disease with no ischemia, it is appropriate simply to follow the patient and to modify the risk factors for atherosclerosis if they exist. All three of the currently available modalities are appropriate in individual patients, including medical management, percutaneous balloon angioplasty, and surgical revascularization. In ambiguous cases, the available studies suggest no benefit from aggressive strategies; therefore, a conservative approach that minimizes side effects and complications of treatment is best.

REFERENCES

1. Gruentzig, AR, Myler, RK, Hanna, ES, et al: Coronary transluminal angioplasty (abstr). Circulation 56(Suppl III):84, 1977.
2. Gruentzig, AR, Senning, A, and Siegenthaler, WE: Nonoperative dilatation of coronary artery stenosis: Percutaneous transluminal coronary angioplasty (PTCA). N Engl J Med 301:61, 1979.
3. Kannel, WB and Feinleib, M: Natural history of angina pectoris in the Framingham Study: Progress and survival. Am J Cardiol 29:154, 1972.
4. Heliovaana, M, Karvoren, MJ, Punsar, S, et al: Importance of coronary risk factors in the presence or absence of myocardial ischemia. Am J Cardiol 50:1248, 1982.
5. Weiner, DA, Ryan, TJ, McCabe, CH, et al: Prognostic importance of a clinical profile and exercise test in medically treated patients with coronary artery disease. J Am Coll Cardiol 3:772, 1984.
6. Reeves, TJ, Oberman, A, Jones, WB, et al: Natural history of angina pectoris. Am J Cardiol 33:423, 1979.
7. Proudfit, WJ, Bruschke, AVG, MacMillan, JP, et al: Fifteen year survival study of patients with obstructive coronary artery disease. Circulation 68:986, 1983.
8. Mock, MB, Ringquist, I, Fisher, LD, et al: Circulation 66:562, 1982.
9. Califf, RM, Tomabechi, Y, Lee, K, et al: Outcome in one vessel coronary artery disease. Circulation 67:283, 1983.
10. Brushke, AVG, Proudfit, WL, and Jones, FM: Progress study of 590 consecutive nonsurgical cases of coronary disease followed 5–9 years. Arteriographic correlations. Circulation 47:1147, 1973.
11. Kouchoukos, NT, Oberman, O, Russell, RO, et al: Surgical versus medical treatment of occlusive disease confined to the left anterior descending coronary artery. Am J Cardiol 35:836, 1975.
12. Brooks, N, Cattall, M, Jennings, K, et al: Isolated disease of left anterior descending coronary artery: Angiographic and clinical study of 218 patients. Br Heart J 47:71, 1982.
13. Cohn, PF, Harris, P, Barry, WH, et al: Prognostic importance of anginal symptoms in angiographically defined coronary artery disease. Am J Cardiol 47:233, 1981.
14. Theroux, P, Waters, DD, Halphen, C, et al: Prognostic value of exercise testing soon after myocardial infarction. N Engl J Med 301:341, 1979.
15. Schuster, EH and Bulkley, BH: Early post-infarction angina: Ischemia at a distance and ischemia in the infarct zone. N Engl J Med 305:1101, 1981.
16. Lanager, A, Freeman, MR, and Armstrong, PW: ST segment shift in unstable angina: Pathophysiology and association with coronary anatomy and hospital outcome. J Am Coll Cardiol 13:1495, 1989.

17. Falcone, C, De Servi, S, Pomma, E, et al: Clinical significance of exercise-induced silent myocardial ischemia in patients with coronary artery disease. J Am Coll Cardiol 9:295, 1987.
18. Weiner, DA, Ryan, TJ, McCabe, CH, et al: Significance of silent myocardial ischemia during exercise testing in patients with coronary artery disease. Am J Cardiol 59:625, 1987.
19. Chatterjee, K: Ischemia: Silent or manifest: Does it matter? J Am Coll Cardiol 13:1503, 1989.
20. Erikssen, J and Thavlow, E: Followup of patients with asymptomatic myocardial ischemia. In Rutishauser, W and Roskamm, H (eds): Silent Myocardial Ischemia. Berlin, Springer-Verlag, 1984, pp 156–164.
21. Cohn, PF: Asymptomatic coronary artery disease. Modern Concepts Cardiovasc Dis 50:55, 1981.
22. DeWood, MA: Long-term prognosis of patients with and without silent ischemia (abstr). Circulation 74:II-59, 1986.
23. Walters, GL, Assey, ME, Hendrix, GH, et al: Increased incidence of myocardial infarction in patients with exercise induced silent myocardial ischemia (abstr). Circulation 74:II-58, 1986.
24. Varnauskas, E and European Coronary Surgery Study Group: Survival, myocardial infarction, and employment status in a prospective randomized study of coronary bypass surgery. Circulation 72:V-90, 1985.
25. Myers, WO, Davis, K, Foster, ED, et al: Surgical survival in the coronary artery surgery study (CASS) registry. Ann Thorac Surg 40:246, 1985.
26. Ellis, SG, Fisher, L, Dushman-Ellis, S, et al: Comparison of 3–5 year mortality and infarction rates after angioplasty (PTCA) or medical therapy for 1 or 2 vessel left anterior descending disease. Circulation 76:IV-392, 1987.
27. Loop, FD, Lytle, BW, Cosgrove, DM, et al: Influence of the internal mammary artery graft on 10-year survival and other cardiac events. N Engl J Med 314:1, 1986.
28. Barner, HB, Swartz, MT, Mudd, JG, et al: Late patency of the internal mammary artery as a coronary bypass conduit. Ann Thorac Surg 34:408, 1982.
29. Zeff, RH, Kongtahworn, C, Iannone, LA, et al: Internal mammary artery versus saphenous vein graft to the left anterior descending coronary artery. Prospective randomized study with 10-year follow-up. Ann Thorac Surg 45:533, 1988.
30. Detre, K, Holubkov, R, Kelsery, S, et al: Percutaneous transluminal coronary angioplasty in 1985–1986 and 1977–1981: The National Heart, Lung, and Blood Institute Registry. N Engl J Med 318:256, 1988.
31. Ellis, SG, Roubin, GS, King, SB III, et al: Angiographic and clinical predictors of acute closure after native vessel coronary angioplasty. Circulation 77:372, 1988.
32. Simon, R, Amede, I, Herman, G, et al: Coronary angioplasty of lesions adjacent to the left main: Results and risks. Circulation 74 (Suppl II):193, 1986.
33. Haraphorgse, M and Rossall, RE: Subacute left main coronary stenosis following percutaneous transluminal coronary angioplasty. Cath Cardiovasc Diag 13:401, 1987.
34. Bourana, MG and Noble, J. Complication rate of coronary arteriography: A review of 5250 cases studied by a percutaneous femoral technique. Circulation 53:106, 1976.
35. Slack, JD, Pinkerton, CA, Van Tassel, JW, et al: Left main coronary artery dissection during percutaneous transluminal angioplasty. Cath Cardiovasc Diag 12:255, 1986.
36. Meier, B: Kissing balloon coronary angioplasty. Am J Cardiol 53:918, 1984.

Commentary

By Melvin D. Cheitlin, M.D.

Decision making in therapy is easiest when the therapy has been proved to be effective in achieving important goals for the patients and can be applied with low morbidity and mortality. The problem of the asymptomatic patient with a left anterior descending coronary artery lesion, addressed in this chapter by Chatterjee and Srebro, is one that occurs not infrequently in practice. When surgery was the only alternative to medical therapy, the decision was easier. The uncertainties of definite benefit of revascularization in these patients, well described in this chapter, combined with the certain morbidity of a thoracotomy, weighed heavily against surgical bypass and argued for medical therapy and observation. The development of PTCA with its high initial success rate and low mortality and morbidity makes the decision not to recommend revascularization more difficult. This is especially true if *ischemia,* as defined by ST segment and changes in T wave either spontaneously occurring or precipitated by exercise, is present, especially since evidence is becoming convincing that this *silent ischemia* may have a prognostic significance similar to angina.[1]

In practice many angiographers consider the presence of a high-grade, proximal coronary arterial obstruction, especially in the left anterior descending coronary artery, an indication for angioplasty with or without ischemia. Against this opinion is evidence from the large randomized studies of surgical versus medical management, that bypass of a single-vessel obstruction in symptomatic patients has no advantages over medical management, either in survival or in avoiding myocardial infarction. As stated, it is unlikely (although still possible) that the prognosis would be worse in asymptomatic patients with the same pathophysiologic situation as in symptomatic patients. Because we are considering the asymptomatic patient, the goals of therapy must be the avoidance of future morbidity or mortality.

Although controversial, there is evidence that not all patients lumped into "single-vessel disease" have the same prognosis and that symptomatic patients with high-grade proximal lesions of the left anterior descending coronary artery are at higher risk than either those with more distal lesions of the left anterior descending coronary artery or those with proximal right coronary artery or left circumflex coronary artery lesions.[2,3] Kouchoukas and colleagues[4] reported a benign prognosis with medical management in single-vessel left anterior descending disease. Califf and colleagues[2] reported the annual mortality of patients with proximal left anterior descending coronary artery disease to be 2 percent per year compared with 0.4 percent per year mortality for patients with distal left anterior descending coronary artery lesions. The mortality even in the patients with proximal lesions is low, and

42

the vast majority of the patients were symptomatic. There is some evidence, however, that patients with proximal left anterior descending coronary arterial lesions can benefit from bypass surgery compared with those medically managed.[2] With the use of the internal mammary artery as a conduit, long-term patency has proved to be excellent, and if it is accepted that in the asymptomatic patient with evidence of ischemia by noninvasive testing that the prognosis is similar to that of patients with angina, a case could be made for bypass surgery in these patients.

There is no study that randomizes the asymptomatic patient with left anterior descending coronary artery obstruction to medical versus surgical therapy. The unrandomized portion of the CASS study[5] indicates that symptomatic patients with single left anterior descending coronary artery disease and left ventricular dysfunction do better with bypass surgery than with medical therapy. The only nonrandomized study with PTCA, that of Ellis and colleagues,[6] showed no difference in survival in patients with one- or two-vessel disease involving the left anterior descending artery, between PTCA (95 percent survival) and medical therapy (93 percent survival) at five years. On subgroup analysis the patients with ejection fractions less than 50 percent had a better survival after PTCA.

Balanced against these possible survival benefits of revascularization in the symptomatic patients with left anterior descending coronary artery disease are the definite problems of PTCA. It is appropriate to use the NHLBI Registry data,[7] because these data are more likely to be representative of what can be expected in the usual facility doing PTCA than individual reports from university centers. In this registry the incidence of PTCA-related complications in single-vessel disease was death in 0.2 percent, nonfatal myocardial infarction in 3.5 percent, and need for emergency bypass surgery in 2.9 percent. The chance of one of these adverse events occurring is 5.5 percent. Combining this with an additional 3.9 percent occlusion rate and a 3.5 percent prolonged anginal rate, a 10 percent failure to achieve successful PTCA rate, and a late restenosis rate of 25 to 35 percent of patients with some of these requiring second procedures or even bypass surgery, the attractiveness of starting an asymptomatic patient down this therapeutic pathway diminishes somewhat. Furthermore, consideration must be given to the presence or absence of collateral vessels. If collateral vessels are present, there is probably a protective situation for the patient with a proximal left anterior descending lesion that would make extensive infarction less likely and, therefore, would mitigate against revascularization in the asymptomatic patient.

With all of these factors considered, Chatterjee and Srebro have done what all practicing physicians must do: Decide on an action even before all the facts are in. They have accepted the evidence, as I do, that patients with a large volume of ischemic myocardium are at increased risk of an adverse event whether or not they have the subjective symptom of angina pectoris and that this risk can be reduced by revascularization. This is especially compelling when reduced left ventricular function is present either at rest or with exercise, indicating a reduced reserve of myocardium and significant amount of ischemic myocardium. I therefore opt to believe that PTCA is indicated in such patients, and when PTCA is not possible, that bypass surgery using the internal mammary artery is justified.

REFERENCES

1. Weiner, DA, Ryan, TJ, McCabe, CH, et al: Significance of silent myocardial ischemia during exercise testing in patients with coronary artery disease. Am J Cardiol 59:725, 1987.

2. Califf, RM, Tomabechi, Y, Lee, K, et al: Outcome in one vessel coronary artery disease. Circulation 67:283, 1983.
3. Brooks, N, Cattall, M, Jennings, K, et al: Isolated disease of left anterior descending coronary artery: Angiographic and clinical study of 218 patients. Br Heart J 47:71, 1987.
4. Kouchoukas, NT, Oberman, O, Russell, RO, et al: Surgical versus medical treatment of occlusive disease compared to the left anterior descending coronary artery. Am J Cardiol 35:836, 1975.
5. Myers, WO, Davis, K, Foster, ED, et al: Surgical survival in the Coronary Artery Surgery Study (CASS) Registry. Ann Thorac Surg 40:246, 1985.
6. Ellis, SG, Fisher, L, Dushman-Ellis, S, et al: Comparison of 3–5 year mortality and infarction rates after angioplasty (PTCA) or medical therapy for 1- or 2-vessel left anterior descending disease. Circulation 76:IV–392, 1987.
7. Detre, K, Holubkov, R, Kelsery, S, et al: Percutaneous transluminal coronary angioplasty in 1985–1986 and 1977–1981: The National Heart, Lung and Blood Institute Registry. N Engl J Med 318:256, 1988.

CHAPTER 3

How Should We Manage Continuing Asymptomatic Ischemia in Patients Treated for Angina Pectoris?

Khether E. Raby, M.D.
Andrew P. Selwyn, M.D.

Treatment for coronary artery disease has made impressive progress over the last decade. Successes have included primary risk factor prevention schemes, such as antismoking campaigns, trials of lipid-lowering agents, and a variety of medical and surgical regimens that have been shown to reduce risk of morbidity and mortality. It can be argued, however, that revascularization procedures have played the most significant role in altering our approach to the patient with coronary artery disease.[1]

Recognition and quantification of coronary artery disease have relied heavily so far on spontaneous or inducible symptoms, and directing treatment at symptoms alone is the traditional approach. In most patients, angina is common and, when present, is easy to recognize and quantify. It is present in a wide range, from mild to severe, with a rough correlation with anatomic severity of coronary artery disease. Severity of symptoms along with anatomy is what ultimately guides the most aggressive interventions, specifically revascularization, which is highly effective in relieving symptoms and improving the quality of life.

More recently, coronary artery bypass surgery has emerged as the treatment of choice in selected, high-risk cohorts for reasons other than symptom control. In patients with left main coronary artery disease, or multivessel coronary artery disease and impaired left ventricular function, revascularization clearly improves prognosis and thus prolongs life.[2,3] In addition to these findings, it has been clearly established that transient myocardial ischemia is the mechanism by which coronary artery disease causes permanent damage and subsequent death. It also has become clear that a significant proportion of myocardial ischemia is asymptomatic. Given the potential of revascularization to improve the prognosis of a sizable population of patients at high risk, it has now become important not to rely on symptoms alone as a measure of coronary artery disease activity. Indeed, a fresh approach is needed that may have to aim therapy at all ischemia, both with and without symptoms.

As will be shown in this review, asymptomatic ischemia is common, and it is detectable in totally asymptomatic patients with coronary artery disease as well as patients with angina pectoris. It correlates at least as well as angina with anatomic severity of disease. Most important, however, is that measuring *all* ischemic episodes is a readily available and noninvasive index of prognosis and risk, and is independent of anatomical severity of coronary arterial obstruction. We also hope to show that in patients with various manifestations of coronary artery disease such as myocardial infarction, impaired left ventricular fucntion, and multivessel stenoses, ischemia regardless of symptoms is a vitally important and additional independent risk factor that should be addressed in any rational treatment plan.

ASYMPTOMATIC ISCHEMIA IN A POPULATION AT RISK

The special role of asymptomatic ischemia in a population at risk has been described in various settings. Several important early studies provided evidence that symptoms may be unreliable in estimating disease activity and frequently fail to give warning of impending adverse events. During the 14-year follow-up of the Framingham population, it was observed that 40 percent of patients with documented myocardial infarctions were not hospitalized. One third of these had unrecognized events discovered later in life, and 40 percent died suddenly. Most importantly, the silent infarction patients showed the same adverse prognosis on long-term follow-up that was found in patients who were symptomatic.[4] In a study of 15 survivors of out-of-hospital ventricular fibrillation, Sharma and colleagues[5] found that all patients had significant coronary artery disease at diagnostic cardiac catheterization. Twelve out of 15 had asymptomatic ST depression and regional wall motion abnormalities during exercise testing consistent with inducible ischemia (Fig. 3–1).

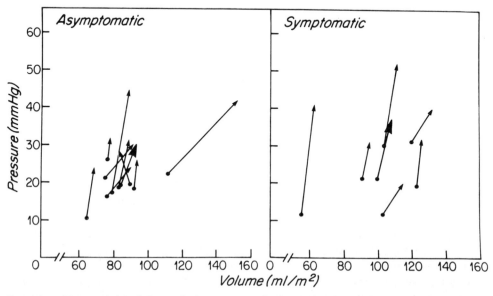

Figure 3–1. Changes in the left ventricular pressure-volume relation from rest to exercise in patients with out-of-hospital ventricular fibrillation. (From Sharma, et al[5] with permission.)

In the postmyocardial infarction population, independent studies have shown that ST segment depression during limited exercise testing as well as ambulatory electrocardiogram (ECG) monitoring was predictive of a high-mortality risk at one year of follow-up; interestingly, symptoms did not independently contribute to these findings.[6] Since then, numerous studies using the new technique of ambulatory ECG monitoring have shown that up to 75 percent of all strictly defined ischemic events occurred without symptoms.[7,8]

The aforementioned data suggest that asymptomatic ischemia occurs in an important fraction of patients who have sustained infarctions, or are otherwise at high risk, in whom symptomatic ischemia alone may not adequately reflect their total ischemic burden. Can asymptomatic ischemia be prospectively and reliably measured? Does it correlate with the anatomic severity of coronary artery disease, and how does it affect prognosis?

DETECTION OF ASYMPTOMATIC ISCHEMIA:
CORRELATION WITH ANATOMY AND PROGNOSIS

The detection of ischemia in totally asymptomatic patients is subject to an important caveat: Diagnostic testing has a significantly greater predictive accuracy when the prior likelihood of disease is high. It is for this reason that "positive" results in exercise testing and ambulatory ECG monitoring are of little use in screening homogeneous populations without risk factors for coronary artery disease.[9] On the other hand, noninvasive testing in a population with risk factors for coronary disease as defined by the Framingham criteria can provide a more sensitive means for assessing the risk of future adverse events.[10] Interestingly, it appears that symptoms are not a necessary marker of important ischemia.

Asymptomatic, exercise-induced ischemia elicited retrospectively in survivors of ventricular fibrillation correlates strongly with diffuse coronary artery disease.[5] Several exercise test trials have established the importance of this technique in assigning risk of adverse future events in a population at risk.[11-13] Bruce and coworkers[11] showed that the development of ST segment depression during exercise identified a subgroup of patients with significantly higher risk of adverse coronary events. Of note is that this group as well as others included many patients with inducible ST segment depression who were asymptomatic at rest and/or during exercise. Nevertheless, these patients demonstrated the same incremental risk as those with symptoms. In another study that carefully examined the importance of symptoms in a positive exercise test, Lindsey and Cohn[14] concluded that, in a cohort of 44 asymptomatic and 78 symptomatic patients, there was no obvious difference in risk factors, coronary anatomy, or left ventricular function. Similar findings were reported by Ouyang and colleagues,[6] who found no differences between symptomatic and asymptomatic patients in exercise testing, anatomy, and functional status after myocardial infarction. The same pattern held true in thallium studies; for example, Ladenheim and associates[15] showed in more than 1600 patients that the number of hypoperfused segments, the magnitude of hypoperfusion, and the peak heart rate—regardless of symptoms—were strong predictors of anatomy and future adverse events. Studies of patients with known coronary artery disease who underwent exercise radionuclide ventriculography have shown that the cohort with ST depression and a fall in exercise ejection fraction was associated with a significant increased risk of future coronary events. This group could not be

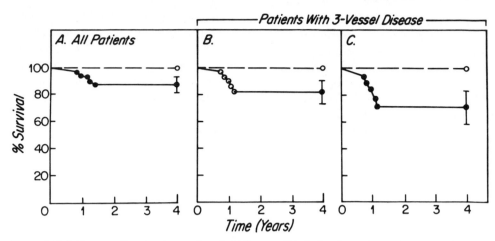

Figure 3–2. Influence of anatomic severity of CAD, reversible ischemia, and exercise capacity on survival. Survival curves are shown for: *A*) patients with three-vessel disease (closed circles, solid line) as
compared with those with one or two-vessel disease (open circles, dotted line); *B*) patients with three-
vessel disease and an increased ejection fraction or a negative ST segment response to exercise (open
circles, dotted line) as compared with those with three-vessel disease and both decreased ejection fraction
and a positive ST segment response with exercise (closed circles, solid line); and *C*) patients with three-
vessel disease and a decrease in ejection fraction during exercise, a positive ST segment response, and
exercise capacity of 120W or less (closed circles, solid line) as compared with all other patients with
three-vessel disease (open circles, dotted line). (From Bonow, et al[16] with permission.)

separated on the basis of coronary anatomy alone, and, again, the absence of symptoms was common and did not alter the prediction of risk[16,17] (Fig. 3–2).

MYOCARDIAL ISCHEMIA DURING DAILY LIFE

With the development of ambulatory ECG monitoring came an entirely new
perspective on the detection and significance of asymptomatic ischemia. In patients
with coronary artery disease, careful analytic criteria and strict definitions of ST
depression have made this technique a reliable, reproducible measure of the ambulatory ischemia of daily life. Ambulatory monitoring has shown that although ischemia is present in patients who are asymptomatic but at risk for coronary artery
disease, it strongly cross-correlates with traditional measures of coronary artery disease activity (that is, it is present predominantly in patients with coronary artery
disease and symptoms). Moreover, these traditional measures seem to severely
underestimate ischemic activity.[18–21] Important ambulatory ischemia is more frequently detected in patients with symptoms and positive exercise test results and
unstable angina, and it is less frequently detected in patients with stable angina
alone or with few symptoms.[22] In all instances, ambulatory monitoring has shown
that a significant proportion of the ischemia of daily life is asymptomatic.[18–22]

Early studies have shown that ambulatory ischemia correlates with anatomic
severity of coronary artery disease in a manner analogous to other noninvasive
tests. Studies are now available in many settings that confirm the prognostic impact
of asymptomatic ischemia. First, two separate groups have demonstrated that
ambulatory ischemia in patients with unstable angina was frequently asymptomatic

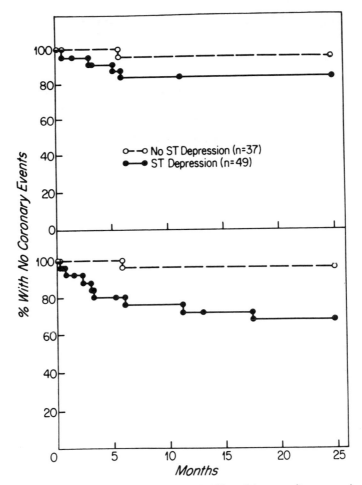

Figure 3–3. Kaplan-Meier curves comparing the probability of *(top panel)* not experiencing an acute ischemic event (i.e., death, myocardial infarction, unstable angina), and *(bottom panel)* progressive ischemic event (i.e., acute events or revascularization for worsening symptoms) during follow-up for the 37 patients without ST segment depression (open circles, dotted lines) and the 49 patients with ST segment depression (closed circles, solid lines), as detected by ambulatory monitoring. (From Rocco, et al[25] with permission.)

and was an independent predictor of subsequent infarction or need for revascularization.[23,24] Similarly, in populations with chronic stable angina and positive exercise test results, ambulatory ischemia provided independent, incremental information for predicting future adverse coronary events, and it was most often asymptomatic[25,26] (Fig. 3–3). Our group has recently used ambulatory monitoring in evaluating patients scheduled to undergo elective peripheral vascular surgery and has found that preoperative ambulatory ischemia is almost exclusively asymptomatic and is the strongest independent predictor of postoperative adverse coronary events.[27] Lastly, ambulatory monitoring of patients early after myocardial infarction revealed frequent asymptomatic ischemia that is, again, an independent predictor of adverse outcome.[28]

TREATMENT OF ASYMPTOMATIC ISCHEMIA: DOES
REVASCULARIZATION WORK?

As the aforementioned evidence suggests, ischemia as measured by any non-invasive method seems to affect prognosis and predict adverse coronary events. Moreover, in every study discussed, asymptomatic ischemia appears to be at least as important as symptomatic ischemia, particularly in identifying patients at high risk. There is evidence to suggest that relief of symptomatic ischemia clearly reduces coronary risk and improves prognosis. Numerous well-designed randomized trials of coronary artery bypass surgery show improved risk profiles and decreased mortality in selected high-risk groups.[1-3] Several beta blocker trials have established these drugs as a major medical intervention that reduces mortality and risk of infarction.[29,30] Although similar data do not exist for calcium channel blockers and nitrates, these agents have also been shown to effect a modest reduction in the symptomatic ischemic burden.[31,32] In a different approach, the Multiple Risk Factor Intervention Trial (MRFIT)[33] showed an objective reduction in risk of future coronary events via coronary risk factor intervention but only in subjects with evidence of ischemia in the electrocardiogram.

In some of the aforementioned studies, the reduction of symptomatic ischemia translated into a reduction of the risk of death and future adverse events. Several trials have demonstrated that asymptomatic ischemia—as measured by exercise testing, radionuclide angiography, and ambulatory monitoring—responds to traditional medical therapy and primary coronary risk factor reduction schemes in ways analogous to symptomatic ischemia.[34-36] Because it also appears clear that asymptomatic ischemia exerts equivalent effects on risk, it seems intuitively reasonable that treatment of asymptomatic ischemia should afford the same degree of risk reduction as symptomatic ischemia. The notion needs rigorous testing.

The issue of revascularization in particular, however, is more complex. First, we have already discussed that, for the majority of patients undergoing coronary artery bypass surgery or percutaneous transluminal coronary angioplasty, the indication remains symptomatic relief that is otherwise unattainable with medical therapy, and improvement of life-style. In the patient who has uncontrolled symptoms despite medical therapy, therefore, the issue is settled and more objective quantification of ischemia is of interest but not necessary. What of the patient who has controlled or no symptoms but evidence of high risk?

There does exist a group of patients at higher risk for death as defined by their coronary anatomy and left ventricular function, many of whom have little or no symptoms, and it appears clear that surgery in these patients offers better survival.[2,3] In addition, it is those patients with objective evidence of important ischemia that appear to derive the greatest benefit from surgery.[3] Is this benefit equivalent in symptomatic and asymptomatic ischemia? In reviewing the CASS registry, Weiner and associates[2] determined that anatomy and/or left ventricular function alone was not as precise in predicting surgical benefit and had to be accompanied by evidence of reversible ischemia. In addition, benefit was afforded regardless of symptoms, inasmuch as any inducible ischemia proved an excellent marker (Fig. 3–4). These findings were recently confirmed by Varnauskas[3] and the European coronary surgery study group.

Is ambulatory ischemia an equivalent marker of surgical benefit? Little evidence yet exists to answer this question. A recent trial by Egstrup[37] prospectively monitored 36 patients scheduled for elective coronary artery bypass surgery.

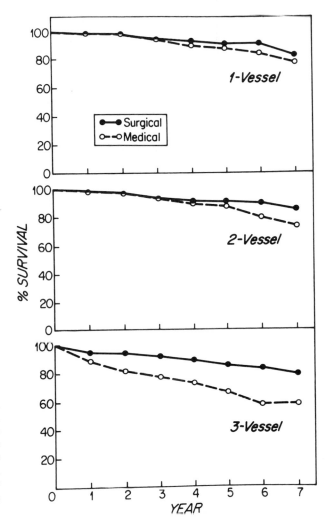

Figure 3–4. Cumulative survival rates for medical and surgical patients with at least 1 mm of ST-segment depression on exercise and who could exercise only to stage I or less, and had single-, double-, or triple-vessel coronary disease (From Weiner, et al[2] with permission.)

Ambulatory ischemia was common preoperatively, and its reduction postoperatively was documented in 24 patients (67 percent) and was associated with a much improved prognosis. Conversely, 12 patients (33 percent) who had persistent postoperative ischemia remained at higher risk for coronary events over a brief follow-up period, including one episode of sudden death. These data suggest that revascularization effectively reduces ambulatory ischemia and that ambulatory ischemia is a potential marker for surgical benefit in an unselected population.

Although asymptomatic ischemia appears to be an excellent marker for high risk, and its disappearance postoperatively a marker for a favorable outcome, it is also clear from the aforementioned discussion that the implications of ischemia are greatly modified by coronary anatomy and left ventricular function. *All three factors provide important, independent information relevant to assessing indications for revascularization rationally.* There remains little argument that patients with left main or three-vessel coronary artery disease with impaired ventricular function and evidence of ischemia, regardless of symptoms, have a longer survival with surgery. In mildly symptomatic and asymptomatic patients with two-vessel disease the situation is less clear. The presence of ventricular dysfunction sways the decision toward surgery. More importantly, we believe that there is enough evidence to suggest that in such patients, any evidence of persistent ischemia should be treated as persistent symptoms and, hence as a piece of evidence when seeking indication for surgery. Finally, patients with single-vessel disease and no significant symptoms are very rarely surgical candidates. However, based on the evidence that any ischemia is an independent marker of adverse outcome, and that revascularization appears to reduce such ischemia, we believe again that asymptomatic ischemia, particularly severe ischemia, should be considered as symptoms. In such cases, transluminal angioplasty may be the method of choice.[38]

CONCLUSION

It appears clear from available data that symptomatic ischemia as a traditional measure of the severity of coronary artery disease is an incomplete quantification of the overall ischemic burden in a given population. Symptoms may seriously underestimate ischemia, particularly in patients who have sustained myocardial infarctions, who have impaired left ventricular function, or who have high-risk coronary anatomy. It is clear also that asymptomatic ischemia is common and equivalent to symptomatic ischemia as a prognostic indicator. Preliminary data suggest that asymptomatic ischemia, both inducible and ambulatory, is equally responsive to conventional therapy, including revascularization procedures, and that this translates to an equivalent reduction of risk.

How should one approach the patient with controlled angina pectoris who has prolonged episodes of "silent" ischemia? Because asymptomatic ischemia is an important predictor of future adverse outcome, such a patient is at increased risk for death, infarction, or need for revascularization. We recommend that when the evidence is severe—early positive stress test, fall in ejection fraction, extensive perfusion defects, increased lung uptake, and 60 minutes or more of ischemia during monitoring—the patient should have delineation of coronary anatomy, with surgery recommended as a life-prolonging measure for left main coronary artery disease or three-vessel coronary artery disease with decreased left ventricular function. In the cases with lower-risk anatomy, asymptomatic ischemia is still a marker for future adverse outcome, and we believe that failure to eradicate such ischemia with medical therapy should be regarded as an indication for revascularization, with transluminal angioplasty to be used as an alternative to surgery in anatomically appropriate cases.

REFERENCES

1. Rahimtoola, SH: A perspective on the three large multicenter randomized clinical trials of coronary bypass surgery for chronic stable angina. Circulation 72(Suppl):123, 1985.
2. Weiner, DA, Ryan, TJ, McCabe, CH, et al: Significance of silent myocardial ischemia during exercise testing in patients with coronary artery disease. Am J Cardiol 59:725, 1987.
3. Varnauskas, E: Twelve-year follow-up of survival in the randomized European coronary surgery study. N Engl J Med 319:332, 1988.
4. Kannel, WB, McNamara, P, Feinleib, M, et al: The unrecognized myocardial infarction: Fourteen-year follow-up experience in the Framingham study. Geriatrics 25:75, 1970.
5. Sharma, B, Asinger, R, Francis, CS, et al: Demonstration of exercise-induced painless myocardial ischemia in survivors of out-of-hospital ventricular fibrillation. Am J Cardiol 59:740, 1987.

6. Ouyang, P, Shapiro, EP, Chandra, NC, et al: An angiographic and functional comparison of patients with symptomatic and asymptomatic treadmill ischemia early post myocardial infarction. Am J Cardiol 59:730, 1987.

7. Schang, ST, Jr and Pepine, CJ: Transient asymptomatic ST-segment depression during daily activity. Am J Cardiol 39:396, 1977.

8. Selwyn, AP, Fox, F, Eves, M, et al: Myocardial ischemia in patients with frequent angina pectoris. Br Med J 2:1594, 1978.

9. Berman, DS, Rozanski, A, and Knoebel, SB: The detection of silent ischemia; cautions and precautions, editorial. Circulation 75:101, 1987.

10. Levy, D and Kannel, WB: Cardiovascular risks: New insights from Framingham. Am Heart J 116:266, 1988.

11. Bruce, RA, Hossack, KF, Darouen, TA, et al: Enhanced risk assessment for primary coronary heart disease events by maximal exercise testing: 10 years of experience of the Seattle Heart Watch Study. J Am Coll Cardiol 2:656, 1983.

12. Froelicher, VF, Thompson, AJ, Longo, MR, Jr, et al: Value of exercise testing for screening asymptomatic men for latent coronary artery disease. Prog Cardiovasc Dis 18:265, 1976.

13. Giagnoni, E, Secchi, MB, Wu, SC, et al: Prognostic value of exercise EKG testing in asymptomatic, normotensive subjects: A prospective matched study. N Engl J Med 309:1085, 1983.

14. Lindsey, HE, Jr and Cohn, PF: "Silent" myocardial ischemia during and after exercise testing in patients with coronary artery disease. Am Heart J 95:441, 1978.

15. Ladenheim, ML, Pollock, BH, Rozanski, A, et al: Extent and severity of myocardial hypoperfusion as predictors of prognosis in patients with suspected coronary artery disease. J Am Coll Cardiol 7:464, 1986.

16. Bonow, RO, Kent, KM, Rosing, DR, et al: Exercise-induced ischemia in mildy symptomatic patients with coronary artery disease and preserved left ventricular function. N Engl J Med 311:1339, 1984.

17. Bonow, RO, Bacharach, SL, Green, MV, et al: Prognostic implications of symptomatic versus asymptomatic (silent) myocardial ischemia induced by exercise in mildly symptomatic and in asymptomatic patients with angiographically documented coronary artery disease. Am J Cardiol 60:778, 1987.

18. Deanfield, JE, Ribiero, P, Oakley, K, et al: Analysis of ST segment changes in normal subjects: Implications for ambulatory monitoring in angina pectoris. Am J Cardiol 54:1321, 1984.

19. Gallino, A, Chierchia, S, Smith, G, et al: Computer system for analysis of ST segment changes on 24 hour Holter monitor tapes: Comparison with other available systems. J Am Coll Cardiol 4:245, 1984.

20. Campbell, S, Barry, J, Rocco, MB, et al: Features of the exercise test that reflect the activity of ischemic heart disease out of hospital. Circulation 74:72, 1986.

21. Deanfield, JE, Selwyn, AP, Chierchia, S, et al: Myocardial ischaemia during daily life in patients with stable angina: Its relation to symptoms and heart rate changes. Lancet 2:753, 1983.

22. Cohn, PF: Silent myocardial ischemia: Classification, prevalence, and prognosis. Am J Med 79(Suppl 3A):3, 1985.

23. Gottlieb, SO, Weisfeldt, ML, Ouyang, P, et al: Silent ischemia as a marker of early unfavorable outcome in patients with unstable angina. N Engl J Med 314:1214, 1986.

24. Nademanee, K, Intarachol, V, and Josephson, MA: Prognostic significance of silent ischemia in patients with unstable angina. J Am Coll Cardiol 10:1, 1987.

25. Rocco, MB, Nable, EG, Campbell, S, et al: Prognostic importance of myocardial ischemia detected by ambulatory monitoring in patients with stable coronary artery disease. Circulation 78:877, 1988.

26. Stern, S, Gavish, A, Zin, D, et al: Clinical outcome of silent myocardial ischemia. Am J Cardiol 61:16F, 1988.

27. Raby, KE, Goldman, L, Creager, MA, et al: Correlation between preoperative ischemia and major cardiac events in peripheral vascular surgery. N Engl J Med 321:1296, 1989.

28. Gottlieb, SO, Gottlieb, SH, Ascuff, SC, et al: Silent ischemia on Holter monitoring predicts mortality in high risk, post infarction patients. JAMA 259:1030, 1988.

29. Pederson, TR and the Norwegian Multicenter Study Group: Six-year follow-up of the Norwegian multicenter study on timolol after acute myocardial infarction. N Engl J Med 313:1055, 1985.

30. Beta Blocker Heart Attack Study Group: The beta-blocker heart attack trial. JAMA 246:2073, 1981.

31. Gibson, RS, Boden, WE, Theroux, P, et al: Diltiazem and reinfarction in patients with non-Q-wave myocardial infarction. N Engl J Med 315:423, 1986.

32. Rapport, E: Influence of long acting nitrate therapy on the risk of reinfarction, sudden death, and total mortality in survivors of acute myocardial infarction. Am Heart J 110:276, 1985.
33. Multiple Risk Factor Intervention Trial Research Group: Exercise electrocardiogram and coronary heart disease mortality in the Multiple Risk Factor Intervention Trial. Am J Cardiol 55:16, 1985.
34. Cohn, PF, Brown, EJ, Swinford, R, et al: Effect of beta-blockade on silent regional left ventricular wall motion abnormalities. Am J Cardiol 57:521, 1986.
35. Dargie, HJ, Lynch, PG, Krikler, DM, et al: Nifedipine and propranolol, a beneficial drug interaction. Am J Med 71:676, 1981.
36. Cohn, PF and Lawson, WE: Effect of nifedipine on out-of-hospital silent myocardial ischemia in asymptomatic men with coronary artery disease. Am J Cardiol 61:908, 1988.
37. Egstrup, K: Asymptomatic myocardial ischemia as a predictor of cardiac events after coronary artery bypass grafting for stable angina pectoris. Am J Cardiol 61:248, 1988.
38. Kent, KM: Transluminal coronary angioplasty in asymptomatic or mildly symptomatic patients. Circulation 75(Suppl II):45, 1987.

Commentary

By Melvin D. Cheitlin, M.D.

Evidence that myocardial ischemia, whether symptomatic or asymptomatic, is predictive of future ischemic events is presented in Raby's and Selwyn's chapter. It is unclear whether the number and length of episodes of ischemia as detected by ambulatory electrocardiography recording give risk information independent of evidence of ischemia obtained by other techniques, such as exercise testing with or without thallium perfusion scintigraphy. If so, it will be important to perform ambulatory electrocardiography even if the patient has been stratified according to risk by exercise testing.

The evidence that eliminating symptomatic ischemia by medicine or by revascularization diminishes the risk is also tenuous. Certainly in some subgroups the risk is lessened after revascularization, and this decrease in risk is apparently greater than the effect of anti-ischemic medical therapy as shown by the various randomized, controlled trials of medical versus surgical management. That the risk is lowered in those patients with silent ischemia is less clear. How many patients declared low risk by stress testing in fact had prolonged episodes of silent ischemia is also not apparent. That almost all patients with silent ischemia have angina and ischemia on exercise testing is generally agreed upon. Once the patient is shown to have this marked ischemia by stress testing with ST segment depression occurring at low double product, coronary arteriography is done, and patients who have an anatomic situation that could benefit from surgery or angioplasty are usually revascularized. If the absence of silent ischemia in this "high-risk group" predicts a good prognosis, that is, if we could factor this "high-risk group" again into a lower and even higher-risk group, we could avoid doing coronary arteriography on some of these patients.

The benefit from decreases in total ischemic burden accomplished by medical management is not clear. Knowing whether medical therapy in patients who are "high risk" by stress testing decreases the ischemic burden is important, as is knowing whether in those patients in whom this happens, the excess of ischemic events is occurring in the group in whom medical therapy was not eliminating the silent ischemia. The answers to these questions remain for future investigation; until then, therapy to eliminate all evidence of ischemia remains a hope, a *best guess,* and an act of faith.

CHAPTER 4

How Should Intravenous Thrombolytic Agents for Acute Myocardial Infarction Be Selected?

Eric J. Topol, M.D.

Over the past five years, there has been considerable evolution in the development, clinical trial experience, and widescale use of intravenous thrombolytic agents for acute myocardial infarction. By the end of 1989, it is likely that four thrombolytic agents will be approved by the United States Food and Drug Administration (FDA) for use: streptokinase (SK), tissue plasminogen activator (t-PA), anisoylated plasminogen streptokinase activator complex (APSAC), and urokinase (UK). Within the next few years, several other agents will also become available. As in the treatment of many other diseases, such as in the choice of an antihypertensive or antibiotic agent, the therapeutic choice for clinicians is becoming increasingly complex over time. The purpose of this chapter is to provide a critical appraisal of all the current data for intravenous thrombolytic agents.

HISTORICAL PERSPECTIVE

Although Herrick[1] described coronary thrombosis in 1912, the first application of thrombolytic therapy for acute myocardial infarction did not occur until the 1950s.[2] Streptokinase, a protein derived from streptococcal bacteria, was first given to a patient for treatment of pleural effusion in 1948.[3] Early clinical studies with streptokinase administered intravenously yielded discouraging results, most likely due to the low dose employed and the late initiation of therapy.[4] Urokinase was introduced nearly a decade later, and although this enzyme is a naturally occurring fibrinolytic enzyme and is relatively nonantigenic, it did not become very popular

57

owing to concern over hemorrhagic events and the increased expense. Schroder and colleagues[5] initiated high-dose, brief duration intravenous streptokinase, an important advance in the transformation of use of this agent for systemic administration, in the early 1980s. In 1984, the first patient was treated with intravenous recombinant t-PA, a product of a new molecular biology.[6] By late 1987, both intravenous t-PA and SK were approved by the FDA.

THE IDEAL AGENT

To evaluate current thrombolytic agents, it is helpful to understand what would be the preferred characteristics of a therapeutic fibrinolytic enzyme. For coronary artery thrombolysis, the desired agent would be capable of lysing in a rapid time frame (e.g., <5 min) and be effective in all patients. Establishment of infarct vessel patency in 100 percent of patients with acute coronary occlusion is clearly a far-reaching but important goal.

Once patency has been achieved, no reocclusion should occur, thereby preventing reinfarction or recurrent ischemic events. Beyond the objectives of an open, stabilized artery is the need to avoid any side effects. First, bleeding complications need to be eliminated, which may be possible only by direct tissue-specific targeting of thrombolysis. An example would be an agent directed only to receptors in the left anterior descending coronary artery in a patient with evolving anterior wall myocardial infarction. This theoretical potential may never be realized, but the lack of target specificity will set up the potential for dissolution of physiologic fibrin or *hemostatic plugs*. Second, the ideal agent should have *no* antigenicity. This important property would account for eliminating allergic reactions, such as drug rash, fever, serum sickness, or anaphylactoid events. In addition, such an agent would not have intrinsic immunogenicity, primary or secondary resistance would not occur, and there would be no concern over repeat administration. By not activating kinins or the complement system, the avoidance of directly inducing hypotension is a worthwhile feature in the setting of acute myocardial infarction.[7] Third, a key practical issue is one of cost. Certainly in this era of cost consciousness in health care, the ideal agent should be very inexpensive. It is clear that none of the currently available fibrinolytic agents or those under investigation truly approach the description of the ideal one.

There are other features in which uncertainty exists as to their relative merit. An example is whether the agent should have a long biologic and plasma half-life, enabling bolus administration. Although this represents a convenience and may facilitate prehospital therapy, the other concern is the lack of control over the effect. If a patient developed serious bleeding during the course of an infusion with a short half-life agent, the cessation of the infusion might be accompanied by a less significant hemorrhagic event. Furthermore, all patients with acute myocardial infarction need to have intravenous access so that whereas a bolus therapy may be viewed as simple, it certainly is not requisite.

The debate over fibrin selectivity as a desirable characteristic is currently unsettled. The difference in mechanism of circulating versus plasmin-bound plasminogen is represented in Figure 4–1. Whereas an agent with absolute or relative fibrin selectivity appears to achieve more rapid infarct vessel patency, by 24 hours a definite *catch-up* phenomenon has been observed in the recent randomized intravenous prourokinase (scu-PA) versus streptokinase trial.[8] In Table 4–1, the basic fea-

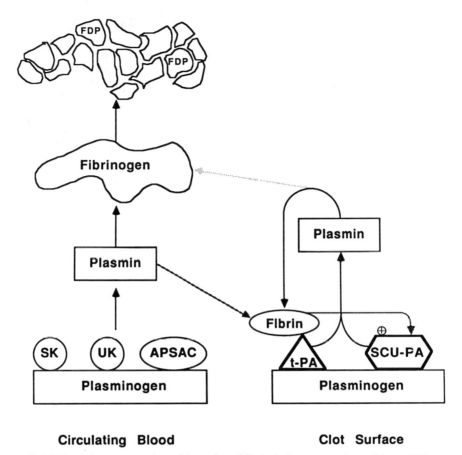

Figure 4–1. Schematic representation of the action of fibrinolytic enzymes. Streptokinase (SK) and uro-kinase (UK), and acylated plasminogen-streptokinase activator complex (APSAC) work predominantly on circulating plasminogen; tissue-type plasminogen activator (t-PA) and single-chain urokinase plas-minogen activator (SCU-PA) are relatively clot-selective. (From Topol EJ, Heart & Lung: The Journal of Critical Care, 16:760–774, 1987, with permission.)

Table 4–1. Basic Comparisons of Relative Fibrin Selective and Nonselective Agents

	Fibrin Selectivity	Fibrin Nonselectivity
Agents	t-PA, scu-PA	SK, UK, APSAC
Infarct vessel patency at 90 min	75%	50–65%
Infarct vessel patency at 24 hr	85%	85%
Velocity of reperfusion	More rapid	Slow, but *catch-up* phenomenon
Fibrinogen breakdown	Moderate	Extensive
Reocclusion	Probably increased*	Probably lower*
Bleeding complications	No difference	No difference
Time dependency	Relatively no	Yes (efficacy ↓ after 3–4 hr)

*Definitive randomized studies comparing the agents with acute and convalescent phase coronary angiography with more than 90% follow-up are currently lacking.

APSAC = anisoylated plasminogen streptokinase activator complex, scu-PA = single chain urokinase (prourokinase) plasminogen activator, SK = streptokinase, t-PA = tissue plasminogen acti-vator, UK = urokinase.

tures of the two classes of agents are compared. Of note, the term *fibrin selectivity* refers only to the potential of the agent under experimental conditions, inasmuch as both t-PA and scu-PA induce moderate fibrinogenolysis at the doses commonly used for treatment of acute myocardial infarction. In contrast is the earlier achievement of infarct vessel patency for fibrin-selective agents versus likely improvement in sustained patency for the others, with no difference in bleeding complications evident between the two classes of agents. When t-PA was introduced, it was expected that a lesser bleeding complication rate would result.[6,9-12] Later, a higher rate of serious intracranial hemorrhage was observed at an increased dose of t-PA.[13] Marder and Sherry,[14] and Pitt[15] have postulated that t-PA may induce an increased frequency of hemorrhagic events owing to its increased fibrinolytic potency. This issue has not yet been resolved but is a central one in the controversy between the two classes of agents. From the available data base, it can be concluded that the extensive fibrinogenolysis routinely induced by nonselective agents is not associated with a higher rate of intracerebral bleeding compared with t-PA.[16]

PROFILES OF THE THOMBOLYTIC AGENTS

Streptokinase

The first agent that was introduced as a thrombolytic, streptokinase, has been the subject of the most extensive clinical investigation to date (Table 4-2). This protein binds indirectly to circulating plasminogen to set up its subsequent activation of systemic fibrinolysis. As a bacterial-derived protein, it is antigenic and therefore results in drug rash, fever, serum sickness, and anaphylactoid reactions.[17,18] A related problem is the direct induction of hypotension via activation of kinins and the complement system. At times, the hypotensive effect can be serious and require intervention with vasopressor agents.[19] Its half-life is relatively long (18 min) and, at the conventional 1.5 million unit dose, this agent results in marked fibrinogenolysis.

Streptokinase's track record in the large-scale mortality *megatrials* has been extremely good. There have been two such trials: the Gruppo Italiano per lo Studio della Streptochinasi nell'Infarto Miocardico (GISSI) and the International Studies of Infarct Survival (ISIS-2).[20,21] The GISSI Trial was the first landmark study to document the survival benefit of intravenous thrombolytic therapy.[20] In this trial,

Table 4-2. Characteristics of Thrombolytic Agents

	SK	t-PA	APSAC	UK	PUK
Plasminogen binding	Indirect	Direct	Indirect	Direct	Indirect
Time dependent (>3 hr)	Yes	No	Yes	Yes	?
Hemostatic breakdown	4+	1-2+	3+	3+	2+
Hypotension	Yes	No	Yes	No	No
Half-life	18 min	4 min	95 min	14 min	?
Allergic reactions	Yes	No	Yes	No	No
Approximate cost/dose	$200/1.5 mill U	$2200/100 mg	$1400/30 mg	$2200/3 mill U	?

APSAC = anisoylated plasminogen streptokinase activator complex, PUK = prourokinase, SK = streptokinase, t-PA = tissue plasminogen activator, UK = urokinase.

Table 4–3. Mortality Trials of Intravenous Thrombolytic Agents

Trial Acronym	Reference	Agent	ECG	Time Window (hr)	ASA	Hep	N	Treatment %	Control %
GISSI	20	SK	Y	12	N	N	11,806	10.7	13.0
ISIS-2	21	SK	N	24	Y	N	17,187	9.2	12.0
ISAM	22	SK	Y	6	Y*	Y	1,741	5.1	6.5
ASSET	23	t-PA	N	5	N	Y†	5,011	7.2	9.8
AIMS	24	APSAC	Y	6	N	N	1,004	6.3	12.1

*ASA 0.5 g given initially followed by Coumadin
†Heparin given for 24 hours only
AIMS = APSAC Intervention Mortality Study, APSAC = anisoylated plasminogen streptokinase activator complex, ASA = aspirin, ASSET = Anglo Scandinavian Study of Early Thrombolysis, GISSI = Gruppo Italiano per lo Studio della Streptochinasi nell'Infarto Miocardico, Hep = heparin, ISAM = intravenous streptokinase and myocardial infarction, ISIS-2 = International Study of Infarct Survival, SK = streptokinase, t-PA = tissue plasminogen activator.

over 11,800 patients were randomized to high-dose intravenous streptokinase or conventional therapy. In contrast to some subsequent trials, the investigators required an entry 12-lead electrocardiogram, used a 12-hour maximal time window of symptom duration, and did not protocolize adjunctive therapy such as aspirin or heparin (Table 4–3). Overall, an 18 percent mortality reduction was demonstrated, with the most striking advantage for patients who were treated within one hour from symptom onset. After six hours of symptom duration, no survival benefit was shown.

The ISIS-2 Trial was even larger; the number of patients enrolled was over 17,000.[21] This was a randomized trial of both streptokinase and aspirin, using a 2 × 2 factorial design. In ISIS, the time window was up to 24 hours, no ECG was required for entry, and aspirin was given to half the patients. Beyond confirmation of the mortality reduction for streptokinase, the ISIS study extended the GISSI findings by showing clearcut benefit up to 24 hours for patients with inferior infarction, advanced age (age >75), and significant hypotension or hypertension at the time of entry.[21] Of note, these results supporting apparent benefit for ISIS-2 subgroups are problematic and must be interpreted with caution, as duly noted by the investigators. The sample size was not adequate for the comparisons, nor was it calculated on the basis of these subgroup analyses, many of which are post hoc. Nonetheless, the largest reperfusion trial to date has provided the most evidence for survival advantage for varied patient groups and expanded applications (e.g., late entry, elderly).

Of fundamental importance in ISIS-2 was the first evidence of the vital role of prompt administration of aspirin, which had an independent, substantial effect on mortality reduction and was additive to the benefit derived from streptokinase alone. The mortality risk reduction for aspirin alone was 21 percent, streptokinase alone 26 percent, but 39 percent for the combination. A randomized trial of other thrombolytics with or without aspirin has not and probably will not be performed. Empirically, however, early administration of aspirin is now frequently given to patients with evolving myocardial infarction no matter which thrombolytic they receive.

The effects of intravenous streptokinase on global ventricular function are

Table 4–4. Randomized Studies of Intravenous Thrombolytic
Agents for Evaluation of Left Ventricular Function

Trial	Reference	N	Time Assessed (d)	Method	Ejection Fraction (%) Thrombolytic	Placebo
Streptokinase vs Placebo						
ISAM	14	848	21	C	56.8	53.9
Western Washington	25	368	10	C	54.3	50.7
White, et al	26	219	21	C	59.0	53.0
t-PA vs Placebo						
Guerci	65	138	10	N	53.2	46.4
National Heart Foundation	66	144	7	C	57.7	51.7
TICO	67	126	21	C	61.0	54.0
Van de Werf	64	721	14	C	50.7	48.5
TPAT	68	115	9	N	53.6	47.8
APSAC vs Placebo						
Bassand (APSIM)	84	230	14	C	52 ± 13	47 ± 13
Meinertz	83	331	14	C	53 ± 15	54 ± 15
t-PA vs UK						
GAUS	87	246	7	C	53 ± 12(t-PA)	52 ± 14(UK)
t-PA vs SK						
PAIMS	92	171	12	E	56 ± 10(t-PA)	52 ± 11(SK)
White, et al	91	271	21	C	58 ± 12(t-PA)	58 ± 12(SK)

All differences (thrombolytic vs placebo) of global ejection fraction were significant ($p < 0.05$) except the Western Washington Study ($p = 0.056$).

C = Contrast, radiographic, E = echocardiography, N = radionuclide, APSAC = anisoylated plasminogen streptokinase activator complex, APSIM = APSAC Intervention Mortality Study, GAUS = German Activator Urokinase Study, ISAM = intravenous streptokinase for acute myocardial infarction, PAIMS = Plasminogen Activator Italian Multicenter Study, SK = streptokinase, TICO = thrombolysis in coronary occlusion, t-PA = tissue plasminogen activator, TPAT = tissue plasminogen activator: Toronto, UK = urokinase.

summarized in Table 4–4. In the Intravenous Streptokinase in Acute Myocardial Infarction (ISAM) Trial,[22] only patients who underwent left ventriculography are included in the table. The three placebo-controlled streptokinase trials all showed benefit of convalescent phase ejection fraction, ranging from 2 to 6 points.[22,25,26] As can be seen in Table 4–4, the magnitude of functional recovery, as calculated by subtracting the mean value of placebo group from the streptokinase group patients, is similar to that with the other thrombolytic agents.

Early angiographic reperfusion and patency of the infarct-related artery is a third important end point, each of which has been evaluated for intravenous streptokinase in several studies.[27–43] Reperfusion refers to actual demonstration of infarct vessel recanalization after angiographic confirmation of total occlusion (TIMI Grade 0 or 1 flow pattern).[27] In contrast, patency is established as an end point without prior confirmation of occlusion. Patency values therefore tend to be higher, owing to a 15 to 20 percent incidence of an open vessel at baseline angiography. This observation is related to either spontaneous recanalization or the lack of there ever having been total occlusion.

Overall, the pooled results for streptokinase indicate a 42 percent reperfusion rate and a 51 percent patency rate. In considering the finding of an open vessel as

Table 4–5. Intravenous Streptokinase: Early Angiographic
Reperfusion and Patency Studies

	Reference	Dose (mill U)	Symptom Duration (hr)	Time to Angio (min)	% Open (N/N)
		Streptokinase			
TIMI Phase I	27	1.5	4.8	90	31 (37/119)
Hillis	28	1.5	4.5	90	32 (11/34)
Spann	29	0.85–1.5	3.5	60	49 (21/43)
Rogers	30	1.0	6.5	75	44 (7/16)
Neuhaus	31	1.7	3.7	60	60 (24/40)
de Marneffe	32	1.5	3.6	60	80 (8/10)
Pooled			4.4		42 (116/275)
		Patency			
Schwartz	33	1.5	2.5	90	45 (25/55)
Verstraete	34	1.5	2.6	90	55 (34/62)
Cribier	35	1.5	3.1	60	52 (11/21)
Brochier	36	1.5	2.8	125	56 (24/43)
Monnier	37	1.5	2.5	150	64 (7/11)
TIMI	38	1.5	4.7	90	42 (61/146)
Stack	39	1.5	3.0	90	44 (95/216)
Lopez-Sendón	40	1.5	2.9	90	58 (14/24)
Miller	41	1.5	<4.0	NR	70 (53/76)
Vogt	42	1.5	NR	NR	72 (21/31)
Taylor	43	0.85	3.2	60	77 (17/22)
Pooled			3.0		51 (362/707)

NR = not reported.
TIMI = Thrombolysis in myocardial infarction.

a function of the time to therapy, there does not appear to be as good an inverse relationship as one would expect. With the impressive first-hour mortality reduction observed in GISSI,[20] it has been proposed that streptokinase is more effective when administered earlier in the course of the event. Indeed, in TIMI-1 there was a fall-off for patency achieved with streptokinase over time of symptom duration,[27] which suggests that streptokinase exhibits time dependency for its coronary thrombolytic effect. The collective angiographic reperfusion and patency data (Table 4–5) for streptokinase can be compared with the other agents in a similar way, as provided in Table 4–6 for t-PA and Table 4–7 for APSAC.

Tissue Plasminogen Activator

The recombinant form of t-PA has been administered to patients only over the past five years, but during this period of time there has been intense clinical investigation involving over 15,000 patients enrolled in prospective trials. A serine protease enzyme, t-PA has marked affinity to the fibrin-plasminogen complex. By virtue of this property, the fibrinolytic effect can occur locally, without the development of free, circulating plasmin and thus the theoretic basis for fibrin selectivity. However, with the doses commonly used for coronary thrombolysis, alpha-2 antiplasmin is overridden, plasminemia occurs, and there is fibrinogen and plasminogen depletion, and some systemic hemostatic effect. Although the extent

Table 4–6. Intravenous t-PA: Early Angiographic Reperfusion and Patency Studies

	Reference	Type	Dose	Time (hr) of Symptoms	Time of Angio (min)	Open Vessel
			Reperfusion			
Collen	9	DC	0.5–0.75 mg/kg	4.7	90	75 (25/33)
TIMI-1	27	DC	50 mg	4.8	90	62 (70/113)
Williams	44	DC	50 mg	4.8	90	68 (25/37)
Gold	45	DC	0.4–0.75 mg/kg	3.0	60	83 (24/29)
TIMI-B	46	SC	70 mg	4.6	90	71 (59/83)
TIMI-C	47	SC	100 mg	4.6	90	68 (42/62)
Pooled				4.4	—	69 (245/357)
			Patency			
Verstraete	48	DC	0.75 mg/kg	3.4	90	61 (38/66)
Verstraete	34	DC	0.75 mg/kg	3.0	90	70 (43/61)
Verstraete	49	DC	40 mg	2.5	90	66 (78/119)
Topol	50	SC	1.25 mg/kg	4.0	90	71 (27/38)
Topol	51	SC	150 mg	3.9	90	75 (288/386)
Topol	52	SC	1.5 mg/kg	2.8	90	79 (104/132)
Simoons	53	SC	100 mg	2.6	90	89 (160/180)
Johns	54	SC	1 mg/kg	<6.0	90	76 (52/68)
TIMI-2A	55	SC	70–100 mg	2.9	120	75 (144/192)
McNeill	56	SC	100 mg	2.3	90	82 (14/17)
Neuhaus	57	SC	100 mg	<6.0	90	69 (43/62)
Neuhaus	58	SC	70 mg	2.8	90	86 (30/35)
Miller	59	SC	100 mg	<4.0	90	83 (80/96)
Pooled				3.0	—	76 (1101/1444)

DC = double chain, SC = single chain, TIMI = thrombolysis in myocardial infarction.

Table 4–7. Intravenous APSAC: Early Angiographic Reperfusion and Patency Studies

	Reference	Dose	Time (hr) of Symptoms	Time of Angio (min)	Open Vessel (%,N)
			Reperfusion		
Bonnier	76	30 U	2.5	90	64 (23/36)
DeWilde	77	30 U	<3.0	90	67 (10/15)
Marder	78	5–30 U	4.1	90	60 (9/15)
Timmis	79	30 U	3.3	90	53 (8/15)
Anderson	75	30 U	<6.0	90	51 (59/115)
Pooled					56 (109/196)
			Patency		
Kasper	80	30 U	2.5	90	84 (42/50)
Brochier	81	30 U	<6.0	90	72 (28/39)
Monassier	82	30 U	<6.0	90	74 (37/50)
Belik-Van Wely	83	30 U	<4.0	90	76 (75/99)
Lopen-Sendón	84	30 U	2.9	90	90 (18/20)
Vogt	85	30 U	2.6	90	76 (23/30)
Pooled			2.7		77 (223/288)

of fibrinogenolysis with t-PA is, in part, proportional to the dose, there is an idio-syncratic phenomenon of hemostatic protein depletion.[60] There is a modest inverse correlation of fibrinogen breakdown after t-PA with clinical bleeding events.[61]

With biotechnologic expression of this human enzyme via the Chinese hamster ovary cell line, there has been no antigenicity reported. Patients have not developed antibodies to t-PA after first exposure,[62] but there is a very limited experience and screening in patients who have been treated with a second dose of t-PA months or years later. Without apparent immunogenicity, t-PA has not resulted in any febrile reactions, rash, serum sickness, or anaphylactoid events that could not be attributed to other medications or conditions. There is some activation of the complement system,[63] but t-PA does not directly induce hypotension most likely related to lack of kinin release. Certainly hypotension occurs after t-PA administration, but this is due to the activation of cardiovascular reflexes, most notably the Bezold-Jarisch, substantial myonecrosis, or concomitant medical treatment.

There has been one placebo-controlled large-scale trial designed to examine t-PA's effect on mortality reduction. In the Anglo-Scandinavian Study of Early Thrombolysis (ASSET), more than 5000 patients were randomly assigned to therapy or placebo. Enrollment was performed without a qualifying electrocardiogram, like in ISIS-2,[21] but the time window was five hours, and all patients received 24 hours of intravenous heparin but no aspirin was protocolized (see Table 4-3). Despite the important interstudy design differences, the 26 percent overall reduction of mortality is comparable with GISSI[20] and ISIS-2[21], as shown in Figure 4-2.

META ANALYSIS

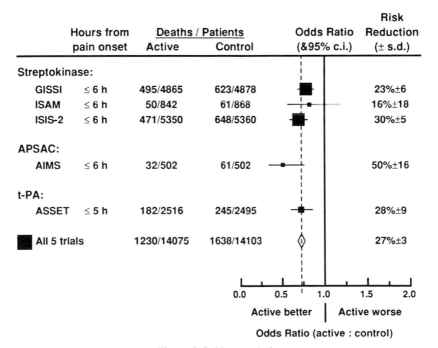

Figure 4-2. Meta analysis.

In the randomized t-PA versus placebo trial of 721 patients designed by Van de Werf and others, there was a 50 percent mortality reduction at 14 days.[64] This benefit, however, was not statistically significant at the 5 percent alpha error level, and the trial was not designed in sample size to acquire meaningful mortality reduction data. Nonetheless, the benefit was observed in spite of a very low placebo group mortality (<6 percent; all patients did receive aspirin and heparin).

There have been five randomized placebo-controlled trials of t-PA that were performed chiefly to consider the agent's preservation of left ventricular function.[64,68] The trials are summarized in Table 4–4 and demonstrate a range of 2.2 to 7.0 ejection fraction point improvement. The most recent study, TPAT,[68] was the first randomized trial of the Burroughs-Wellcome, predominantly two-chain t-PA preparation, which showed benefit for cardiac function. In the other four studies, the Genentech double[65] or single-chain preparation[66,67] or both[64,65] (over the course of the study) were used. As noted in Table 4–4, the extent of functional recovery is similar to that reported in the parallel streptokinase trials.[14,25,26]

The cumulative angiographic infarct vessel reperfusion and patency data base for t-PA is presented in Table 4–6. In a large number of patients, the early reperfusion rate of 69 percent and patency rate of 76 percent reflect the high thrombolytic potency of t-PA, and these data compare favorably with streptokinase. The achievement of reperfusion with t-PA appears to be relatively time independent.[7] Even when t-PA was combined with high doses of intravenous urokinase[69] or heparin,[52] a patency rate above 80 percent could not be achieved. This may be interpreted as that the coronary thrombolytic effect of t-PA is maximal, inasmuch as there has yet to be an agent to yield higher early patency rates in large series of patients. Weight-adjusted dosing of t-PA (1.5 mg/kg over 3–4 hrs, max 135 mg) appears to yield the most rapid recanalization[7] and may also decrease bleeding in lightweight individuals, as well as reduce reocclusion in patients weighing more than 90 kg.[70]

APSAC

The anisoylated plasminogen activator streptokinase complex (APSAC) is an acyl derivative of streptokinase. The change in molecular structure of the catalytic site results in a very prolonged plasma half-life because this agent requires deacylation prior to plasminogen activation. The advantage of APSAC is the ability to administer it as a bolus and to achieve therapeutic results comparable to the other agents[24] (see Fig. 4–2). This feature of convenience may be of particular benefit as out-of-hospital thrombolytic therapy[71–74] becomes more commonplace. The dose of APSAC is a uniform one of 30 mg (or units). It is given over 2 to 4 minutes. With antigenic features in common with streptokinase, APSAC's side effect profile of fever, rash, anaphylactoid reactions, and hypotension is quite similar to the parent agent in published clinical studies.[36,40,42,75–84]

The primary randomized controlled trial of APSAC is the APSAC Intervention Mortality Study (AIMS).[24] In this study of 1004 patients treated with intravenous APSAC 30 U or placebo, there was a 50 percent mortality risk reduction at 30 days postinfarction. This is the highest risk reduction thus far reported in a reperfusion trial of this size and, in fact, the study was stopped prematurely by its policy board because of this substantial effect. As seen in Figure 4–2, however, the 95 percent confidence intervals for risk reduction in AIMS overlap with those of the other thrombolytic mortality trials. By subgroup analysis, the mortality reduction appeared to be independent of age and time of symptom duration. In AIMS, no serious bleeding events occurred. Another smaller (313 patients) randomized APSAC trial reported by Meinertz and coworkers[83] also has demonstrated mortality reduction. The APSIM study[84] compared APSAC to heparin for evaluation of left ventricular function. As shown in Table 4–4, an improvement of global ejection fraction for APSAC was confirmed in this study. The data in Table 4–7 summarize early angiographic findings for reperfusion and patency. These values of 56 and 77, respectively, compare favorably with those for streptokinase and the patency rate is very similar to that of t-PA. There are, however, considerably fewer patients studied with APSAC, such that the statistical power of this observation is less. In the trial by Anderson and colleagues,[75] a time dependency for APSAC was observed for decreased coronary thrombolytic effect in patients with ≥ 4 hours of symptoms.

Urokinase

The naturally occurring plasminogen activator urokinase (u-PA, UK) was introduced as a therapeutic agent in the 1960s.[85] Although approved for intracoronary use in the early 1980s, there has been considerably less clinical research with this agent, compared with SK, t-PA, or APSAC.

However, urokinase is nonantigenic, thus avoiding allergic reactions, resistance, and direct induction of hypotension. Like APSAC, the agent can be given as a bolus.[86] There has not been a placebo-controlled mortality trial for UK, but this no longer would be ethically possible for patients presenting early with ST segment elevation infarction and no contraindication to thrombolytic intervention. The major urokinase trial performed to date is the German Activator Urokinase Study (GAUS),[87] in which 3.0 million units of UK versus t-PA (70 mg given over 90 min) yielded not only an equivalent high rate of angiographic patency at 90 and 120 minutes of therapy but also equivalent left ventricular function (Table 4–4). Time dependency (>3 hr of symptom duration) was observed for urokinase in GAUS. The reocclusion rate in patients not undergoing coronary angioplasty tended to be lower for UK than for t-PA. In a recent angiographic patency study by Califf and colleagues,[88] a 64 percent rate was achieved with 3 million units of urokinase. There are several ongoing randomized trials of UK for left ventricular function.

Prourokinase

Prourokinase (scu-PA) is the single chain proenzyme that ultimately is cleaved to urokinase, but it, too, is a naturally occurring plasminogen activator with a unique yet incompletely described mechanism.[89] It has similar features to t-PA, including lack of antigenicity, a short half-life, and relative fibrin selectivity. Of the five agents, it is the least well studied to date in clinical trials. Two studies have evaluated early angiographic reperfusion and patency. Using varying doses of the kidney cell line preparation, Loscalzo and coworkers[90] demonstrated reperfusion at 90 minutes in 23 of 44 patients (53 percent). In this study, with serial angiography after control injections, an appreciable time lag to vessel patency was noted. The Prourokinase in Myocardial Infarction (PRIMI) trial investigators used the recombinant glycosylated form of scu-PA in a randomized trial comparing it with intravenous streptokinase for infarct vessel patency at 60 minutes, 90 minutes, and 24 hours.[8] At 90 minutes in 378 patients the patency rate for prourokinase was 71 percent compared with 64 percent for streptokinase.

COMPARATIVE FEATURES

From the discussion of the profiles of the various agents, it can be seen that all are effective in achieving infarct vessel patency in the majority of patients. t-PA clearly achieves a higher early patency rate than that of streptokinase, but there is definitely a catch-up phenomenon between 90 minutes and 24 hours after initiation of therapy. Clinical benefit in terms of mortality reduction or cardiac function for t-PA over streptokinase has yet to be proven in a direct, comparative trial. Two recent trials have compared the two agents for effect on left ventricular function. In the trial by White and associates,[91] 271 patients were randomized and had contrast left ventriculography at three weeks. The ejection fraction was identical for the two treatment groups; both t-PA and SK resulted in a 58 ± 12 percent value. The Plasminogen Activator Italian Multicenter Study (PAIMS) group studied 170 patients randomly assigned to t-PA or SK with two-dimensional echocardiography at two weeks.[92] The ejection fraction for the t-PA and streptokinase groups was 56 and 51 percent, by two-dimensional echocardiography, respectively. Overall, it is clear that there are no substantial differences between these two thrombolytic agents for recovery of ventricular function.

The comparative effect on mortality reduction is the focus of ongoing large-scale clinical investigation. Of the five completed randomized trials designed to examine mortality differences, meta-analysis demonstrates very similar effects (Fig. 4–2). The heterogeneous inclusion criteria, time window, electrocardiographic criteria, and adjunctive therapy make such intertrial comparisons difficult. In the GISSI-2 trial, approximately 20,000 patients are being randomized to receive t-PA and aspirin or SK and aspirin, with a subrandomization to subcutaneous heparin or no heparin (Fig. 4–3). The anticipated completion date is late 1989. Similarly, in the ISIS-3, patients will receive combination therapy of a thrombolytic agent plus aspirin, but this study group will enroll 30,000 patients and examine the relative mortality risk reduction of t-PA versus SK versus APSAC (Fig. 4–4). The ISIS-3 trial will probably not complete enrollment until early in 1991.

In the meantime, what data can be used to choose between t-PA and SK, the only currently FDA-approved intravenous thrombolytics for acute myocardial infarction? Although the four direct t-PA versus SK comparative studies showed no differences in left ventricular function, a 29 percent further mortality reduction for t-PA is evident by meta-analysis (see Table 4–8). This reduction is not statisti-

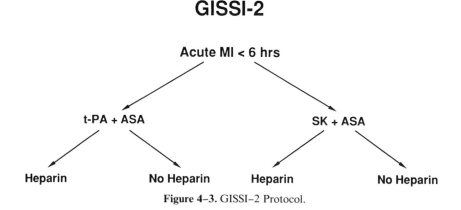

Figure 4–3. GISSI–2 Protocol.

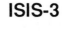

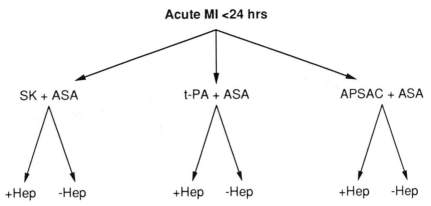

30,000 pts; Endpoint 5 wk. Vascular Mortality

Figure 4–4. ISIS–3 Protocol.

Table 4–8. Meta-analysis of Mortality in Streptokinase *versus* Tissue Plasminogen Activator: Randomized Studies

| | | Intention-to-Treat | |
	Reference	SK	t-PA
TIMI-1	27	14/159	12/157
ECSG-1		3/64	3/65
PAIMS	92	7/85	4/86
White, et al	91	10/136	5/135
		34/444	24/443
		7.6%	5.4%
		29%	
		Actual Treatment	
TIMI-1	27	12/147	7/143
ECSG-1		3/64	3/65
PAIMS	92	7/85	4/86
White, et al	91	10/136	5/135
		32/432	19/429
		7.4%	4.4%
		40.5%	

ECSG = European Cooperative Study Group, PAIMS = Plasminogen Activator Italian Multicenter Study, SK = streptokinase, TIMI = thrombolysis in myocardial infarction, t-PA = tissue plasminogen activator.

Table 4–9. Intracranial Bleeding Complications and
Stroke in Major Reperfusion Trials

	t-PA		
	N	Rx	%
	Intracranial Bleed		
TAMI 1–4	758	ASA, Hep	0.6
TIMI-2	2742	ASA, Hep	0.5
ECSG 4,5	722	ASA, Hep	0.8
	Stroke		
ASSET	2512	Hep × 24 hr	1.0

	SK		
	Intracranial Bleed		
ISAM	859	ASA, Hep	0.5
WWIVST	191	Hep	0.5
	Stroke		
GISSI	5860	—	1.1%
ISIS-2	8377	± ASA	0.8%

ASSET = Anglo-Scandinavian Study of Early Thrombolysis
 ASA = Aspirin
 ECSG = European Cooperative Study Group
 GISSI = Gruppo Italiano per lo Studio della Streptochinasi nell'Infarto Miocardico
 ISAM = Intravenous Streptokinase in Acute Myocardial Infarction
 Hep = Heparin
 ISIS = International Study of Infarct Survival
 SK = Streptokinase
 TAMI = Thrombolysis and Angioplasty in Myocardial Infarction
 TIMI = Thrombolysis in Myocardial Infarction
 t-PA = Tissue plasminogen activator
 WWIVST = Western Washington Intravenous Streptokinase Trial

cally significant but indicates a trend in favor of t-PA, perhaps reflecting the advantage of early infarct vessel recanalization. Of course, this paramount end point of survival benefit will be effectively compared only in the large-scale trials of GISSI-2 and ISIS-3.

Besides efficacy, the comparative side effects of t-PA and SK are important to consider. The avoidance of immunogenicity, allergic reactions, and primary or secondary resistance are all desirable features in favor of t-PA. The lack of idiosyncratic hypotension induced by t-PA is also a noteworthy advantage. There has been considerable debate regarding the bleeding complications and relative risk.

In two of the four direct comparative trials, a slight advantage in a decreased frequency of extracranial bleeding events was conferred for t-PA.[27,34,91,92] In the large-scale trials of GISSI-1, ISIS-2, and ASSET patients with stroke were not characterized by computerized axial tomographic (CAT) scanning. Thus, only the overall stroke rate can be derived, but it cannot be categorized into hemorrhagic or embolic (Table 4–9). The intracranial hemorrhage rate for t-PA was clearly increased and high for patients receiving 150 mg in the TIMI-2 trial.[96]

In this largest t-PA trial to date, the incidence of hemorrhagic stroke was 0.5

percent for 2742 patients receiving 100 mg.[93] As shown in Table 4–9, the overall data set for intracranial hemorrhage are relatively similar for t-PA versus SK, especially when one considers that adjunctive therapy with aspirin and heparin has been more frequent in the t-PA trials. In addition, there has been more extensive CAT scanning and detailed surveillance in trials with this agent. For example, in TIMI, a head CAT scan was routinely performed for any patient with a new neurologic deficit; in GISSI and ISIS-2 this was the exception rather than the rule.

Finally, a discussion of the relative merits of t-PA versus SK cannot be complete without mention and emphasis of the costs of these agents. There is a 10-fold higher price for t-PA: $2200 versus approximately $200 for streptokinase. This cost differential has fueled the heated controversy of the choice between agents. Were their costs equivalent, there would be no controversy and probably no need for the GISSI-2 or ISIS-3 trials. The advantages of t-PA insofar as timely restoration of infarct vessel patency and lack of antigenicity would be more greatly apparent.

The large price differential is most unfortunate because it has imposed a strain on the health care system with respect to hospitals absorbing the cost.[94] It is likely, however, that over time and with the introduction of APSAC and other t-PA products, the price attached to the first t-PA commercially available will decrease substantially. At the present, from the data presented, it is obvious t-PA is not cost effective: t-PA does not open 10 times as many infarct vessels as SK, nor does it result in 10 times as much cardiac function or survival benefit.

CONCLUSION

With the advantage of lack of antigenicity, t-PA is a more efficient coronary thrombolytic agent than SK. There has been no trial that has yet demonstrated superiority of t-PA over SK in terms of mortality reduction or improvement of cardiac function. Other new agents, such as APSAC, high-dose urokinase regimens, prourokinase, or new mutants,[95,96] may also find their place in the future. The intelligent selection of an intravenous thrombolytic agent for acute myocardial infarction can be done only on the basis of well-designed, carefully performed, ongoing clinical trials. For the time being, selection should be based on practical considerations, including familiarity, concern over antigenicity or hypotension, need for prompt infarct vessel patency, and, unfortunately, cost.

REFERENCES

1. Herrick, JB: Clinical features of sudden obstruction of the coronary arteries. JAMA 59:2015, 1912.
2. Fletcher, AP, Alkjaersig, N, Smyrniotis, FE, et al: The treatment of patients suffering from early myocardial infarction with massive and prolonged streptokinase therapy. Trans Assoc Am Physicians 71:289, 1958.
3. Tillett, WS and Sherry, S: The effect in patients of streptococcal fibrinolysin (streptokinase) and streptococcal desoxyribonuclease on fibrinous, purulent, and sanguinous pleural exudations. J Clin Invest 28:173, 1949.
4. European Working Party: Streptokinase in recent myocardial infarction: A controlled multicenter trial. Br Med J 3:325, 1971.
5. Schroder, R, Biamino, G, Leitner, E-RV, et al: Intravenous short-term infusion of streptokinase in acute myocardial infarction. Circulation 67(3):536, 1983.
6. Collen, D, Topol, EJ, Tiefenbrunn, AJ, et al: Coronary thrombolysis with recombinant human tissue-type plasminogen activator: A prospective, randomized, placebo-controlled trial. Circulation 70:1012, 1984.

7. Topol, EJ: Advances in thrombolytic therapy for acute myocardial infarction. J Clin Pharmacol 27:735, 1987.
8. Meyer, J, Bar, F, Barth, H, et al: International double-blind randomized trial of intravenous r-scu-PA vs streptokinase in acute myocardial infarction (PRIMI). Circulation 78(Suppl II):II303, 1988.
9. Collen, D: Systemic thrombolytic therapy of acute myocardial infarction? Circulation 68:462, 1983.
10. Sobel, BE: Pharmacologic thrombolysis: Tissue-type plasminogen activator. Circulation 76(Suppl II):II39, 1987.
11. Sobel, BE, Gross, RW, and Robison, AK: Thrombolysis, clot selectivity, and kinetics. Circulation 70:160, 1984.
12. Bergmann, SR, Fox, KAA, Ter-Pogossian, MM, et al: Clot-selective coronary thrombolysis with tissue-type plasminogen activator. Science 220:1181, 1983.
13. Braunwald, E, Knatterud, GL, Passamani, ER, et al: Announcement of protocol change in thrombolysis in myocardial infarction trial. J Am Coll Cardiol 9:467, 1987.
14. Marder, VJ and Sherry, S: Thrombolytic therapy: Current status (Part One). N Engl J Med 318:1512, 1988. (Part Two). N Engl J Med 318:1585, 1988.
15. Pitt, B: Clot-specific thrombolytic agents: Is there an advantage? J Am Coll Cardiol 12:588, 1988.
16. Topol, EJ and Califf, RM: TPA backlash. J Am Coll Cardiol 13:1477–80, 1989.
17. Noel, J, Rosenbaum, LH, Gangadharan, V, et al: Serum sicknesslike illness and leukocytoclastic vasculitis following intracoronary arterial streptokinase. Am Heart J 113:395, 1987.
18. Hoffman, JJML, Fears, R, Bonnier, JJRM, et al: Significance of antibodies to streptokinase in coronary thrombolytic therapy with streptokinase or APSAC. Fibrinolysis 2:203, 1988.
19. Lew, AS, Laramee, P, Cercek, B, et al: The hypotensive effect of intravenous streptokinase in patients with acute myocardial infarction. Circulation 72(6):1321, 1985.
20. Gruppo Italiano per lo Studio della Streptochinasi nell'Infarto Miocardico (GISSI): Effectiveness of intravenous thrombolytic treatment in acute myocardial infarction. Lancet 1:397, 1986.
21. ISIS-2 (Second International Study of Infarct Survival) Collaborative Group: Randomised trial of intravenous streptokinase, oral aspirin, both, or neither among 17,187 cases of suspected acute myocardial infarction: ISIS-2. Lancet 2:349, 1988.
22. Schroder, R, Neuhaus, K-L, Leizorovicz, A, et al: A prospective placebo-controlled double-blind multicenter trial of intravenous streptokinase in acute myocardial infarction (ISAM): Long-term mortality and morbidity. J Am Coll Cardiol 9:197, 1987.
23. Wilcox, RG, von der Lippe, G, Olsson, CG, et al: Trial of tissue plasminogen activator for mortality reduction in acute myocardial infarction. Lancet 2:525, 1988.
24. AIMS Trial Study Group: Effect of intravenous APSAC on mortality after acute myocardial infarction: Preliminary report of a placebo-controlled clinical trial. Lancet 1:545, 1988.
25. Kennedy, JW, Martin, GV, Davis, KB, et al: The Western Washington intravenous streptokinase in acute myocardial infarction randomized trial. Circulation 77:345, 1988.
26. White, HD, Norris, RM, Brown, MA, et al: Effect of intravenous streptokinase on left ventricular function and early survival after acute myocardial infarction. N Engl J Med 317:850, 1987.
27. The TIMI Study Group: The thrombolysis in myocardial infarction (TIMI) trial. N Engl J Med 312:932, 1985.
28. Hillis, LD, Borer, J, Braunwald, E, et al: High dose intravenous streptokinase for acute myocardial infarction: Preliminary results of a multicenter trial. J Am Coll Cardiol 6:957, 1985.
29. Spann, JF, Sherry, S, Carabello, BA, et al: Coronary thrombolysis by intravenous streptokinase in acute myocardial infarction: Acute and follow-up studies. Am J Cardiol 53:655, 1984.
30. Rogers, WJ, Mantle, JA, Hood, WP, Jr, et al: Prospective randomized trial of intravenous and intracoronary strepokinase in acute myocardial infarction. Circulation 68:1051, 1983.
31. Neuhaus, KL, Tebbe, U, Sauer, G, et al: Hochdosierte intravenose Kurzinfusion von Streptokinase beim acuten Myocardinfarkt. In Trübestein, G and Etzel, F (eds): Fibrinolytische Therapie. FK Schattauer Verlag, Stuttgart/New York, p 475, 1983.
32. de Marneffe, M, Van Thiel, E, Ewalenko, M, et al: High-dose intravenous thrombolytic therapy in acute myocardial infarction: Efficiency, tolerance, complications and influence on left ventricular performance. Acta Cardiol 40:183, 1985.
33. Schwartz, F, Hofmann, M, Schuler, G, et al: Thrombolysis in acute myocardial infarction: Effect of intravenous followed by intracoronary streptokinase application on estimates of infarct size. Am J Cardiol 53:1505, 1984.
34. Verstraete, M, Bory, M, Collen, D, et al: Randomized trial of intravenous recombinant tissue-type plasminogen activator versus intravenous streptokinase in acute myocardial infarction. Lancet 1:842, 1985.

35. Cribier, A, Berland, J, Saoudi, N, et al: Intracoronary streptokinase, heparin or intravenous strep-tokinase in acute infarction: Preliminary results of a prospective randomized trial with angiographic evaluation in 44 patients. Haemostasis 16(Suppl 3):122, 1986.

36. Brochier, ML, Quillet, L, Kulbertus, H, et al: Intravenous APSAC versus intravenous streptokinase in evolving myocardial infarction. Drugs 3(Suppl 3):140, 1987.

37. Monnier, P, Sigwart, U, Vincent, A, et al: Anisoylated plasminogen streptokinase activator complex versus streptokinase in acute myocardial infarction: Preliminary results of a randomized study. Drug 33(Suppl 3):175, 1987.

38. Chesebro, JH, Knatterud, G, Roberts, R, et al: Thrombolysis in Myocardial Infarction (TIMI) Trial, Phase I: A comparison between intravenous tissue plasminogen activator and intravenous strepto-kinase. Circulation 76:142, 1987.

39. Stack, RS, O'Connor, CM, Mark, DB, et al: Coronary perfusion during acute myocardial infarction with a combined therapy of coronary angioplasty and high-dose intravenous streptokinase. Circu-lation 77:151, 1988.

40. Lopez-Sendón, J, Seabra-Gomes, R, Martin Santos, F, et al: Intravenous anisoylated plasminogen streptokinase activator complex (APSAC) versus intravenous streptokinase (SK) in myocardial infarction (AMI). A randomized multicentre trial. Eur Heart J 9(Suppl A):10, 1988.

41. Miller, HI, Roth, A, Parades, A, et al: A comparison of early thrombolytic therapy with streptoki-nase and tissue plasminogen activator in acute myocardial infarction. Eur Heart J 9(Suppl A):215, 1988.

42. Vogt, P, Schaller, MD, Monnier, P, et al: Systemic thrombolysis in acute myocardial infarction: Bolus injection of APSAC versus infusion of streptokinase. Eur Heart J 9(Suppl A):213, 1988.

43. Taylor, GJ, Mikell, FL, Moses, HW, et al: Intravenous versus intracoronary streptokinase therapy for acute myocardial infarction in community hospitals. Am J Cardiol 54:256, 1984.

44. Williams, DO, Borer, J, Braunwald, E, et al: Intravenous recombinant tissue-type plasminogen acti-vator in patients with acute myocardial infarction: A report from the NHLBI thrombolysis in myo-cardial infarction trial. Circulation 73:338, 1986.

45. Gold, HK, Leinbach, RC, Garabedian, HD, et al: Acute coronary reocclusion after thrombolysis with recombinant human tissue-type plasminogen activator: Prevention by a maintenance infusion. Circulation 73:347, 1986.

46. The TIMI Study Group Special Report: The thrombolysis in myocardial infarction (TIMI) trial. N Engl J Med 312:932, 1985.

47. Mueller, HS, Rao, AK, Forman, SA, et al: Thrombolysis in myocardial infarction (TIMI): Com-parative studies of coronary reperfusion and systemic fibrinogenolysis with two forms of recombi-nant tissue-type plasminogen activator. J Am Coll Cardiol 10:479, 1987.

48. Verstraete, M, Brower, RW, Collen, D, et al: Double-blind randomised trial of intravenous tissue-type plasminogen activator versus placebo in acute myocardial infarction. Lancet 2:965, 1985.

49. Verstraete, M, Arnold, AEF, Brower, RW, et al: Acute coronary thrombolysis with recombinant human tissue-type plasminogen activator: Initial patency and influence of maintained infusion on reocclusion rate. Am J Cardiol 60:231, 1987.

50. Topol, EJ, Morris, DC, Smalling, RW, et al: A multicenter, randomized, placebo-controlled trial of a new form of intravenous recombinant tissue-type plasminogen activator (Activase) in acute myo-cardial infarction. J Am Coll Cardiol 9:1205, 1987.

51. Topol, CJ, Califf, RM, George, BS, et al: A randomized trial of immediate versus delayed elective angioplasty after intravenous tissue plasminogen activator in acute myocardial infarction. N Engl J Med 317:581, 1987.

52. Topol, EJ, George, BS, Kereiakes, DJ, et al: A randomized controlled trial of intravenous tissue plasminogen activator and early intravenous heparin in acute myocardial infarction. Circulation 79:281–286, 1989.

53. Simoons, ML, Arnold, AER, Betriu, A, et al: Thrombolysis with rt-PA in acute myocardial infarc-tion: No beneficial effects of immediate PTCA. Lancet 1:197, 1988.

54. Johns, JA, Gold, HK, Leinbach, RC, et al: Prevention of coronary artery reocclusion and reduction in late coronary artery stenosis after thrombolytic therapy in patients with acute myocardial infarc-tion. Circulation 78:546, 1988.

55. TIMI Research Group: Immediate vs delayed catheterization and angioplasty following thrombo-lytic therapy for acute myocardial infarction. JAMA 260:2849, 1988.

56. McNeill, AJ, Shannon, JS, Cunningham, SR, et al: A randomized dose ranging study of recombi-nant tissue plasminogen activator in acute myocardial infarction. Br Med J 296:1768, 1988.

57. Neuhaus, K, Tebbe, U, Gottwik, M, et al: Intravenous recombinant tissue plasminogen activator

(rt-PA) and urokinase in acute myocardial infarction: Results of the German Activator Urokinase Study (GAUS). J Am Coll Cardiol 12:581, 1988.

58. Neuhaus, KL, Tebbe, U, Gottwik, M, et al: Intravenose Infusion von recombinant tissue plasminogen Activator (rt-PA) und Urokinase beim akuten Myokardinfarkt: Zwischenergebnisse der GAUS Studie (German Activator Urokinase Study). Klin Wschr 66:102, 1988.

59. Miller, HI, Roth, A, Parades, A, et al: A comparison of early thrombolytic therapy with streptokinase and tissue plasminogen activator in acute myocardial infarction. Eur Heart J 9(Suppl A):215, 1988.

60. Topol, EJ: Coronary angioplasty for acute myocardial infarction. Ann Intern Med 109:970, 1988.

61. Califf, RM, Topol, EJ, Stump, D, et al: Hemorrhagic complications associated with the use of intravenous tissue-plasminogen activator in the treatment of acute myocardial infarction. Am J Med 85:353, 1988.

62. Jang, I-K, Vanhaecke, J, De Geest, H, et al: Coronary thrombolysis with recombinant tissue-type plasminogen activator: patency rate and regional wall motion after 3 months. J Am Coll Cardiol 8:1455, 1986.

63. Bennett, WR, Yawn, DH, Migliore, PJ, et al: Activation of the complement system by recombinant tissue plasminogen activator. J Am Coll Cardiol 10:627, 1987.

64. Van de Werf, F and Arnold, AER: Intravenous tissue plasminogen activator and size of infarct, left ventricular function, and survival in acute myocardial infarction. Br Med J 297:1374, 1988.

65. Guerci, AD, Gerstenblith, G, Brinker, JA, et al: A randomized trial of intravenous tissue plasminogen activator for acute myocardial infarction with subsequent randomization to elective coronary angioplasty. N Engl J Med 317:1613, 1987.

66. National Heart Foundation of Australia Coronary Thrombolysis Group: Coronary thrombolysis and myocardial salvage by tissue plasminogen activator given up to 4 hours after onset of myocardial infarction. Lancet 1:203, 1988.

67. Topol, EJ, Califf, RM, George, BS, et al: Insights derived from the thrombolysis and angioplasty in myocardial infarction (TAMI) trials. J Am Coll Cardiol 12:24A, 1988.

68. Armstrong, PW, Baigrie, RS, Daly, PA, et al: Tissue plasminogen activator Toronto (TPAT): Randomized trial in myocardial infarction. J Am Coll Cardiol 13:1469–76, 1989.

69. Topol, EJ, Califf, RM, George, BS, et al: Coronary arterial thrombolysis with combined infusion of recombinant tissue-type plasminogen activator and urokinase in acute myocardial infarction. Circulation 77:1100, 1988.

70. Topol, EJ, George, BS, Kereiakes, DJ, et al: Comparison of two dose regimens of intravenous tissue plasminogen activator for acute myocardial infarction. Am J Cardiol 61:723, 1988.

71. Villemant, D, Barriot, P, Riou, B, et al: Achievement of thrombolysis at home in cases of acute myocardial infarction. Lancet 1:228, 1987.

72. Dudley, CRK: Thrombolysis at home. Lancet 2:1459, 1987.

73. Herve, C, Gaillard, M, Castaigne, A, et al: Thrombolysis at home. Lancet 2:1278, 1987.

74. Weiss, AT, Fine, DG, Applebaum, D, et al: Prehospital coronary thrombolysis: A new strategy in acute myocardial infarction. Chest 92:124, 1987.

75. Anderson, JL, Rothbard, RL, Hackworthy, RA, et al: Multicenter reperfusion trial of intravenous anisoylated plasminogen streptokinase activator complex (APSAC) in acute myocardial infarction: Controlled comparison with intracoronary streptokinase. J Am Coll Cardiol 11:1153, 1988.

76. Bonnier, HJRM, Visser, RF, Klomps, HC, et al: Comparison of intravenous anisoylated plasminogen streptokinase activator complex and intracoronary streptokinase in acute myocardial infarction. Am J Cardiol 62:25, 1988.

77. DeWilde, P, Taeymans, Y, Demoor, D, et al: Intravenous thrombolysis with BRL 26921 in acute myocardial infarction. Presented at the International Symposium on Cardiovascular Pharmacotherapy, Geneva, (abstr 96), 1985.

78. Marder, VJ, Rothbard, RL, Fitzpatrick, PG, et al: Rapid lysis of coronary artery thrombi with anisoylated plasminogen: Streptokinase activator complex. Treatment by bolus intravenous injection. Ann Intern Med 104:304, 1986.

79. Timmis, AD, Griffin, B, Crick, JCP, et al: An interim report of a double-blind placebo controlled recanalization study of anisoylated plasminogen streptokinase activator complex in acute myocardial infarction. Drugs 33(Suppl 3):146, 1987.

80. Kasper, W, Meinertz, T, Wollschlaeger, H, et al: Coronary thrombolysis during acute myocardial infarction by intravenous BRL 26921, a new anisoylated plasminogen streptokinase activator complex. Am J Cardiol 58:416, 1986.

81. Monassier, JP, Borchier, M, Charbonnier, B, et al: Eminase versus streptokinase á la phase aiguë de l'infarctus du myocarde: Étude randomisée (étude I.R.S. II). 14e Congrès de Cardiologie de langue francaise 25, 1987.
82. Relik-Van Wely, L, van der Pol, JMJ, Visser, RF, et al: A preliminary report on the angiographic assessed patency and reocclusion in patients treated with APSAC for acute myocardial infarction (AMI). A Dutch Multicentre Study. Eur Heart J 9(Suppl A):8, 1988.
83. Meinertz, T, Kasper, W, Schumacher, M, et al: The German multicenter trial of anisoylated plasminogen streptokinase activator complex versus heparin for acute myocardial infarction. Am J Cardiol 62:347, 1988.
84. Bassand, JP, Machecourt, J, Cassagnes, J, et al: A multicenter double-blind trial of intravenous APSAC versus heparin in acute myocardial infarction. Final report of the APSIM study. J Am Coll Cardiol 11:232A, 1988.
85. Lippschutz, EJ, Ambrus, JL, Ambrus, CM, et al: Controlled study of the treatment of coronary occlusion with urokinase-activated human plasmin. Am J Cardiol 16:93, 1965.
86. Mathey, DG: Urokinase. In Topol, EJ (ed): Acute Coronary Intervention. Alan R. Liss, New York, pp 25–34, 1987.
87. TIMI Research Group: Immediate vs delayed catheterization and angioplasty following thrombolytic therapy for acute myocardial infarction. JAMA 260:2849, 1988.
88. Califf, RM, Wall, TC, Tcheng, JE, et al: High-dose urokinase for acute myocardial infarction results in high rate of sustained infarct artery patency. Circulation 78(Suppl II):II304, 1988.
89. Stump, DC and Collen, D: Single-chain urokinase-type plasminogen activator. In Topol, EJ (ed): Acute Coronary Intervention. Alan R. Liss, New York, pp 49–60, 1987.
90. Loscalzo, J, Wharton, TP, Kirshenbaum, JM, et al: Relative clot-selective coronary thrombolysis with prourokinase. Circulation 79:776–82, 1989.
91. White, HD, Rivers, JT, Maslowski, AH, et al: Comparison of tissue plasminogen activator and streptokinase for preservation of left ventricular function after a first myocardial infarction. N Engl J Med 320:817–21, 1989.
92. Magnani, B, for the PAIMS Investigators: Plasminogen Activator Italian Multicenter Study (PAIMS): Comparison of intravenous recombinant single-chain human tissue-type plasminogen activator (rt-PA) with intravenous streptokinase in acute myocardial infarction. J Am Coll Cardiol 13:19, 1989.
93. TIMI Study Group: Comparison of invasive and conservative strategies following intravenous tissue plasminogen activator in acute myocardial infarction: Results of the Thrombolysis in Myocardial Infarction (TIMI) II Trial. N Engl J Med 320:618–27, 1989.
94. Rich, MW: TPA: Is it worth the price? Am Heart J 114:1259, 1987.
95. Gheysen, D, Lijnen, HR, Pierard, L, et al: Characterization of a recombinant fusion protein of the finger domain of tissue-type plasminogen activator with a truncated single chain urokinase-type plasminogen activator.
96. Pannekoek, H, de Vries, C, and van Zonneveld, A: Mutants of human tissue-type plasminogen activator (t-PA): Structural aspects and functional properties. Fibrinolysis 2:123, 1988.

Commentary

By Melvin D. Cheitlin, M.D.

In this chapter Topol discusses the relative merits of the various fibrinolytic agents available at present for use in the lysis of intracoronary thrombi in the patient with acute myocardial infarction. The most experience currently is with streptokinase[1] and recombinant t-PA (rt-PA),[2] although a large body of information about APSAC[3] and urokinase is accumulating. There is little question that overall there appears to be a higher reperfusion rate for rt-PA than for streptokinase. There is also a time dependency with streptokinase in which lysis occurs more frequently in the younger thrombi and less frequently as the thrombus matures, whereas this does not appear to be evident with rt-PA. The other advantage of rt-PA over strep-tokinase—that is, clot selectivity that could result in lesser incidence of bleeding at the doses needed in acute myocardial infarction—is less evident in the studies reported. Most of the bleeding is associated with puncture sites related to the coronary arteriogram. With the TIMI-2B study,[5] which provides powerful evidence for coronary arteriography being necessary after fibrinolysis only if there is residual evidence of ischemia, the requirement for arterial punctures should decrease, and probably there will be fewer overall instances of bleeding. As long as the total dose of rt-PA is kept below 150 mg, the evidence suggests that the risk of intracranial bleeding is low and is similar with each of the agents.

Although the patency rate increases with streptokinase and finally equals that with rt-PA the later after onset that the coronary arteriogram is done, rt-PA probably opens the artery faster at the doses used in the studies. Because early opening of the vessel is probably the important factor in reperfusion, this should be an important difference between the two fibrinolytic agents. From results thus far, APSAC seems to have an incidence of reperfusion almost equal to urokinase and rt-PA.[6]

The most important result of fibrinolytic therapy in acute myocardial infarction is not simply the opening of the coronary artery, because after 24 hours the patency rate may be similar with all of the agents. Rather, the important result of reperfusion therapy is the myocardial salvage achieved by opening the artery in a timely fashion. The surrogate evidence for myocardial salvage may be found in most of the studies in the acute and late mortality and in recovery of myocardial function compared with placebo, and it is in these end points that we must look for differences among the agents. In these areas there is little proof that one agent has a clear advantage over another. With regard to left ventricular function, the ejection fraction is probably statistically greater after reperfusion compared with placebo, although in most studies the control group has a surprisingly good ejection fraction, meaning that the commonly encountered large acute anterior myocardial infarctions have not been included in these studies. To date there is only one large study comparing streptokinase and rt-PA, that of White and colleagues,[7] in which the mean ejection fraction with streptokinase was exactly the same as that with rt-PA.

The difference in mortality between streptokinase and rt-PA also is difficult to judge from the studies reported thus far. Although in many cases the absolute mortality is lower in the rt-PA studies than in the streptokinase studies, frequently the mortality in the control group is also lower in the rt-PA studies. This is the case, for instance, in the GISSI study,[1] in which the streptokinase mortality was 10.7 percent and the control mortality was 13 percent, an overall reduction of 18 percent in mortality of the treatment group over the control group. In the ASSET study,[2] however, the mortality in the rt-PA group was 7.2 percent and the control mortality was 9.8 percent, which represents a 27 percent reduction in mortality. Topol presents a meta-analysis combining four studies that compared streptokinase and rt-PA and showed a 29 percent reduction in mortality of rt-PA over streptokinase. The difference in cumulative mortality, however, is 7.6 percent for streptokinase and 5.4 percent for rt-PA, which was not statistically significant. In addition, with the variations in the onset to time of treatment, the variability of time windows allowed in each of the studies, the different groups of patients included in the study, and the number of first infarctions versus multiple infarctions, it is obvious that we can draw no conclusions about relative reduction in mortality with different fibrinolytic agents from the studies reported thus far. In almost all studies of fibrinolytic agents in patients with acute myocardial infarction in which the drug was compared to a placebo, the absolute difference in mortality was two to three percent in favor of the drug. In other words, for every 100 patients treated, two to three fewer deaths occurred in the patients treated with fibrinolytic agents. Mortality issues and possibly also the issues of improvement in ventricular function still await the large trials that compare agents directly—the GISSI-2 and the ISIS-3 studies.

Other considerations are important. Clearly, if another course of fibrinolytic agent is needed, the patient who has had streptokinase should receive either urokinase or rt-PA. Also, the activation of kinins, which can result in hypotension, is a potential disadvantage for streptokinase as compared with rt-PA.

Finally, one comparative difference between the agents that is not in doubt is the issue of cost, with the present cost of rt-PA being considerably greater than that of streptokinase. Inasmuch as there is no compelling evidence that rt-PA is better than streptokinase in the important outcome issues—those of survival and residual left ventricular function—the cost must be an important consideration, and in this regard streptokinase has a distinct advantage.

REFERENCES

1. Gruppo Italiano per lo Studio della Streptochinasi nell' Infarcto Miocardico (GISSI): Effectiveness of intravenous thrombolytic treatment in acute myocardial infarction. Lancet 1(8478):397, 1986.
2. Wilcox, RG, von der Lippe, G, Olsson, CG, et al: Anglo-Scandinavian Study on Early Thrombolysis (ASSET) Study Group: Trial of tissue plasminogen activator for mortality reduction in acute myocardial infarction. Lancet 2:525, 1988.
3. AIMS Trial Study Group: Effect of intravenous APSAC on mortality after acute myocardial infarction: Preliminary report of a placebo-controlled clinical trial. Lancet 1:545, 1988.

4. Neuhaus, K, Tobbe, U, Gottwik, M, et al: Intravenous recombinant tissue plasminogen activator (rt-PA) and urokinase in acute myocardial infarction: Results of the German Activator Urokinase Study (GAUS). J Am Coll Cardiol 12:581, 1988.
5. The TIMI Study Group: Comparison of invasive and conservative strategies after treatment with intravenous tissue plasminogen activator in acute myocardial infarction. N Engl J Med 320:618, 1989.
6. Bonnier, HJRM, Visser, RF, Klomps, HC, et al: Comparison of intravenous anisoylated plasminogen streptokinase activator complex and intracoronary streptokinase in acute myocardial infarction. Am J Cardiol 62:25, 1988.
7. White, HD, Rivers, JT, Maslowski, AH, et al: Effect of intravenous streptokinase as compared with that of tissue plasminogen activator on left ventricular function after first myocardial infarction. N Engl J Med 320:817, 1989.

CHAPTER 5

Should Asymptomatic Patients with Coronary Artery Disease and Nonsustained Ventricular Tachycardia Be Treated with Antiarrhythmic Drugs?

Laurence M. Epstein, M.D.
Melvin M. Scheinman, M.D.

Perhaps the most challenging dilemma facing clinicians today is the prevention of sudden cardiac death (SCD). With the advent of coronary care units[1-3] and the emergency response system,[4-6] cardiac arrest became a treatable problem. Closed chest cardiopulmonary resuscitation,[7] direct current defibrillation,[8] and electrical cardioversion[9] were employed with success. Despite these and other advances, SCD remains the leading cause of death, claiming between 200,000 and 400,000 people per year in the United States.[10] Studies have shown that in most cases SCD is caused by ventricular fibrillation[11-19] and that the vast majority of these patients have underlying coronary artery disease (CAD).[17,20-22] Although SCD is the first manifestation of CAD in up to 20 percent of patients,[21,23-26] nearly 75 percent of patients suffering SCD have had previous evidence of coronary artery disease.[23,26,27] It is well known that patients with sustained ventricular tachycardia and those suffering *aborted* sudden death are at high risk for SCD.[6,15,18] It remains a major challenge to identify additional patient groups at high risk for SCD and, once these patients are identified, to initiate an effective and safe prophylactic therapy.

This chapter focuses on one subgroup of those patients: stable, asymptomatic patients with underlying coronary artery disease and nonsustained ventricular tachycardia (NSVT). We will not consider those patients with drug- or electrolyte-induced ventricular arrhythmias, nor patients with a long QT syndrome or ongoing active myocardial ischemia. The latter patients represent different populations with different therapeutic approaches.

The following questions are addressed in this chapter: (1) Are these patients truly at increased risk for SCD? (2) Within this population is there a particular subgroup at higher risk and how do we identify them? (3) And finally, once identified, is there an effective, safe therapy? Unfortunately, most of these questions lack a definitive answer. We will present a review of the current understanding of this problem and address the issue of whether asymptomatic patients with coronary artery disease and nonsustained ventricular tachycardia should be treated with anti-arrhythmic drugs.

WHAT IS NONSUSTAINED VENTRICULAR TACHYCARDIA?

There is no universally accepted definition, yet before we can proceed we must define nonsustained ventricular tachycardia. Variations exist for many parameters, including the minimal and maximal number of beats, duration, and minimal rate. For the purposes of this chapter we will define NSVT as more than or equal to three consecutive ventricular complexes, at a rate more than or equal to 100 beats per minute (BPM), lasting less than 30 seconds, and not causing hemodynamic compromise.

ARE ASYMPTOMATIC PATIENTS WITH CORONARY ARTERY DISEASE AND NONSUSTAINED VENTRICULAR TACHYCARDIA AT INCREASED RISK?

With the advent of coronary care units came continuous electrocardiographic monitoring in the setting of acute myocardial infarctions. This and the development of ambulatory electrocardiographic monitoring allowed physicians to observe what precipitated and occurred during a cardiac arrest. Tachyarrhythmias, and specifically ventricular fibrillation, has been found to be the causative arrhythmia in the majority of patients who died suddenly during monitoring (Fig. 5–1).[28-44] Prior to death, many of these patients were found to have frequent and complex ventricular ectopy.[34,36,42-44] These findings and experience in coronary care units[1-3] suggested that patients with coronary artery disease and frequent or complex ventricular ectopy were at an increased risk of sudden cardiac death.

The absence or presence of ventricular ectopy alone was too nonspecific a finding. Ventricular ectopy could be demonstrated in up to 90 percent of patients with coronary artery disease if monitored long enough.[45] In an effort to better predict which patients were at highest risk Lown and Wolf[46] in 1971 developed a system (Table 5–1) for classifying ventricular ectopy. Throughout the 1970s and 1980s the role of ventricular ectopy in patients with coronary artery disease as a risk factor

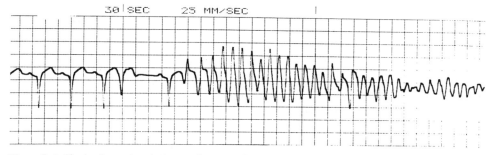

Figure 5–1. Single-channel ambulatory electrocardiographic recording of a patient suffering sudden cardiac death due to a ventricular tachyarrhythmia.

Table 5–1. Lown Classification

0	no ventricular ectopic beats
1	occasional, isolated VPB
2	frequent VPB, (>1/min or 30/hr)
3	multiform VPB
4	repetitive VPB
	a. couplets
	b. salvos
5	R on T

VPB = ventricular premature beat.

for mortality and SCD was evaluated.[47–67] Unfortunately a variety of methods were used and studies varied as to patient populations (varying time after infarction), degree of underlying heart disease (presence or absence of heart failure), form and length of electrocardiographic monitoring (single 12-lead ECG versus 1 to 24 hours of continuous monitoring on one or more occasions), and classification of ventricular ectopy. It is difficult, therefore, to compare findings and to pool data for analysis. The majority of studies support the hypothesis that the presence of frequent (more than or equal to 30 per hour) premature ventricular complexes is an independent predictor of mortality and a higher incidence of SCD.[47–64] There are, however, a few studies[65–67] that are at variance, finding that the frequency of ventricular ectopic complexes serves as a marker for the severity of underlying heart disease alone and that the latter is the more powerful risk factor.

Some studies[57–64,66–86] considered the role of complex ventricular ectopy (including NSVT) as a risk factor along with the frequency of ventricular ectopy. The populations studied, methods employed, and incidence of NSVT are reviewed in Table 5–2. The incidence of NSVT in these patients ranged from 0.1 percent to 30 percent and varied with the patient population studied, and the length, frequency, and type of monitoring employed. The findings of those studies that eval-

Table 5–2. NSVT during Electrocardiographic Monitoring: Incidence

Study (Year)	Patients (Number)	Population	Monitoring (Hours)	Frequency[a]	NSVT[b]	Incidence NSVT (%)
Moss[57] (1971)	100	3 weeks post MI	6	×1	≥3 VPC	4.0
Tuminaga[58] (1973)	2035	>3 months post MI	12 lead ECG	×1	≥2 VPC	0.5
Kolter[59] (1973)	160	male survivors of MI, no CHF	10–12	4–5×	≥3 VPC	2.5
Vismara[60] (1975)	64	5–14 days post MI	10	×1	≥3 VPC	7.8
Ryan[68] (1975)	81	>6 months post MI	24	×1	≥3 VPC	20
Luria[61] (1976)	143	post MI	8	×1	≥3VPC	NA
VanDurme[69] (1976)	150	1–12 months post MI	8	1×/ month	≥3 VPC	15

Table 5–2. NSVT during Electrocardiographic Monitoring: Incidence (*Continued*)

Study (Year)	Patients (Number)	Population	Monitoring (Hours)	Frequency[a]	NSVT[b]	Incidence NSVT (%)
Rehnqvist[62] (1977)	100	3 weeks post MI	6	×1	≥3 VPC	1.0
Ruberman[63] (1971)	1739	post MI	1	×1	NA	C
Schulze[64] (1977)	81	2 weeks post MI	24	×1	NA	C
DeSoyza[67] (1978)	56	3 weeks post MI	24	×1	≥3 VPC ≥120 BPM	4.3
Anderson[70] (1978)	915	pre discharge post MI	6	mean ×5.5	≥3 VPC ≥100 BPM	7.2
Myburg[71] (1978)	175	post MI	6	multiple	≥3 VPC	12.6
Moss[72] (1979)	940	pre discharge post MI	6	×1	≥3 VPC	0.1
Møller[73] (1980)	100	post MI	24	×4	≥3 VPC ≥100	19.0
DeBusk[66] (1980)	90	post MI	12	×1–4	≥3 VPB	4.0
Taylor[85] (1980)	106	10–14 days post MI	24	×1	≥3 VPB	13.2
Ruberman[74] (1980)	416	angina, no MI	1	×1	≥2 VPC ("runs")	29.2
Follansbee[75] (1980)	518	various symptoms	24	×1	≥3 VPC	7.1
	183	CAD	"	"	"	5.5
Kleiger[76] (1981)	289	2wk–12mo post MI	10	×9	≥3 VPC	30.0
Bigger[77] (1981)	430	2 weeks post MI	24	×1	≥3 VPC	11.6
Bigger[86] (1981)	400	10–20 days post MI	24	×1	≥3 VPC	11.8
Ruberman[78] (1981)	1739	post MI	1	×1	NA	C
Bigger[79] (1981)	428	10–20 days post MI	24	×1	≥3 VPC	11.6
Califf[80] (1982)	395	CAD, undergoing angiography	24	×1	≥3 VPC	5.3
Braat[81] (1983)	33	7 days post anterior MI	24	×1	NA	C
Bigger[82] (1984)	766	post MI	24	×1	≥3 VPC	12.1
Mukharji[83] (1984)	533	10 days post MI	24	×1	NA	NA
Maisel[84] (1985)	777	pre discharge post MI	24	×1	≥3 VPC	?6.4

a = definition of nonsustained ventricular tachycardia, b = frequency of monitoring, VPC = ventricular premature complex, NA = not available, C = NSVT grouped with other complex arrhythmias (i.e., multiform bigeminy, couplets, R on T), MI = myocardial infarction, CAD = coronary artery disease, BPM = beats per minute, CHF = congestive heart failure.

Table 5–3. NSVT during Electrocardiographic Monitoring: Outcome

Study (Year)	End Point	Incidence[a]	NSVT Risk[b]	NSVT Independent[c]	Complex[d] Only
Tuminaga (1973)	SCD	1/10	No	No	—
Kolter (1973)	SCD	2/3	Yes	No	—
Vismara (1975)	SCD	2/5	NA	NA	Yes
VanDurme (1976)	SCD	9/23	Yes	NA	—
Rehnqvist (1977)	SCD	1/1	NA	NA	Yes
Ruberman (1977)	Death	NA	NA	NA	Yes
Schulze (1977)	SCD	NA	NA	NA	Yes
DeSoyza (1978)	Death	0/2	No	NA	—
Anderson (1978)	Death	11/66	No	No	—
Myburg (1978)	Death	6/22	Yes	NA	—
Møller (1980)	SCD	0/19	No	No	—
DeBusk (1980)	Coronary event	NA	NA	NA	No
Taylor (1980)	Death	3/14	Yes	No	No
Ruberman (1980)	Death	NA	NA	NA	No
Kleiger (1981)	SCD	4/88	No	No	—
Bigger (1981)	Death	22/55	Yes	NA	—
Bigger (1981)	Death	NA	NA	NA	Yes
Ruberman (1981)	Death	NA	NA	NA	Yes
Bigger	Death	15/50	Yes	NA	—
(1981)	SCD	11/50	No	NA	—
Califf (1982)	SCD	7/21	Yes	No	—
Braat (1983)	Death	NA	NA	NA	No
Bigger (1984)	SCD	15/88	Yes	Yes	—
Mukharji (1984)	SCD	NA	NA	NA	Yes
Maisel (1985)	Death	?3/58	No	NA	—

a = number of patients with end point/number of patients with NSVT, b = significant increased risk of end point if NSVT present, c = NSVT independent predictor of end point when other variables considered, d = analysis for all complex ventricular arrhythmias only (i.e., NSVT, multiform, couplets, bigeminy, R on T), NA = not available, SCD = sudden cardiac death.

uated the risk of death and/or SCD in these patients can be found in Table 5–3. The presence of complex ventricular arrhythmias (NSVT, multiform, bigeminy, couplets, and R on T) was a significant risk factor for subsequent mortality and/or SCD in 7 of 11 studies.[60,62–64,66,74,78,81,83,85,86]

In 14 studies NSVT was separated from other complex ventricular arrhythmias for risk analysis. The incidence of SCD in patients with CAD and NSVT found on electrocardiographic monitoring varied from 0 to 100 percent in these studies. Nonsustained ventricular tachycardia was found to be a significant, independent risk factor for death in three[74,81,85] and for SCD in two studies.[69,82] It was not a significant and/or independent risk factor for SCD in five studies,[58,59,73,76,79] or mortality in three studies.[70,84,85]

As already noted, it remains unclear whether the presence of NSVT independently identifies those patients with CAD who are at increased risk for SCD, and, as can be seen in Table 5–3, the majority of patients with NSVT and CAD did not experience either spontaneous sustained ventricular tachycardia or SCD. If all patients with CAD and NSVT were treated, the majority would unnecessarily be exposed to potentially toxic and expensive medications. It is therefore important to determine which among these patients are at highest risk for SCD.

DETERMINATION OF RISK FACTORS

In recent years there has been a dramatic expansion in our knowledge of the epidemiology and pathophysiology of sudden cardiac death. This has allowed for the development of newer techniques to identify patients at increased risk. In this section we will explore some of these noninvasive and invasive techniques and their specific relevance to our patient population.

NONINVASIVE TECHNIQUES

Continuous Ambulatory Monitoring

Due to reports[43] that found that patients suffering SCD while undergoing continuous electrocardiography (ECG) monitoring had longer and more rapid episodes of ventricular tachycardia (VT) prior to death than those without SCD, many clinicians believe that patients with prolonged, frequent, or rapid bursts of NSVT are at higher risk of subsequent sustained VT and SCD. Although the rationale for this approach is evident, it is not supported by the majority of available data. Studies[70,73,75,79,87–91] (Table 5–4) have shown that the rate, duration (number of beats), and frequency of NSVT are not predictive of future spontaneous or induc-

Table 5–4. Characteristics of NSVT

Study (Year)	Patients (Number)	Population	NSVT[a]	1 Episode Only (%)	3 Beats Only (%)	Significant Characteristic[b]
Winkle[87] (1977)	23	NSVT on Holter (clinical/ research)	≥3 VPC	NA	49	NA
Anderson[70] (1978)	915 66	post MI/ NSVT	≥3 VPC ≥100 BPM	74	47	No
Møller[73] (1980)	100 19	post MI/ NSVT	≥3 VPC ≥100 BPM	84	16	No[c]
Follansbee[75] (1980)	518 37	various/ NSVT	≥3 VPC	35	64	No
Bigger[79] (1981)	428	post MI	≥3 VPC	27	29	No
Buxton[88] (1983)	83	NSVT undergoing EPS	≥3 VPC	NA	30[d]	No
Veltri[89] (1985)	33	NSVT undergoing EPS	≥3 VPC ≥100 BPM	27	70[d]	No
Speilman[90] (1985)	58	NSVT undergoing EPS	≥3 VPC ≤15 seconds	NA	NA	No
Batsford[91] (1986)	81	NSVT undergoing EPS	NA	NA	NA	No

a = definition of NSVT, b = any characteristic of NSVT being a significant predictor of mortality or SCD, c = no patient with NSVT suffered SCD, d = 3–5 beats, NA = not available, MI = myocardial infarction, VPC = ventricular premature complex, BPM = beats per minute, EPS = electrophysiologic study.

ible sustained ventricular tachycardia during electrophysiologic studies or of SCD. Of interest, a significant percentage of patients had only a single episode of NSVT, and the longest episode in many patients was only three beats. Therefore, unfortunately characteristics of the spontaneous NSVT cannot be used to predict outcome in these patients, and treatment should not be based on these findings.

Recently the significance of silent myocardial ischemia found during ambulatory monitoring has been evaluated. Patients with and without angina who have silent myocardial ischemia appear to have an increased mortality and a higher risk of SCD.[92] However, the relationship of silent myocardial ischemia and ventricular tachyarrhythmias requires further study.

Evaluation of Cardiac Function

A variety of methods are available to determine cardiac function (i.e., echocardiography, ventriculography, nuclear studies). It has been well established that the finding most predictive of mortality following myocardial infarction is cardiac function. Marchlinski and coworkers[93] showed that in patients post-myocardial infarction (MI), 5 of 11 (45.5 percent) with ejection fraction (EF) less than 40 percent suffered SCD, whereas this occurred in only one of 26 (3.8 percent) of patients with EF greater than or equal to 40 percent. Roy and associates[94] also found that, in patients post MI the mean ejection fraction was significantly lower (29 percent versus 46 percent) in patients who died, suffered SCD, or had spontaneous sustained ventricular tachycardia. The presence of a left ventricular aneurysm was also a significant risk factor for SCD or sustained ventricular tachycardia. It is clear, therefore, that left ventricular (LV) dysfunction identifies patients with a higher mortality and risk of SCD.

Many studies have shown that patients with poor LV function have increased ventricular ectopy;[64,65,75,76,82,84] others have shown that patients with frequent or complex ventricular ectopy and poor LV function have an excess mortality. In the studies that evaluated patients with frequent ventricular premature complexes (VPCs), complex ventricular ectopy, and NSVT, the presence of poor LV function greatly increased mortality and the risk of SCD.[56,63,64,75,78,80,82,83] Conversely, patients with good LV function, regardless of ventricular ectopic activity, did well. For example, Schulze and associates[64] found that in patients with complex ventricular arrhythmias, SCD occurred only in those with an EF less than or equal to 40 percent.

Therefore, patients with poor LV function and NSVT have a significantly increased risk of death and SCD, and patients with good LV function, regardless of the presence or absence of NSVT, do well. The exact cut-off is not known but is most often defined as an EF of 40 percent. There is also a suggestion that patients with LV aneurysms are at increased risk. Although these findings help define a population of patients who will do well without therapy, the majority of patients with CAD, NSVT, and LV dysfunction also will do well. Again, treating all these patients would subject many patients to antiarrhythmic therapy who would do well without such therapy.

Signal-Averaged Late Potentials

Recently, important insights relating to the mechanisms of ventricular arrhythmias have been made. Both canine infarction models and evidence from clinical sources suggest that reentry is the underlying mechanism of sustained ven-

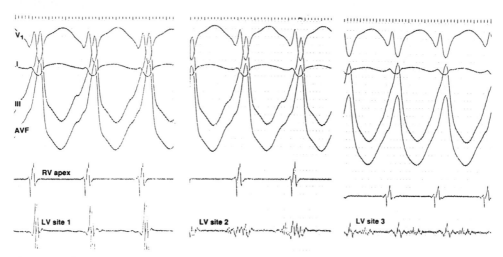

Figure 5-2. Simultaneous recordings of surface ECG leads V1, I, III, AVF and intracardiac electrograms from the right ventricular apex (RV apex) and various left ventricular sites (LV site) in a patient during sustained ventricular tachycardia. *(Site 1)* normal ventricular electrogram, *(Site 2)* fractionated ventricular electrogram, *(Site 3)* Mid-diastolic electrical activity.

tricular tachycardia. Requirements for initiation and maintenance of reentry include slow conduction and unidirectional block. Pathologic analysis of infarcted myocardium revealed islets of viable myocardium interlaced with fibrotic tissue.[99] It has been postulated that this region accounts for slowed conduction and *fractionation* of the depolarizing wavefront.[100] Such fractionated electrograms (Fig. 5–2) have been found in experimental animal models of ischemia and infarction[101–110] and in man.[111,112] Most authors believe that fragmentation of the depolarizing wavefront within these focal, heterogeneous regions leads to fractionated electrograms.[101–107,110,112–120] These fractionated electrograms may or may not arise from the slow conduction zone critical for maintenance of a reentrant arrhythmia.[121,122]

Fragmented electrograms or *late potentials* are not recorded from routine 12-lead ECG recordings. Berbari and associates[123] were the first to describe a technique to record late potentials in animals using amplification and signal averaging of surface recordings, and Fontaine and coworkers[124] were the first to report its use in humans. In 1981, Simson and colleagues[125] described a modification of this technique, which is now the basis for the majority of signal-averaged recorders used in clinical practice (Fig. 5–3). Late potentials are found in up to 90 percent of patients with sustained VT,[126–133] but in only 10 to 30 percent of patients without sustained VT or frequent complex ventricular ectopy.[126,127] It was hoped, therefore, that late potentials would help identify those patients with CAD who were at risk for developing sustained VT and SCD.

Several studies[128,134–136] found that successful surgical removal of tachycardia foci was associated with the loss of late potentials and noninducibility at repeat electrophysiologic study. The presence of late potentials in patients following MI[126–132,137–143] and in those with NSVT[144] placed these patients at higher risk for subsequent spontaneous and induced sustained VT and SCD. Although these findings are encouraging, others found that late potentials were not predictive of SCD[145] or inducible sustained VT in patients with NSVT.[146] The presence of late potentials is not a specific finding because up to one third of patients post MI are found to

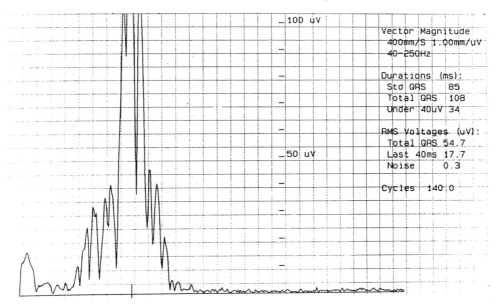

Figure 5–3. Signal-averaged ECG from a patient with ventricular tachycardia.

have late potentials,[126,127,132] but only a small percentage of these patients develop either spontaneous sustained VT or SCD. However, the aforementioned studies did find that the absence of late potentials was associated with a benign prognosis.

Winters and coworkers[147] recently reported on the predictive value of signal-averaged electrograms in patients with NSVT and/or high-grade ventricular ectopy undergoing electrophysiologic testing in a group of patients with predominantly CAD. Abnormal signal-averaged recordings were found in 22 of 53 patients (40 percent). Eleven (55 percent) of the patients with abnormal recordings had inducible VT, whereas only 1 of the 31 normal patients (3 percent) was inducible. At follow-up, only 2 of the 30 noninducible patients without late potentials had an arrhythmic event, one of which was related to an acute MI. Different characteristics of late potentials may have prognostic importance (i.e., duration of signal-averaged QRS, duration of low-amplitude signals, and amplitude of the root mean square voltage of the terminal 40msec), but these data are too preliminary to allow for integration into clinical practice.

Therefore, abnormal signal-averaged recordings showing late potentials appear to be a marker for the substrate in which sustained VT may develop. At present the role of signal-averaged recordings in patients with CAD and NSVT appears to be similar to that of evaluation of LV function, aiding in the selection of patients who should undergo further invasive testing and defining which patients are at low risk of future arrhythmic events.

INVASIVE TECHNIQUES

Electrophysiologic Testing (Programmed Stimulation)

Programmed electrical stimulation (PES) of the heart in humans was introduced in 1967.[148,149] Programmed electrical stimulation has been shown to be useful in predicting long-term outcome and efficacy of antiarrhythmic therapy in patients suffering cardiac arrest and for recurrent sustained VT.[150-158] Although its value in determining appropriate drug therapy for patients with cardiac arrest and sustained VT has been proven, its role in predicting which patients are at risk for these events is still evolving.

Patients with aborted sudden death and induced sustained VT during PES are thought to be at high risk for recurrent sustained VT.[150,158] Although the risk of SCD in patients with NSVT is much lower than in those with sustained ventricular arrhythmias, it seemed logical to assume that patients with NSVT and inducible VT are at high risk for recurrent sustained VT and SCD. To evaluate this hypothesis, electrophysiologic testing was performed in patients with CAD. Unfortunately, these studies vary widely as to stimulation protocol (stimulation strength, number of extrastimuli used, number of right ventricular sites, or use of an isoproterenol infusion) and patient population, and therefore they are difficult to compare. Additionally, because 12-lead ECGs of spontaneous NSVT usually are not available, the relationship of induced arrhythmias to spontaneous arrhythmia is uncertain. In addition, the sensitivity and specificity of PES is less in patients with NSVT compared with those with sustained VT. It is also of concern that in most studies patients received a variety of antiarrhythmic medications in a random fashion, and therefore all the results to date must be evaluated within these limitations.

Predictors and Incidence of a Positive Test

Roy and associates[94] performed electrophysiologic testing and monitoring in 320 patients following an acute MI. The grade of ventricular ectopy was no different in inducible and noninducible patients, but patients who had induced sustained VT had a significantly lower EF than those who did not. In 1986, Roy and associates[159] showed that findings at repeat electrophysiologic testing 4 to 12 months after infarction correlated well with acute studies in 21 patients, but they found no correlation between inducibility and SCD. Hamer and colleagues[160] studied 70 patients post MI at *high risk* (i.e., congestive heart failure, ventricular ectopy, or conduction abnormalities). Of seven patients with Lown class IV arrhythmias found on Holter, three were noninducible, two had inducible sustained VT, and two had inducible NSVT. In this small group of patients, inducibility was predictive of SCD. Richards and coworkers[161] reported similar findings.

There have been several reports[95-98,148,162-165] of patients with NSVT or high-grade ventricular ectopy undergoing electrophysiologic testing, and they are reviewed in Table 5-5. In the six[88,90,91,97,163,164] studies that included patients with a variety of underlying heart conditions, the incidence of induced sustained VT varied widely from 0 to 22 percent, as did the incidence of inducible NSVT (10 to 62 percent). As can be seen in the table, the highest rate of induced sustained ventricular tachycardia was found in the studies with *aggressive* stimulation protocols. The study[163] with no inducible sustained VT used the strictest definition for this finding. In three[88,90,97] of the six studies, variables relating to inducibility were evaluated. Two studies[88,97] found an EF less than 40 percent, and one[165] found the presence of an LV aneurysm to be predictive of inducibility, although one study found no significant difference in EF between inducible and noninducible patients.

Eight studies[89,95,96,98,147,162,165,167] reported results for patients with CAD. Again, the range of patients with inducible sustained ventricular tachycardia varied from 20 to 57 percent and correlated in part with stimulation protocol employed and the definition of sustained ventricular tachycardia. Seven studies[89,95,96,98,147,162,165]

Table 5-5. Electrophysiologic Studies

Study (Year)	Patients (Number)	Population	Stimulation Protocol[a]	Definition Positive[b]	Inducible VT(%)	Predictors[c]
Vandepol[163] (1980)	29	Symptomatic NSVT	S3, mult RV LV	VTs = >1 min VTn = ≥3/ <60 sec	VTs 0% VTn 62%	NA
Swerdlow[164] (1982)	41	NSVT various HD	S4, mult RV Iso	NA	VTs 22% VTn 32% VF 7%	NA
Buxton[88] (1983)	83	NSVT various HD	S4, mult RV Iso, LV	VTs = >30 sec VTn = ≥3/ <30 sec	VTs 18% VTn 33%	EF <40% LV aneurysm
Gomes[97] (1984)	73	High grade vent. ectopy	S3, mult RV	VTs = >30 sec	VTs 18%	EF <40%
	37	NSVT		VTn = ≥5/ <30 sec	VTn 10% S + N 34%	
Greenberg[165] (1984)	25	NSVT CAD	S4, mult RV	VTs = >30 sec VTn = >5/ <30 sec	VTs 20% VTn 36%	EF = NS
Spielman[98] (1985)	30	NSVT CAD/EF <50	S4, mult RV	VTs = ≥15 sec VTn = ≥6/ <15 sec	VTs 50% VTn 17%	LV aneurysm
Veltri[90] (1985)	33	NSVT various HD	S3, mult RV LV	VTs = ≥30 sec VTn = <3/ <30 sec	VTs 21% VTn 21%	EF = NS
Buxton[89] (1986)	56	NSVT CAD	NA	NA	VTs 43% VTn 32%	EF = NS
Batsford[91] (1986)	81	NSVT various HD	NA	NA	VTs 21% VTn 45%	NA
Klein[95] (1986)	22	NSVT (≥5 beats) CAD	S4, mult RV	VTs = ≥15 sec VTn = NA	VTs 50% VTn NA	LV aneurysm
Zheutlin[167] (1986)	57	Complex vent. ectopy CAD	S3, mult RV	VT = ≥6 beats	VT 46%	NA
Buxton[162] (1987)	62	NSVT CAD	S4, mult RV	VTs = >30 sec VTn = ≥3/ <30 sec	VTs 45% VTn 24%	EF <40% LV aneurysm Trend (NS)
Sulpizi[96] (1987)	35	NSVT CAD	S4, mult RV LV	VTs = >15 beats VTn = 3–15 beats	VTs 57% VTn NA	EF <50%
Winters[147] (1988)	49	NSVT CAD	S3, mult RV	VTs = >30 sec VTn = ≥3/ <30 sec	VTs 16% VTn 10%	Trend for lower EF (NS)

a = programmed stimulation protocol; S3 = double extrastimuli; S4 = triple extrastimuli; mult RV = multiple right ventricular sites; Iso = isoproterenol; LV = left ventricular stimulation; b = definition of inducible arrhythmia; VTs = sustained ventricular tachycardia, in all cases definition also includes hemodynamic compromise; VTn = nonsustained ventricular tachycardia; c = predictor of inducibility; EF = ejection fraction, LV = left ventricle; NS = nonsignificant; S+N = grouped sustained and nonsustained ventricular tachycardia; VT = induction of defined tachycardia; VF = ventricular fibrillation; NSVT = nonsustained ventricular tachycardia; HD = heart disease; CAD = coronary artery disease; vent = ventricular; NA = not available.

evaluated EF and/or the presence of LV aneurysm as predictors of inducibility. One[96] found a significant increase in inducibility for patients with an EF less than 50 percent, and two[147,162] reported a trend for lower EFs in inducible patients, whereas two[89,165] found EF not to be significant. In two studies,[95,98] an LV aneurysm was present in significantly more inducible patients than in noninducible patients; a similar trend was seen in one other study.[162]

Clearly, the percentage of patients with inducible sustained ventricular tachycardia varied widely among these studies. This percentage increases with more aggressive stimulation protocols, *laxer* definitions for a positive test, underlying CAD, and the presence of an LV aneurysm. Although there is disagreement, it would appear that patients with LV dysfunction were more likely to have inducible sustained VT.

Risk of Inducible Ventricular Tachycardia

The predictive role of electrophysiologic testing in patients with sustained VT was extended to patients with NSVT in the 1980s. Eleven studies[89,91,95–98,147,162,164,166,167] evaluated the risk of SCD and/or spontaneous sustained VT in patients with high-grade ventricular arrhythmias, including NSVT (n = 2) and NSVT alone (n = 9) (Table 5–6).

Table 5–6. Follow-up of Electrophysiologic Studies

Study (Year)	End Point	Noninducible (%)	Sustained VT (%)[a]	All VT (%)[b]	Significant[c]	Other Risk Factors[d]
Swerdlow[164] (1982)	SCD	2/6(12)	NA	3/25(12)	No	NA
Gomes[97] (1984)	SCD	1/53(2)	NA	5/20(25)	Yes	EF <40%
Buxton[98] (1984)	SCD	4/31(13)	4/15(27)	6/52(12)	Yes	EF <40%
Veltri[89] (1985)	SCD or S-VTs	0/19(0) 9/19(21)	3/14(21)	NA	Yes No	None
Buxton[166] (1986)	SCD	2/36(6)	6/24(25)	NA	Yes	NA
Batsford[91] (1986)	SCD or S-VTs	0/28(0)	4/17(24)	9/53(17)	Yes	None
Klein[95] (1986)	SCD or S-VTs	1/11(9)	5/11(45)*	NA	Yes	LV An
Zheutlin[167] (1986)	SCD or S-VTs	0/55(0)	4/33(12)†	NA	Yes	NA
Buxton[162] (1987)	SCD	1/16(6)	7/28(25)	10/43(23)	Yes	EF <40%
Sulpizi[96] (1987)	SCD	3/50(6)	1/9(11)	NA	No	EF <35%
Winters[147] (1988)	SCD or S-VTs	2/40(5)	NA	2/13(15)	Yes	NA

VTs = sustained ventricular tachycardia; VT = ventricular tachycardia; S-VTs = spontaneous VTs; SCD = sudden cardiac death; LV An = left ventricular aneurysm; EF = ejection fraction; * = VTs defined as >15sec; † = VTs defined as ≥6 beats; a = number of patients with end point and inducible VTs vs total of patients with inducible VTs; b = number of patients with end point and any induced VT vs total patients with any induced VT; c = Is inducibility a significant risk factor for the end point? Applies to VTs unless only all VT available; d = other risk factors for the end point.

The definition of a positive test was induction of any VT (nonsustained and sustained) in three studies.[97,147,164] In two,[97,147] a positive test was a significant risk factor for SCD and/or spontaneous sustained VT. Inducible sustained VT was also a significant risk factor in six of eight studies[89,91,95,96,98,162,166,167] in which it defined a positive test, although no patient without inducible sustained VT suffered SCD in one of the conflicting studies.[89] Again, caution must be taken when interpreting these results inasmuch as patients had serial electropharmacologic guided, empiric, or no therapy, often at the discretion of a physician not participating in the study.

As with tests described earlier, a negative result of an electrophysiologic study (as defined above) was predictive of a good outcome in most cases. Veltri and coworkers[89] found a 21 percent incidence of a presumed arrhythmic event (syncope and presyncope) in patients without inducible sustained VT, but none of these patients suffered SCD. The other studies[96,164] that found poor outcomes in greater than 10 percent of patients without induced sustained VT included patients with a variety of underlying heart diseases, including congestive cardiomyopathy. The value of electrophysiologic testing appears to be less sensitive in this subset of patients compared with those with CAD.[168] Therefore, the available data suggest that those patients with NSVT and no inducible ventricular arrhythmia at PES have an excellent prognosis.

OVERALL RISK

Each of the aforementioned methods can be applied to the individual patient with CAD and NSVT to determine his or her overall risk of subsequent sustained VT and/or SCD. As already shown, patients do well with an EF greater than 40 percent and no LV aneurysm, or without late potentials on signal-averaged recordings. Electrophysiologic study further defines those patients who will have a good outcome. These findings have led us to develop an algorithm for evaluating these patients (Fig. 5–4).

The proarrhythmic effects of many antiarrhythmic medications are well known.[169–172] It is our goal, therefore, to subject only patients with a high risk of SCD to such therapy. We initially divide patients according to LV function. Patients with an EF greater than 40 percent have a benign prognosis without specific therapy, whereas patients with an EF less than 40 percent undergo signal-averaged electrocardiograms. Patients with normal signal-averaged ECG recordings are not considered for therapy, whereas patients with abnormal recordings merit further study. Although one may elect to institute Holter-guided therapy at this point, we believe invasive electrophysiologic testing further subdivides those patients at highest risk. If PES is performed and if sustained VT is not induced, no antiarrhythmic therapy is recommended. Only if a patient has inducible sustained VT is he or she considered for therapy. How and what therapy is chosen is the topic of the next section.

TREATMENT

TREATMENT OPTIONS

A wide variety of approved and experimental antiarrhythmic agents are currently available.[173] In addition, a variety of nonpharmacologic methods are available, including use of cardiac surgery, catheter ablation, or insertion of an auto-

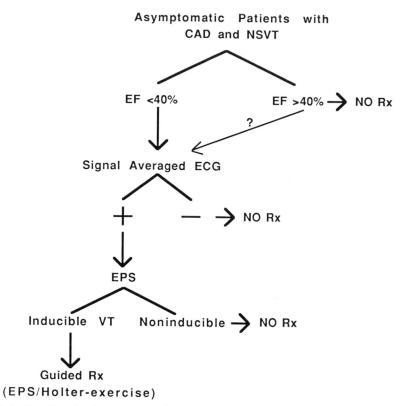

Figure 5–4. Algorithm for the treatment of asymptomatic patients with stable coronary artery disease (CAD) and nonsustained ventricular tachycardia (NSVT). *(See text for explanation.)* EF = ejection fraction; Rx = treatment; EPS = electrophysiologic study.

matic defibrillator.[174] The nonpharmacologic options are reserved currently for those with documented sustained malignant ventricular arrhythmias. If therapy is deemed necessary for patients with NSVT, the current mainstay remains drug therapy. Because most of the treated group will consist of those patients with poor LV function, drugs known to suppress cardiac performance should be avoided (see *Treatment Selection*).

TREATMENT SELECTION

The available data for patients with sustained VT or SCD suggest that an organized therapeutic approach guided either by serial electropharmacologic studies[175] or by Holter-exercise testing[176,177] is more effective than empiric therapy. Presently, only one preliminary study[178] compared both techniques. A larger multi-institutional study is currently underway comparing the efficacy of these two approaches. Presently, there are no studies comparing PES-guided therapy versus Holter-exercise studies in patients with NSVT; therefore, no information is currently available to guide the clinician with regard to the optimal approach to therapy.

Unfortunately, no prospective randomized study of therapy in patients with NSVT and induced sustained VT exists. Until such a study is done, our therapy is based on inferential data. In 1987, Buxton and associates[162] showed that in patients with CAD and NSVT, SCD occurred in two of 16 (11 percent) patients with inducible sustained VT whose therapy was guided by electrophysiologic study and five of five (100 percent) patients treated with empiric therapy. Gomes and coworkers[97] found that at least one drug prevented induction of VT in 85 percent of patients with NSVT and inducible VT, but they did not report how this related to survival. Five sudden deaths and one episode of sustained VT occurred in their 20 inducible patients. Sulpizi and colleagues[96] found that although antiarrhythmic therapy prevented the induction of sustained VT in eight of nine patients, only 44 percent remained on therapy during all or most of the follow-up period. Of note is the fact that none of these patients suffered SCD during follow-up.

Because most of the patients deemed appropriate for drug therapy will have impaired LV performance, the clinician should avoid those drugs that further impair ventricular function. These drugs include disopyramide, flecainide, and beta-adrenergic blocking agents. In addition, the proarrhythmic effects of both encainide and flecainide are enhanced in those patients with depressed LV function and should, therefore, be avoided.[173,179] If the patient's arrhythmia is found to respond to intravenous lidocaine, then a trial with tocainide or mexiletine would appear to be reasonable. If the patient has suffered a recent MI or the ventricular arrhythmia is exercised or catecholamine induced, then trials of beta-blocker agents with careful monitoring for worsening heart failure would appear to be appropriate. Trials of drugs in the class IA family (quinidine, procainamide, and disopyramide) should be initiated in the hospital in order to detect those at risk for development of polymorphous VT. Several beneficial noncontrolled trials of low-dose amiodarone in patients with congestive heart failure and NSVT have been reported.[180,181] The possible efficacy and toxicity of this agent must be considered prior to initiation of amiodarone therapy. In addition, low-dose amiodarone (200 mg per day or less) therapy appears to be well-tolerated.

CONCLUSION

The available data preclude definitive recommendations regarding therapy of asymptomatic patients with CAD and NSVT. Nevertheless, a great deal of information has become available with regard to assessment of a subset of those patients who appear to be at higher risk for malignant ventricular arrhythmias or SCD. The clinical profile of the high-risk patient with NSVT includes presence of LV dysfunction, a low-amplitude late potential recorded with the signal-averaged ECG, as well as those with inducible sustained VT during programmed electrical stimulation. As a result of these studies, we propose the following algorithm for the management of asymptomatic patients with CAD and NSVT (Fig. 5–4). Those who have reasonably good LV function (i.e., EF greater than or equal to 40 percent) should not be treated (except perhaps for those with low-amplitude late potentials, who should undergo further study). In addition, those without late potentials, even with poor LV function, appear to have a benign prognosis and do not merit antiarrhythmic therapy. For those remaining in the high-risk group, therapy at present may be guided by either Holter-exercise or programmed stimulation studies because it is not clear which of the two methodologies is superior. One advantage of performing a baseline PES is to define further a subset of patients who do not appear to require antiarrhythmic treatment; namely, those in whom sustained VT is not inducible. It should be appreciated that these formulations are based in part on an incomplete data base and undoubtedly will change as our knowledge in this area expands. Finally, it is worthy of emphasis that the proposed algorithm is valid only for patients with CAD because fewer studies of patients without CAD are available and in the latter group the specificity of PES (in terms of replicating the spontaneous rhythm) is poor and data regarding the role of signal-averaged ECG are incomplete.

REFERENCES

1. Lown, B, Fakhro, AM, Hood, BW, et al: The coronary care unit: New perspectives and direction. JAMA 199:188, 1967.
2. Lown, B, Klein, MD, and Hershberg, DI: Coronary and precoronary care. Am J Med 46:705, 1969.
3. Lawrie, DM, Higgens, MR, Goodman, MJ, et al: Ventricular fibrillation complicating acute myocardial infarction. Lancet 2:523, 1968.
4. Training technics for the coronary care unit. Second Bethesda Conference of the American College of Cardiology, December 11,12, 1965. Washington DC. Am J Cardiol 17:736, 1966.
5. Pantridge, JF and Geddes, JS: A mobile intensive-care unit in the management of myocardial infarction. Lancet 2:271, 1967.
6. Baum, RS, Alvarez, H, III, and Cobb, LA: Survival after resuscitation from out-of-hospital ventricular fibrillation. Circulation 50:1231, 1974.
7. Kovwenhoven, WB, Jude, JR, and Knickerbocker, GG: Closed chest cardiac massage. JAMA 173:1064, 1960.
8. Lown, B, Neuman, J, Amarasingham, R, et al: Comparison of alternating current with direct current electroshock across the closed chest. Am J Cardiol 10:223, 1962.
9. Lown, B, Amarasingham, R, and Neuman, J: New method of terminating cardiac arrhythmias. JAMA 182:548, 1962.
10. Corday, E: Symposium on indentification and management of the candidate for sudden cardiac death—an introduction. Am J Cardiol 39:813, 1977.
11. Lown, B, Vassaux, C, Hood, WB, Jr, et al: Unresolved problems in coronary care. Am J Cardiol 20:494, 1967.
12. Hinkle, LE and Thaler, HT: Clinical classification of cardiac death. Circulation 65:457, 1982.
13. Panidis, IP and Morganroth, J: Initiating events of sudden cardiac death. Cardiovascular Clinics 15 (3):81, 1985.
14. Cobb, LA, Conn, RD, Samson, WE, et al: Prehospital coronary care: The role of a rapid response mobile intensive coronary care system. Circulation 44(Suppl II):45, 1971.
15. Schaffer, WA and Cobb, LA: Recurrent ventricular fibrillation and modes of death in survivors of out-of-hospital ventricular fibrillation. N Engl J Med 293:260, 1975.
16. Cobb, LA, Baum, RS, Alvarez, H, et al: Resuscitation from out-of-hospital ventricular fibrillation: 4 year follow-up. Circulation 51,52:111, 1975.
17. Weaver, WD, Lurch, GS, Alvarez, HA, et al: Angiographic findings and prognostic indicators in patients resuscitated from sudden cardiac deaths. Circulation 54:895, 1976.
18. Eisenberg, MS, Halstrom, A, and Bergner, L: Long-term survival after out-of-hospital cardiac arrest. N Engl J Med 306:1340, 1981.
19. Myerberg, RJ, Keffler, KM, Zaman, L, et al: Survivors of prehospital cardiac arrest. JAMA 274:1485, 1982.
20. Reichenbach, DO, Moss, NS, and Myer, E: Pathology of the heart in sudden cardiac death. Am J Cardiol 39:865, 1977.
21. Kannel, WB, Doyle, JJ, McNamara, PM, et al: Precursors of sudden coronary death: Factors related to the incidence of sudden death. Circulation 51:606, 1975.
22. Perper, JA, Kuller, LH, and Cooper, M: Atherosclerosis of coronary arteries in sudden unexpected deaths. Circulation 52:111, 1973.
23. Kuller, L, Lilienfield, A, and Fischer, R: Epidemiological study of sudden death due to arteriosclerotic heart disease. Circulation 34:1056, 1966.
24. Kuller, LH: Sudden death—definition and epidemiologic considerations. Prog Cardiovasc Dis 23:1, 1980.

25. Bashe, WR, Jr, Baba, N, Keller, ND, et al: Pathology of atherosclerotic heart disease in sudden death: II. The significance of myocardial infarction. Circulation 51,52(Suppl III):63, 1975.
26. Doyle, JJ, Kannel, WB, McNamara, RM, et al: Factors related to the suddenness of death from coronary disease: Combined Albany-Framingham studies. Am J Cardiol 37:1073, 1976.
27. Kuller, LH, Cooper, M, and Perper, J: Epidemiology of sudden death. Arch Intern Med 129:1972.
28. Milner, PG, Platia, EV, Reid, PR, et al: Holter monitoring recording at the time of sudden cardiac death. Circulation 68(Suppl III):106, 1983.
29. Kempf, JC, Jr and Josephson, ME: Sudden cardiac death recorded on ambulatory electrocardiogram. Circulation 68(Suppl III):355, 1983.
30. Roelandt, J, Klootwijk, P, and Lubsen J: Prodromal and lethal arrhythmias in sixteen sudden death patients documented with long-term ambulatory electrocardiography (LAE). Circulation 68(Suppl III):356, 1983.
31. Bleifer, SB, Bleifer, DJ, Hansmann, DR, et al: Diagnosis of occult arrhythmias by Holter electrocardiography. Prog Cardiovasc Dis 16:569, 1974.
32. Gradman, AH, Bell, PA, and DeBusk, RF: Sudden death during ambulatory monitoring: Clinical and electrocardiographic correlations: Report of a case. Circulation 55:210, 1977.
33. Pool, J, Kunst, K, and VanWermekerken, JL: Two monitored cases of sudden death outside the hospital. Br Heart J 40:627, 1978.
34. Boudoulas, H, Dervenagas, S, Schaal, SF, et al: Malignant premature beats in ambulatory patients. Ann Intern Med 91:723, 1979.
35. Salerno, D, Hodges, SM, Graham, E, et al: Fatal cardiac arrest during continuous ambulatory monitoring. N Engl J Med 305:700, 1981.
36. Panidis, IP and Morganroth, J: Holter monitoring and sudden cardiac death. Cardiovasc Reviews and Reports 5:283, 1984.
37. Lahari, A, Balasubramanian, V, and Raftery, EB: Sudden death during ambulatory monitoring. Br Heart J 1:1676, 1979.
38. Klein, RC, Vera, Z, Mason, DJ, et al: Ambulatory Holter monitor documentation of ventricular tachycardia as mechanism of sudden death in patients with coronary artery disease. Clin Res 27:7A, 1979.
39. Nikolic, G, Bishop, RL, and Singh, JB: Sudden death recorded during Holter monitoring. Circulation 66:218, 1982.
40. Savage, DD, Castilli, WP, Anderson, SJ, et al: Sudden unexpected death during ambulatory electrocardiographic monitoring: The Framingham study. Am J Med 74:148, 1983.
41. Denes, P, Gabster, A, and Huang, SK: Clinical, electrocardiographic and follow-up observations in patients having ventricular fibrillation during Holter monitoring: Role of quinidine therapy. Am J Cardiol 48:9, 1981.
42. Lewis, BH, Antman, EM, and Graboys, TB: Detailed analysis of 24 hour ambulatory electrocardiographic recordings during ventricular fibrillation or torsade de pointes. J Am Coll Cardiol 2:426, 1983.
43. Pratt, CM, Francis, MJ, Luck, JC, et al: Analysis of ambulatory electrocardiograms in 15 patients during spontaneous ventricular fibrillation with special reference to preceding arrhythmic events. J Am Coll Cardiol 2:789, 1983.
44. Panidis, IP and Morganroth, J: Sudden death in hospitalized patients: Cardiac rhythm disturbances detected by ambulatory monitoring. J Am Coll Cardiol 2:798, 1983.
45. Kennedy, HL, Chandra, V, Sayther, KL, et al: Effectiveness of increasing hours of continuous ambulatory electrocardiographic monitoring in detecting maximal ventricular ectopy: Continuous 48 hour study of patients with coronary heart disease and normal subjects. Am J Cardiol 42:925, 1978.
46. Lown, B and Wolf, MA: Approaches to sudden death from coronary heart disease. Circulation 44:130, 1971.
47. Oliver, GC: Ventricular arrhythmias in coronary artery disease and their relationship to sudden death. In Proceedings of the first US-USSR symposium on sudden death. Yalta, October 3–5, 1977, National Institutes of Health, Publication No (NIH) 78-1470:171, 1978.
48. Chaing, BN, Perlman, LV, Ostrander, LD, Jr, et al: Relationship of premature systoles to coronary heart disease and sudden death in the Tecumseh epidemiology study. Ann Intern Med 70:1159, 1969.
49. Wenger, TL, Bigger, JT, Jr, and Merrill, GS: Ventricular arrhythmias in the late hospital phase of acute myocardial infarction. Circulation 51,52(Suppl II)110, 1976.

50. Fitzgerald, JW, Houston, N, and DeBusk, RF: Natural history of ventricular arrhythmias in post infarction patients. Circulation 53,54(Suppl II):10, 1976.
51. Moss, AJ, DeCamilla, J, Engstrom, F, et al: The post hospital phase of myocardial infarction: Identification of patients with increased mortality risk. Circulation 49:460, 1974.
52. Moss, AJ, DeCamilla, J, Mietowski, W, et al: Prognostic grading and significance of ventricular premature beats after recovery from myocardial infarction. Circulation 51,52(Suppl 3):204, 1975.
53. Moss, AJ, DeCamilla, JJ, Davis, HP, et al: Clinical significance of ventricular ectopic beats in the early post hospital phase of myocardial infarction. Am J Cardiol 39:635, 1977.
54. Rehnqvist, N: Ventricular arrhythmias prior to discharge after myocardial infarction. Eur J Cardiol 4:63, 1976.
55. Ruberman, W, Weinblatt, E, Frank, CW, et al: Prognostic value of one hour of ECG monitoring of men with coronary heart disease. J Chron Dis 29:497, 1976.
56. The Multicenter Post Infarction Research Group: Risk stratification and survival after myocardial infarction. N Engl J Med 309:331, 1983.
57. Moss, AJ, Schnitzler, R, Green, R, et al: Ventricular arrhythmias 3 weeks after acute myocardial infarction. Ann Intern Med 75:837, 1971.
58. Tuminaga, S and Blackburn, D: Prognostic importance of premature beats following myocardial infarction: Experience in the coronary drug project. JAMA 223:1116, 1973.
59. Kolter, MN, Tabatznik, B, Mower, MM, et al: Prognostic significance of ventricular ectopic beats with respect to sudden death in the late post infarction period. Circulation 47:959, 1973.
60. Vismara, LA, Amsterdam, EA, and Mason, DJ: Relation of ventricular arrhythmias in the late hospital phase of acute myocardial infarction to sudden death after hospital discharge. Am J Med 59:6, 1975.
61. Luria, MH, Knoke, JD, Margolis, RM, et al: Acute myocardial infarction: Prognosis after recovery. Ann Intern Med 85:561, 1976.
62. Rehnqvist, N and Sjogren, A: Ventricular arrhythmias prior to discharge and one year after myocardial infarction. Eur J Cardiol 5:425, 1977.
63. Ruberman, W, Weinblatt, E, Golberg, J, et al: Ventricular premature beats and mortality after myocardial infarction. N Engl J Med 297:750, 1977.
64. Schulze, RA, Strauss, HW, and Pitt, B: Sudden death in the year following myocardial infarction. Am J Med 62:192, 1977.
65. Bigger, JT, Jr, Heller, CA, Wegner, TL, et al: Risk stratification after acute myocardial infarction. Am J Cardiol 42:202, 1978.
66. DeBusk, RF, Davidson, DM, Houston, N, et al: Serial ambulatory electrocardiography and treadmill exercise testing following uncomplicated myocardial infarction. Am J Cardiol 45:547, 1980.
67. DeSoyza, N, Bennett, FA, Murphy, MC, et al: The relationship of paroxysmal ventricular tachycardia complicating the acute phase and ventricular arrhythmia during the late phase of myocardial infarction to long-term survival. Am J Med 64:377, 1978.
68. Ryan, M, Lown, B, and Horn, H: Comparison of ventricular ectopic activity during 24 hour monitoring and exercise testing in patients with coronary artery disease. N Engl J Med 292:224, 1975.
69. VanDurme, JD and Pannier, RH: Prognostic significance of ventricular dysrhythmias 1 year after myocardial infarction. Am J Cardiol 37:178, 1976.
70. Anderson, KP, DeCamilla, J, and Moss, AJ: Clinical significance of ventricular tachycardia (3 beats or longer) detected during ambulatory monitoring after myocardial infarction. Circulation 57:890, 1078.
71. Myburg, DP and Goldman, AP: Repetitive ventricular ectopic activity in chronic ischemic heart disease. S Afr Med J 53:373, 1978.
72. Moss, AJ, Davis, HT, DeCamilla, J, et al: Ventricular ectopic beats and their relation to sudden death and nonsudden cardiac death after myocardial infarction. Circulation 64:297, 1981.
73. Møller, M, Nielsen, BL, and Fabricius, J: Paroxysmal ventricular tachycardia during repeated 24-hour ambulatory electrocardiographic monitoring of poly myocardial infarction patients. Br Heart J 43:447, 1980.
74. Ruberman, W, Weinblatt, E, and Goldberg, J: Ventricular premature complexes in prognosis of angina. Circulation 61:1172, 1980.
75. Follansbee, WD, Michelson, EL, and Morganroth, J: Nonsustained ventricular tachycardia in ambulatory patients: Characteristics and association with sudden cardiac death. Ann Intern Med 92:741, 1980.
76. Kleiger, RE, Miller, JP, Thanauaro, S, et al: Relationship between clinical features of acute myocardial infarction and ventricular runs 2 weeks after infarction. Circulation 63:64, 1981.

77. Bigger, JT, Jr, Weld, FM, and Rolnitzky, LM: Prevalence and significance of ventricular tachycardia in the late hospital phase of myocardial infarction. Am J Cardiol 47:397, (abstr) 1981.
78. Ruberman, W, Weinblatt, E, Goldberg, JD, et al: Ventricular premature complexes and sudden death after myocardial infarction. Circulation 64:297, 1981.
79. Bigger, JT, Weld, FM, and Rolnitzky, LM: Prevalence, characteristics and significance of ventricular tachycardia (three or more complexes) detected with ambulatory electrocardiographic recording in the late hospital phase of acute myocardial infarction. Am J Cardiol 48:815, 1981.
80. Califf, RM, McKinnis, RA, and Burks, J: Prognostic implication of ventricular arrhythmias during 24 hour ambulatory monitoring in patients undergoing cardiac catheterization for coronary artery disease. Am J Cardiol 50:23, 1982.
81. Braat, H, deZwaan, C, Brugada, P, et al: Value of left ventricular ejection fraction in extensive anterior infarction to predict the development of ventricular tachycardia. Am J Cardiol 52:686, 1983.
82. Bigger, JT, Jr, Fleiss, JL, Kleiger, R, et al: The relationships among ventricular arrhythmias, left ventricular dysfunction, and mortality in the 2 years after myocardial infarction. Circulation 69:250, 1984.
83. Mukarji, J, Rude, RE, Poole, KW, et al: Risk factors for sudden death after acute myocardial infarction: Two-year followup. Am J Cardiol 54:31, 1984.
84. Maisel, AS, Scott, N, Gilpin, E, et al: Complex ventricular arrhythmias in patients with Q wave versus non-Q wave myocardial infarction. Circulation 72:963, 1985.
85. Taylor, GJ, Humphries, JO, Mellits, DE, et al: Predictors of clinical course, coronary anatomy and left ventricular function after recovery from acute myocardial infarction. Circulation 62:960, 1980.
86. Bigger, JT, Jr and Weld, FM: Analysis of prognostic significance of ventricular arrhythmias after myocardial infarction. Br Heart J 45:717, 1981.
87. Winkle, RA, Derrigton, DC, and Schroeder, JS: Characteristics of ventricular tachycardia in ambulatory patients. Am J Cardiol 39:487, 1977.
88. Buxton, AE, Waxman, HL, Marchlinski, FE, et al: Electrophysiologic studies in nonsustained ventricular tachycardia: Relation to underlying heart disease. Am J Cardiol 52:985, 1983.
89. Veltri, EP, Platia, EV, Griffith, LSC, et al: Electrophysiologic stimulation and long-term follow-up in asymptomatic, nonsustained ventricular tachycardia. Am J Cardiol 56:310, 1985.
90. Spielman, SR, Greenspan, AM, Kay, HR, et al: Electrophysiologic testing in patients at high risk for sudden cardiac death. I. Nonsustained ventricular tachycardia and abnormal ventricular function. J Am Coll Cardiol 6:31, 1985.
91. Batsford, WP, Sudbrink, L, Stark, SI, et al: Outcome in nonsustained ventricular tachycardia: Relation to clinical factors, spontaneous and induced ventricular arrhythmias. J Am Coll Cardiol 7:71A, (abstr) 1986.
92. Cohen, PF (ed). Silent Myocardial Ischemia and Infarction. Marcel Dekker, New York, 1986.
93. Marchlinski, FE, Buxton, AE, Waxman, HL, et al: Identifying patients at risk of sudden death after myocardial infarction: Value of the response to programmed stimulation, degree of ventricular ectopic activity and severity of left ventricular dysfunction. Am J Cardiol 52:1190, 1983.
94. Roy, D, Marchand, E, Theroux, P, et al: Programmed ventricular stimulation in survivors of an acute myocardial infarction. Circulation 72:487, 1985.
95. Klein, RC and Mandell, C: Electrophysiologic studies in patients with nonsustained ventricular tachycardia and coronary artery disease: Relation of ventricular aneurysm to inducible tachycardia and prognosis. J Am Coll Cardiol 7:71A, 1986.
96. Sulpizi, AM, Friehling, TD, and Kowey, PR: Value of electrophysiologic testing in patients with nonsustained ventricular tachycardia. Am J Cardiol 59:841, 1987.
97. Gomes, JAC, Hariman, RI, Kany, PS, et al: Programmed electrical stimulation in patients with high-grade ventricular ectopy: Electrophysiologic findings and prognosis for survival. Circulation 70:43, 1984.
98. Buxton, AE, Marchlinski, FE, Waxman, HL, et al: Prognostic factors in nonsustained ventricular tachycardia. Am J Cardiol 53:1275, 1984.
99. Gardner, PI, Ursell, PC, Fenoglio, JJ, et al: Electrophysiologic and anatomic basis for fractionated electrograms recorded from healed myocardial infarcts. Circulation 72:596, 1985.
100. Ideker, RE, Mirvis, DM, and Smith, WM: Late fractionated potentials. Am J Cardiol 55:1614, 1985.
101. El-Sherif, N, Scherlag, BJ, Lazzara, R, et al: Reentrant arrhythmias in the late myocardial infarction period. I. Conduction characteristics in the infarct zone. Circulation 55:686, 1977.

102. El-Sherif, N, Hope, RR, Scherlag, BJ, et al: Reentrant arrhythmias in the late myocardial infarction period. II. Periods of initiation and termination. Circulation 55:707, 1977.

103. Bioneau, JF and Cox, JL: Slow ventricular activation in acute myocardial infarction. A source of reentrant premature ventricular contraction. Circulation 48:702, 1973.

104. Waldo, AL and Kaisar, GA: Study of ventricular arrhythmias associated with acute myocardial infarction in the canine heart. Circulation 47:1222, 1973.

105. Scherlag, BJ, El-Sherif, N, Hope, RR, et al: Characterization and localization of ventricular arrhythmias resulting from myocardial ischemia and infarction. Circ Res 35:372, 1974.

106. Kaplinsky, E, Ogawa, S, Kmetzo, J, et al: Intramyocardial activation in early ventricular arrhythmias following coronary artery ligation. J Electrocardiol 13:1, 1980.

107. Janse, MJ, van Capelle, FLJ, Morsink, H, et al: Flow of "injury" current and patterns of excitation during early ventricular arrhythmias in acute regional myocardial ischemia in isolated porcine and canine hearts. Circ Res 47:151, 1980.

108. Kabell, G, Brachmann, J, Scherlag, BJ, et al: Mechanism of ventricular arrhythmia in multivessel coronary disease: The effect of collateral zone ischemia. Am Heart J 108:447, 1984.

109. Kabell, G, Scherlag, BJ, Hope, RR, et al: Patterns of ectopic activation recorded during pleomorphic ventricular tachycardia after myocardial infarction in the dog. Am J Cardiol 49:56, 1982.

110. Garan, H and Ruskin, JN: Localized reentry: Mechanism of induced sustained ventricular tachycardia in canine model of recent myocardial infarction. J Clin Invest 74:377, 1984.

111. Spear, JF, Horowitz, LN, Moore, EN, et al: Verapamil sensitive slow response activity in infarcted human ventricular myocardium. Circulation 54 (Suppl II):II75, 1976.

112. Josephson, ME, Horwitz, LN, Farshidi, A, et al: Sustained ventricular tachycardia: Evidence for protected localized reentry. Am J Cardiol 42:416, 1978.

113. Han, J: Mechanisms of ventricular arrhythmias associated with myocardial infarction. Am J Cardiol 24:1969.

114. Scherlag, BJ, Helfant, RH, Haft, JI, et al: Electrophysiology underlying ventricular arrhythmias due to coronary ligation. Am J Physiology 219(6):1665, 1970.

115. Josephson, ME, Horowitz, LN, and Farshidi, A: Continuous local electrical activity: A mechanism of recurrent ventricular tachycardia. Circulation 57:658, 1978.

116. Fontaine, G, Guiraudon, G, Frank, R, et al: Modern concepts of ventricular tachycardia. Eur J Cardiol 8:565, 1978.

117. El-Sherif, N, Smith, A, and Evans, K: Canine ventricular arrhythmias in the late myocardial infarction period: Epicardial mapping of reentrant circuits. Circ Res 49:255, 1981.

118. Wit, AL, Allessie, MA, Bonke, FIM, et al: Electrophysiologic mapping to determine the mechanism of experimental ventricular tachycardia initiated by premature impulses: Experimental approach—initial results demonstrating reentrant excitation. Am J Cardiol 49:166, 1982.

119. Josephson, ME and Wit, AL: Fractionated electrical activity and continuous electrical activity: Fact or fiction. Circulation 70:529, 1984.

120. Spielman, SR, Untereker, WJ, Horowitz, LN, et al: Fragmented electrical activity: Relationship to ventricular tachycardia (abstr). Am J Cardiol 47:448, 1981.

121. Waxman, HL and Sung, RJ: Significance of fragmented ventricular electrograms observed using intracardiac recording techniques in man. Circulation 62:1349, 1980.

122. Brugada, P, Abdollah, H, and Wellens, HJJ: Continuous electrical activity during sustained monomorphic ventricular tachycardia: Observations on its dynamic behavior during the arrhythmia. Am J Cardiol 55:402, 1985.

123. Berbari, EJ, Scherlag, BJ, Hope, RR, et al: Recording from the body surface of arrhythmogenic ventricular activity during ST segment. Am J Cardiol 41:697, 1979.

124. Fontaine, G, Frank, R, Gallais Hamonno, F, et al: Electrocardiographie des potentiels tardifs du syndrome de post-excitation. Arch Mal Coeur 71:854, 1978.

125. Simson, MB, Euler, D, Michelson, EL, et al: Detection of delayed ventricular activation on the body surface in dogs. Am J Physiol 241:363, 1981.

126. Simson, MB: Use of signals in the terminal QRS complex to identify patients with ventricular tachycardia after myocardial infarction. Circulation 64:235, 1981.

127. Kanovsky, MS, Falcone, RA, Dresden, CA, et al: Identification of patients with ventricular tachycardia after myocardial infarction: Signal averaged electrocardiogram, Holter monitoring, and cardiac catheterization. Circulation 70:264, 1984.

128. Rozanski, JJ, Mortara, D, Meyerburg, RJ, et al: Body surface detection of delayed depolarizations in patients with recurrent ventricular tachycardia and left ventricular aneurysm. Circulation 63:1172, 1981.

129. Hombach, V, Braun, V, Hopp, HW, et al: The application of the signal averaging technique in clinical cardiology. Clin Cardiol 5:107, 1982.
130. Breithardt, G, Borggrefe, M, Karbenn, U, et al: Prevalence of late potentials in patients with and without ventricular tachycardia. Am J Cardiol 49:1932, 1982.
131. Denes, P, Santarelli, P, Hauser, RG, et al: Quantitative analysis of the high-frequency components of the terminal portion of the body surface QRS in normal subjects and in patients with ventricular tachycardia. Circulation 67:1129, 1983.
132. Breithardt, G, Borggrefe, M, Quantius, B, et al: Ventricular vulnerability assessed by programmed stimulation in patients with and without late potentials. Circulation 68:275, 1983.
133. Denes, P, Uretz, E, and Santarelli, P: Determinants of arrhythmogenic ventricular activity detected on the body surface QRS in patients with coronary artery disease. Am J Cardiol 53:1519, 1984.
134. Breithardt, G, Seipel, L, Ostermeyer, J, et al: Effects of antiarrhythmic surgery on late potentials recorded by precordial signal averaging in patients with ventricular tachycardia. Am Heart J 104:996, 1982.
135. Simpson, MB, Spielman, SR, Horowitz, LN, et al: Effects of surgery for control of ventricular tachycardia on late potentials. Circulation 64(Suppl IV):IV88, 1981.
136. Marcus, NH, Falcone, RA, Harken, AL, et al: Body surface late potentials: Effect of endocardial resection in patients with ventricular tachycardia. Circulation 70:632, 1984.
137. Breithardt, G, Becker, R, Seipel, L, et al: Noninvasive detection of late potentials in man: A new marker for ventricular tachycardia. Eur Heart J 2:1, 1981.
138. Haberl, R, Hoffman, E, and Steinbeck, G: Low-frequency components in patients with delayed ventricular activation. Circulation 72(Suppl III):III6, 1985.
139. Freedman, RA, Gillis, AM, Kern, A, et al: Signal-averaged electrocardiographic late potentials in patients with ventricular fibrillation or ventricular tachycardia: Correlation with clinical arrhythmia and electrophysiologic study. Am J Cardiol 55:1350, 1985.
140. von Leitner, ER, Oeff, M, Loock, D, et al: Value of noninvasively detected delayed ventricular depolarizations to predict prognosis in post myocardial infarction patients. Circulation 68(Suppl III):III83, 1983.
141. Kuchar, D, Thornburn, C, and Sammel, N: Natural history and clinical significance of late potentials after myocardial infarction. Circulation 72(Suppl III):III47, 1985.
142. Dennis, AR, Cody, DV, Fenton, SN, et al: Significance of delayed activation potentials in survivors of myocardial infarction (abstr). J Am Coll Cardiol 1:582, 1983.
143. Kacet, S, Libersa, C, Caron, J, et al: The prognostic value of averaged late potentials in patients suffering from coronary artery disease (abstr). International symposium Ventricular Tachycardias, May 1986.
144. Buxton, AE, Simson, MB, Falcone, R, et al: Signal averaged ECG in patients with nonsustained ventricular tachycardia: Identification of patients with potential for sustained ventricular tachycardia (abstr). J Am Coll Cardiol 3:495, 1984.
145. Breithhardt, G, Schwarzmaier, J, Borggrefe, M, et al: Prognostic significance of late ventricular potentials after myocardial infarction. Eur Heart J 4:487, 1983.
146. Turrito, G, El-Sherif, N, Ursell, S, et al: Comparison of programmed electrical stimulation and the signal averaged electrocardiogram in patients with nonsustained ventricular tachycardia (abstr). Clin Res 34:349A, 1986.
147. Winters, SL, Stewart, D, Targonski, A, et al: Role of signal averaging of the surface QRS complex in selecting patients with nonsustained ventricular tachycardia and high grade ventricular arrhythmias for programmed ventricular stimulation. J Am Coll Cardiol 12:1481, 1988.
148. Durrer, D, Schoo, L, Schuilenburg, RM, et al: The role of premature beats in the initiation and termination of supraventricular tachycardia in the Wolff-Parkinson-White syndrome. Circulation 36:644, 1967.
149. Coumel, P, Cabrol, C, Fabiato, A, et al: Tachycardie permenete par rhythme reciproque. Arch Mal Coeur 60:1830, 1967.
150. Ruskin, JN, DiMarco, JP, and Garan, H: Out-of-hospital cardiac arrest: Electrophysiologic observations and selection of long-term antiarrhythmic therapy. N Engl J Med 303:607, 1980.
151. Kehoe, RF, Zheutlin, T, Mattioni, T, et al: Factors associated with time to arrhythmic recurrence in survivors of ventricular fibrillation (abstr). J Am Coll Cardiol 9:108A, 1987.
152. Morady, F, Scheinman, MM, Hess, DS, et al: Electrophysiologic testing in the management of survivors of out-of-hospital cardiac arrest. Am J Cardiol 51:85, 1983.
153. Roy, D, Wavman, HL, Kienzle, MG, et al: Clinical characteristics and long-term follow-up of 119

survivors of out-of-hospital cardiac arrest: Relation to inducibility at electrophysiologic testing. Am J Cardiol 52:969, 1983.
154. Benditt, DG, Benson, DW, Jr, Klein, MR, et al: Prevention of recurrent sudden cardiac arrest: Role of provocative electropharmacologic testing. J Am Coll Cardiol 2:418, 1983.
155. Skale, BT, Miles, WM, Heger, JJ, et al: Survivors of cardiac arrest: Prevention of recurrence by drug therapy predicted by electrophysiologic testing or electrophysiologic monitoring. Am J Cardiol 57:113, 1986.
156. Mason, JW and Winkle, RA: Electrode-catheter arrhythmia induction in the selection and assessment of antiarrhythmic drug therapy for recurrent ventricular tachycardia. Circulation 58:971, 1978.
157. Horowitz, LN, Josephson, ME, Fardhidi, A, et al: Recurrent sustained ventricular tachycardia. 3. Role of electrophysiologic study in selection of antiarrhythmic regimens. Circulation 58:986, 1978.
158. Wilber, DJ, Garan, H, Finkelstein, D, et al: Out-of-hospital cardiac arrest: Use of electrophysiologic testing in the prediction of long-term outcome. N Engl J Med 318:19, 1988.
159. Roy, D, Marchand, E, Theroux, P, et al: Long-term reproducibility and significance of provokable ventricular arrhythmias after myocardial infarction. J Am Coll Cardiol 8:32, 1986.
160. Hamer, A, Vohra, J, Hunt, D, et al: Prediction of sudden death by electrophysiologic studies in high risk patients surviving acute myocardial infarction. Am J Cardiol 50:223, 1982.
161. Richards, DA, Cody, DV, Denniss, AR, et al: Ventricular instability: A predictor of death after myocardial infarction. Am J Cardiol 51:75, 1973.
162. Buxton, AE, Marchlinski, FE, Flores, BT, et al: Nonsustained ventricular tachycardia in patients with coronary artery disease: Role of electrophisiologic study. Circulation 75:1178, 1987.
163. Vandepol, CJ, Farshidi, A, Speilman, SR, et al: Incidence and clinical significance of induced ventricular tachycardia. Am J Cardiol 45:725, 1980.
164. Swerdlow, CD, Echt, DS, Soderholm-Difatte, V, et al: Limited value of programmed stimulation in patients with unsustained ventricular tachycardia. Circulation 66(Suppl 2):II145, 1982.
165. Greenberg, RM, Volosin, K, Kmonicek, J, et al: Nonsustained ventricular tachycardia: Role of programmed electrical stimulation. Clin Res 32:171A, 1984.
166. Buxton, AE, Marchlinski, FE, Doherty, JU, et al: Nonsustained ventricular tachycardia: Utility of electrophysiologic study to guide therapy. J Am Coll Cardiol 7:71A, 1986.
167. Zheutlin, TA, Roth, H, Chua, W, et al: Programmed electrical stimulation to determine the need for antiarrhythmic therapy in patients with complex ventricular ectopic activity. Am Heart J 111:860, 1986.
168. Gonska, BD, Bethge, KP, and Kreuzer, H: Programmed ventricular stimulation in coronary artery disease and dilated cardiomyopathy: Influence of the underlying heart disease on the results of electrophysiologic testing. Clin Cardiol 10:294, 1987.
169. Ruskin, JN, McGovern, B, Garan, H, et al: Antiarrhythmic drugs: A possible cause of out-of-hospital cardiac arrest. N Engl J Med 309:1302, 1983.
170. Velebit, V, Podrid, P, Lown, B, et al: Aggravation and provocation of ventricular arrhythmias by antiarrhythmic drugs. Circulation 65:886, 1982.
171. Rinkenberger, RL, Prystowsky, EN, Jackman, WM, et al: Drug conversion of nonsustained ventricular tachycardia to sustained ventricular tachycardia during serial electrophysiologic studies: Identification of drugs that exacerbate tachycardia and potential mechanisms. Am Heart J 103:177, 1982.
172. Rae, AP, Kay, HR, Horowitz, LN, et al: Proarrhythmic effects of antiarrhythmic drugs in patients with malignant ventricular arrhythmias evaluated by electrophysiologic testing. J Am Coll Cardiol 12:131, 1988.
173. Zannad, F, Khalife, AK, and Gilgenkrantz: New drugs for the treatment of ventricular tachycardia. In Aliot, E and Lazzara, R (eds): Ventricular Tachycardia: From Mechanisms to Therapy. Martin Nijhoff Publishers, Durdrecht, 1987.
174. Platia, EV (ed): Management of Cardiac Arrhythmias: The Non Pharmacologic Approach. JB Lippincott, Philadelphia, 1987.
175. Zipes, BP and Rahimtoola, SH (eds): State of the art consensus conference on electrophysiologic testing in the diagnosis and treatment of patients with cardiac arrhythmias. Circulation 75(Suppl III), 1987.
176. Graboys, TB, Lown, B, Podrid, PJ, et al: Long term survival of patients with malignant ventricular arrhythmias treated with antiarrhythmic drugs. Am J Cardiol 50:437, 1982.
177. Vlay, SC, Kalman, CH, and Reid, PR: Prognostic assessment of survivors of ventricular tachycardia and ventricular fibrillation with ambulatory monitoring. Am J Cardiol 3:71, 1984.

178. Mitchell, LB, Duff, HJ, Manyari, DE, et al: A randomized clinical trial of the noninvasive and invasive approaches to drug therapy of ventricular tachycardia. N Engl J Med 317:1681, 1987.
179. Herre, JM, Titus, C, Franz, MR, et al: Inefficacy and proarrhythmia of flecainide and encainide in patients with sustained ventricular tachycardia. Circulation 78 (Suppl II): II61, 1988.
180. Cleland, JDJ, Dargie, HJ, and Ford, I: Mortality in heart failure: Clinical variables of prognostic value. Br Heart J 58:572, 1987.
181. Simonten, CA, Daly, P, Kerieakes, D, et al: Survival in severe congestive heart failure treated with the new nonglycosidic nonsympathomimetic oral inotropic agents. Chest 92:118, 1988.

Commentary

By Melvin D. Cheitlin, M.D.

A major effort in following patients with recognized coronary artery disease is the categorization of these patients into groups at low- and high-risk of dying. However, even high-risk groups contain many patients who will do well and in low-risk groups are those who will not. We have no method that absolutely separates these groups and isolates the high-risk individuals. Among the recognized risk factors predicting future complications are low-ejection fraction, the presence of myocardial ischemia, and the presence of ventricular ectopy, especially those with complex ventricular arrhythmias.

In this chapter Epstein and Scheinman discuss the patient with known coronary artery disease who has asymptomatic, nonsustained, ventricular tachycardia (defined as three or more beats of ventricular tachycardia at a rate of 100 beats per minute or greater, lasting less than 30 seconds).

The study of Schultze and colleagues[1] as well as a study from San Francisco General Hospital by Remedios and Rapaport[2] showed that sudden death in patients after myocardial infarction requires both the substrate of poor left ventricular function as well as the trigger of Lown grade III to V ventricular arrhythmias.

In addressing the question of the need for antiarrhythmic therapy for ventricular ectopy in patients with coronary artery disease, the broad experience we have with noninvasive risk stratification must be considered. In most studies we find it possible to divide the population into high- and low-risk categories based solely on the knowledge of ventricular function and the presence or absence of myocardial ischemia. The high-risk group are those in whom residual myocardial function would be severely impaired if another event occurred. Patients with good left ventricular function and minimal or no myocardial ischemia have an excellent prognosis. This ability to define low- and high-risk groups exists even in the absence of any knowledge of the presence or absence of nonsustained ventricular tachycardia.

In the Post-Myocardial Infarction Multihospital Study, the four factors having independent contribution to risk were (1) a history of symptoms before the myocardial infarction, (2) a history of more than bibasilar rales during the infarction, (3) a left ventricular ejection fraction less than 40 percent, and (4) PVCs greater than 10 per hour. In over two thirds of the patients, zero or only one of these factors was present and the mortality was quite low, with one of the factors about 1.5 percent per year, and with two of the factors 2 to 4 percent per year. In a study by Defeyter and colleagues[3] the ability to walk 10 minutes on the treadmill or into stage IV of the Bruce protocol predicted good left ventricular function and little myocardial ischemia. Follow-up in such patients was associated over the next two years with no deaths and only one myocardial infarction, and this predictive accuracy was present not only in the absence of knowledge concerning ventricular arrhythmias but even of knowledge of ST segment response to the exercise. In these patients it is difficult to conceive how there could have been a meaningful contribution to risk stratification by an ambulatory electrocardiogram (ECG), signal-averaged ECG, or even an electrophysiologic study.

Because the literature suggests a higher risk of sudden death in coronary disease patients with complex ectopy, especially ventricular tachycardia, the question of the value of antiarrhythmic therapy is frequently raised in the asymptomatic patient. Antiarrhythmic drugs are frequently prescribed according to the local practice or in an effort to do something that might prevent a sudden death. The proarrhythmic effects of the antiarrhythmic agents plus the side effects and the cost of prolonged therapy must be considered; it is important, therefore, to confine treatment to only those patients most likely to benefit from the antiarrhythmic drugs.

I agree in general with the algorithm set forth by the authors in determining the need for antiarrhythmic therapy. I would add, however, that in patients with known coronary artery disease who have evidence of myocardial ischemia by treadmill testing or dipyridamole thallium perfusion scanning, especially with multiple areas of redistribution on low rate of myocardial oxygen demand, coronary arteriography is necessary even if the patient is asymptomatic. This is in view of the fact that there are anatomic findings such as left main coronary artery disease or situations in which large areas of myocardium are dependent upon flow past a high-grade proximal obstruction or three-vessel disease with reduced left ventricular function, which might be sufficient indications for coronary revascularization.

I would also assert that a problem exists in the algorithm in the insertion of signal-averaged electrocardiography as a means of risk stratification. Inasmuch as the absence of signal-averaged after-potentials identifies patients at low risk of sudden ventricular tachycardia and the presence of signal-averaged after-potentials does not necessarily indicate a patient at extremely high risk, I find little justification for recommending this procedure, especially inasmuch as the availability for obtaining this information is not accessible to the average practitioner. Furthermore, as Epstein and Scheinman admit, the exact features of the after-potentials such as duration, amplitude, and frequency that indicate the likelihood of late development of ventricular tachycardia are not well established. Until studies are done that prove the added value of the new technology above and beyond that which we already can do without it, by looking for the presence of ischemia and evaluating left ventricular function, patients without ischemia and with good left ventricular function probably should not be treated for the presence of runs of nonsustained ventricular tachycardia. The recent experience in the CAST study—a randomized, double-blind, placebo-controlled study evaluating encainide and flecainide in patients after myocardial infarction with decreased ventricular function and ventricular arrhythmias—is instructive.[4] This study was prematurely terminated because of increased mortality in the treated groups.

The goal of identifying patients at very high risk is still important. Efforts to this end of the kind typified by signal-averaged detection of after-potentials is useful and must be continued in order to find their proper place in risk stratification.

REFERENCES

1. Schultze, RA, Jr, Strauss, HW, Pitt, B: Sudden death in the year following myocardial infarction: Relation to ventricular premature contractions in the late-hospital phase and left-ventricular ejection fraction. Am J Med 62:192, 1977.
2. Rapaport E, Remedios P: The high risk patient after recovery from myocardial infarction: Recognition and management. J Am Coll Cardiol 1:391, 1983.
3. Defeyter, PJ, VanEenke, MJ, Dighton, DH, et al: Prognostic value of exercise testing, coronary angiograph, and left ventriculography six to eight weeks after myocardial infarction. Circulation 66:527, 1982.
4. The Cardiac Arrythmia Suppression Trial (CAST) Investigators: Preliminary report: Effect of encanide and flecanide on mortality in a randomized trial of arrhythmia suppression after myocardial infarction. N Engl J Med 321:406, 1989.

CHAPTER 6

Should Patients with Large Anterior Wall Myocardial Infarction Have Echocardiography to Identify Left Ventricular Thrombus and Should They Be Anticoagulated?

Michael D. Ezekowitz, M.D.,Ph.D.
Michael A. Azrin, M.D.

With the demonstration of reliable techniques for the identification of left ventricular thrombi,[1-9] important questions have emerged concerning the potential value of these tests for defining which patient groups are at high risk for embolization and which patients should receive treatment. This chapter will critically review each technique and attempt to define a rational approach to therapy of left ventricular thrombi in the setting of an acute myocardial infarction.

TECHNIQUES FOR DIAGNOSIS OF LEFT VENTRICULAR THROMBI

ECHOCARDIOGRAPHY

It is generally agreed that echocardiography is the technique of choice for the diagnosis of left ventricular clot. It is the least expensive of the available imaging techniques and the most widely available, and it is totally noninvasive and without known danger. Most contemporary two-dimensional echocardiographic instruments are compact and portable, and thus studies can be performed at the patient's bedside in the intensive care unit. Echocardiography also provides important additional information in patients with myocardial infarction. The consensus among

*With support from NIH #1 R01 HL39467-01 and 5 R01 HL39467-02 and VA Merit Review Grant.

investigators is that whereas echocardiography in most cases is superfluous for the diagnosis of acute infarction,[10] it often provides important prognostic information. Several studies have shown an important relationship between the degree of acute left ventricular dysfunction and serious complications such as death, shock, heart failure, and arrhythmias.[11-14] It has been shown that patients with detectable anatomic impairment have four to five times higher risk for major in-hospital complications.[12,13] This functional information is obtainable by a skilled echocardiographer in a few minutes. A baseline study also serves as a frame of reference for specific complications that may occur during the course of hospitalization. In association with Doppler, the detection of mechanical complications such as ventricular septal defect, papillary muscle rupture or dysfunction, myocardial expansion, aneurysm formation and pseudoaneurysm formation, as well as the evaluation of right ventricular infarction, are all possible. In this era of aggressive management of the early infarction with thrombolytic therapy, angioplasty, and even surgery, serial two-dimensional echocardiography is capable of documenting the effects of successful coronary reperfusion and monitoring the recovery of function.

The amount of clinically useful information derived from echocardiography depends almost entirely on the skill of the technologist, the quality of the equipment, and the nature of the population being studied.[15-18] It is widely accepted that it is not possible to obtain satisfactory studies in all cases. However, a skilled operator should obtain adequate images about 80 percent of the time.[9]

Accuracy of Echocardiography

Over the past decade, important studies have defined the accuracy of this technique in identifying thrombi in the left ventricle of the heart. Early studies that were performed using M-mode echocardiography were neither sensitive nor specific for identifying left ventricular thrombus because it is seldom possible to examine the cardiac apex where over 90 percent of the thrombi occur.[15-18] The modality of choice, therefore, is two-dimensional echocardiography. It offers spatial resolution, enabling examination of the apex of the heart in most patients from either the apical or subxyphoid transducer positions. To distinguish thrombus from artifact, it is important to use strict criteria for thrombus diagnosis.[9] The thrombus should (1) be adjacent to (but distinct from) abnormally contracting myocardium, (2) be seen in at least two transducer positions, and (3) be distinguished by a clear thrombus-blood interface. The interior of the thrombus may vary from being highly echogenic to being relatively echo-free if it is homogeneous. The spatial characteristics of the thrombus may be classified as mural, protuberant, or highly mobile.[19-21] The accuracy of two-dimensional echocardiography in diagnosing thrombus has been assessed in five studies (Table 6–1). In one of the largest prospective studies, Visser and coworkers[22] in 1983 found that echocardiography carried a sensitivity of 92 percent and a specificity of 88 percent in 67 patients, of whom 51 underwent left ventricular aneurysmectomy, and an additional 16 patients were studied at autopsy after dying during the acute phase of infarction. In a second study by Ezekowitz and associates,[9] in 53 patients studied prospectively prior to surgery (n = 50) or death (n = 3), the sensitivity and specificity of echocardiography were 77 percent and 93 percent, respectively. In a third study by Stratton and colleagues[23] in which aneurysmectomy and platelet scintigraphy were used as the reference standard, the sensitivity was 95 percent and the specificity 86 percent for 78 patients; and in a fourth study by Starling and associates[24] which included 21 patients undergoing

Table 6–1. Accuracy of Echocardiography for the
Diagnosis of Left Ventricular Thrombus

		Sensitivity	Specificity	Validation
Ezekowitz	('82)	10/13 = 77%	26/27 = 96%	Surgery
Stratton	('82)	21/22 = 95%	48/56 = 86%	Surgery/autopsy/platelet scan
Visser	('83)	24/26 = 92%	36/41 = 88%	Surgery/autopsy
Starling	('83)	10/13 = 77%	8/8 = 100%	Surgery/autopsy
Sheiban	('87)	14/14 = 100%	57/59 = 97%	Surgery

Sensitivity = true positive/(true positive + false negative)
Specificity = true negative/(true negative + false positive)

echocardiography prior to aneurysmectomy, a sensitivity of 77 percent and a specificity of 100 percent were found. More recently, Sheiban and coworkers[25] reported a sensitivity of 100 percent (14 of 14) and a specificity of 97 percent (57 of 59) in a series of 77 patients with surgical validation. The four earlier studies were performed almost five years ago. As reflected in Sheiban's study, the technology of echocardiography has improved significantly. In addition, color Doppler promises to provide additional information[26] by demonstrating flow patterns that might further predict the development of thrombi or emboli. Thus for the vast majority of patients, echocardiography is a very accurate technique for the identification of left ventricular thrombus.

The Optimal Timing for Imaging

The optimal timing for echocardiography in acute myocardial infarction depends not only on when thrombi can be visualized but also on when emboli occur and on the expected effect of therapy. It has long been recognized that most mural thrombi occur very early after myocardial infarction [5,27,29–31] (Fig. 6–1). Asinger and coworkers[5] found that thrombi occurred a mean of 5 ± 3 days after the acute event. Guerct and associates[28] found, in a series of 21 patients with thrombi, that the thrombi occurred 4.3 ± 3 days after the acute event, with 10 seen by the second day and 20 of 21 by the fourth day. Davis and Ireland[29] reported that 23 of 29 patients had thrombi by the third day after acute infarction, and Spirito and colleagues[30] established that approximately half of their patients had thrombi before 48 hours. In a recent study by Domenicucci and coworkers[31] in which serial echocardiography was performed following acute myocardial infarction on 59 patients who were not receiving anticoagulants, thrombi developed 12 ± 47 days after infarction, with a range of 1 to 362 days. Eighty-three percent of the thrombi were seen in the first week, with 5 percent in the first to second weeks and 12 percent after the second week. Thus most left ventricular clots were seen in the first week after acute myocardial infarction; however, more than 15 percent of patients developed thrombi after the first week. Thus thrombi may be first seen at times much later following infarction than was recognized in earlier studies. It is also important to note that very early studies—that is, within the first 48 to 72 hours after the infarct—may fail to identify thrombi that presumably have not yet formed at this stage. In the study by Asinger and associates[5] only 1 of 12 was seen at less than 72 hours, and, similarly, in 3 other studies,[28–30] only about 50 percent of thrombi were identified by 48 hours. Therefore, evaluation in the first few days after infarction

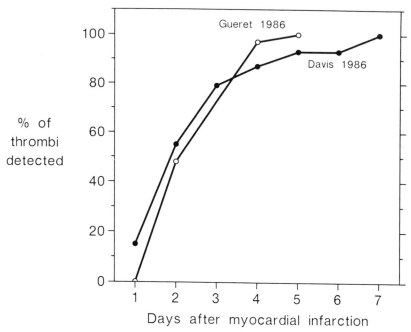

Figure 6-1. This figure depicts two studies defining the time when thrombi were detected by echocardiography after myocardial infarction. A large proportion of thrombi were not detected prior to the second or third day, but at one week nearly all thrombi were visualized. Percent of thrombi detected = number of thrombi detected at a given time/total number of thrombi detected × 100.

will fail to detect a large proportion of thrombi, whereas by the end of the first week, most (though admittedly not all) thrombi can be visualized.

When Do Systemic Emboli Occur Following Acute Myocardial Infarction?

In patients with acute myocardial infarction, the risk of embolization is highest in the first few days and decreases over time, with approximately two thirds of systemic emboli occurring within the first week after the index infarction[19-21,32-42] (Fig. 6-2). In a prospective study, Stratton and Resnick[33] demonstrated that increased embolic risk was not restricted to the immediate postinfarction period but that patients with left ventricular thrombi continue to be at increased risk of embolization as long as 5 years after myocardial infarction, although the risk is less than in the acute period. Thus, the risk of embolization is highest immediately after infarction (emboli may occur as early as the first day) but the presence of thrombus indicates a persistently increased risk in the chronic setting as well.

Stratification of Risks

Because the overall risk of embolization following myocardial infarction is low, it is important to identify subgroups of patients at higher risk of embolization. A number of investigators have identified anterior transmural myocardial infarction as being the major source of intracardiac thrombi and therefore of systemic embolization.[5,8,31,32,42-46] The risk of systemic embolization in patients with inferior myocardial infarction or with subendocardial myocardial infarction is

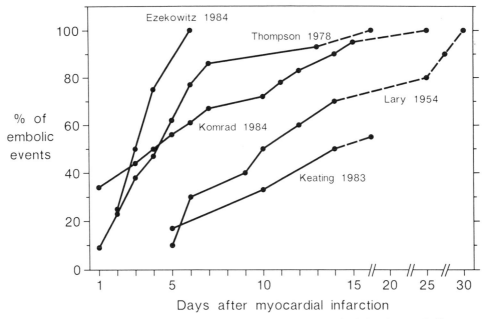

Figure 6–2. This graph defines the embolism rate after acute myocardial infarction. Emboli occur as early as the first day and the risk diminishes after the first week. Percent emboli = number of emobli occurring at a given time/total number of embolic episodes × 100.

small.[5,8,41,42,44,45] Large inferior myocardial infarctions that involve the anteroapical segment should be treated, with regard to intraventricular thrombi and systemic embolization, in the same way as anterior myocardial infarction.

The presence of thrombus indicates a significant risk for subsequent embolization in both the setting of chronic thrombus, as demonstrated by Stratton and Resnick,[33] and in the acute setting, as demonstrated by others.[43,47] In addition, both the morphology and the mobility of the thrombus predict risk for embolization. Several studies have shown a positive correlation between the mobility of the clot, its protuberance into the ventricular cavity, and the risk of subsequent embolization.[19–21,33,46,48] These studies show that the more mobile and protuberant the thrombus, the more likely it is to embolize. An extensive and prospective evaluation of the morphologic characteristics of left ventricular clot by Domenicucci and coworkers[31] demonstrated considerable spontaneous variation in the characteristics of a thrombus at different times and confirmed the observation that had been reported in an earlier case report by Johannessen.[46] Domenicucci and coworkers[31] found that five out of eight mobile thrombi later became nonmobile, whereas 12 originally nonmobile thrombi subsequently became mobile, and 41 percent of thrombi changed from mural to protuberant or vice versa. They also noted that these changes occurred over widely disparate times. Therefore they caution that the analysis of morphologic features of thrombi may have major limitations. Recently, Johannessen and colleagues[48] studied a large group of patients with anterior myocardial infarction and noted that in addition to thrombus mobility and protuberance, patient age (more than 68 years old) was also a significant predictor of subsequent embolization, although this observation is at variance with some previous data.[33]

COMPETING TECHNOLOGY

There are several techniques that compete with echocardiography for accurate diagnosis of intracardiac clot. These are indium-111 (^{111}In) platelet scintigraphy, magnetic resonance imaging, contrast ventriculography, and x-ray tomography.

Platelet Imaging

Working at the Hammersmith Hospital in London, Thakur and associates[49] first chelated ^{111}In with 8-hydroxyquinoline, which permitted the labeling of platelets with an imagable isotope that did not alter the physiologic function of the cells. It was possible, therefore, to inject labeled platelets into patients and theoretically to image hematologically active clot in any location in the body. This technique not only allows identification of thrombus but also reflects its activity.[50,51] In patients with left ventricular aneurysm, this technique has been found to be highly specific, with a figure that approached 100 percent.[9] The sensitivity, however, was lower, that is, 72 percent. This reflects the relative inactivity of clot that is long-standing. Although comparative studies have not been performed in patients with acute infarction, one would anticipate that sensitivity would be higher because of the active formation of clot.

INTERPRETATION OF IMAGES. The interpretation of platelet images is usually decisive. Thrombi are most often represented as a single *hot spot*. Multiple hot spots may be seen, but this is less common. A thrombus may be imaged tangentially, in which case a linear area of increased activity is depicted. Occasionally, in a clot that is laminated against the aneurysm, a doughnut-shape image is seen. In patients with elevated left hemidiaphragms, the spleen may cause difficulty with interpretation of the anterior and right anterior oblique images. The main point of differentiation between splenic activity and thrombus is that the activity related to the spleen characteristically accumulates early, that is, within minutes of injection. Increased activity due to a thrombus tends to be maximal three to four days after injection of the platelet suspension. Occasionally, cardiac myxomas may accumulate platelets on their surface and be mistaken for thrombi.[52] With attention to these caveats, errors in interpretation are unusual.

In a retrospective analysis of 662 images obtained from 64 patients read on two separate occasions by three blinded observers, the intra-observer and inter-observer agreement was 91 percent and 88 percent, respectively.[53] The optimal time for imaging was in the three- to four-day period following the injection of the platelet suspension, and the left anterior oblique projection was the optimal view. For the best diagnostic accuracy, an image obtained on the first day and a second image obtained three or four days later in the left anterior oblique view are usually adequate. In the specific instance of imaging patients during the acute phase of myocardial infarction, multiple imaging views are often used to assist in the localization of the thrombus to a particular chamber because in these patients it is important to distinguish thrombi in the coronary arteries or in the atria from those in the left ventricle.[54–56]

Platelets interact in a dynamic manner at the blood-thrombus interface, and, therefore, platelet scintigraphy might be used as a direct index of thrombus activity. The effect of aspirin on the incorporation of ^{111}In-labeled platelets into cardiac thrombi has been studied.[51,54] Stratton and Ritchie[51] noted that one of six positive platelet scans became negative in patients treated with aspirin and dipyridamole, and that sulfinpyrazone and coumarin adminstration converted three of seven and two of three positive platelet scans, respectively. In another study by Ezekowitz and associates,[54] the *in vitro* and *in vivo* behaviors of platelets were compared in 11 patients with aneurysms and mural thrombi. In all patients, imaging showed that labeled autologous platelets were incorporated into ventricular clot, whether they were treated with aspirin or not. Thus, although *in vitro* platelets from patients on aspirin aggregated abnormally, nevertheless they took part in thrombosis *in vivo*. This study by Ezekowitz and associates suggests a disparity between the *in vivo* behavior of platelets and their *in vitro* function. Thus, antiplatelet drugs may affect the interpretation of platelet scintigraphy in situations specified above.

QUANTIFICATION OF IMAGES. Quantification of intracardiac imaging has met with difficulty. The amount of radioactivity detected depends on the size, shape, and orientation of the object in the area of interest, as well as the distance of the object from the detector and the characteristics of the imaging system itself.[56] Because platelets circulate in the blood, differentiation of circulating platelets from those accumulating on a thrombogenic surface can be difficult because of limitations imposed by inadequate target-to-background ratios and the spatial resolution of most gamma cameras. Attempts to obviate these problems have been made by developing a dual isotope blood pool subtraction technique.[56] This technique assumes that labeled red cells are not taken up by the thrombus, whereas the activity due to the ^{111}In-labeled platelets is found both within the thrombus and the blood. The ratio of activity from technetium 99m- (^{99m}Tc) labeled red cells and ^{111}In-labeled platelets is determined by quantitative imaging of a remote vascular zone by direct analysis of a blood sample. The ratio is used for subtraction of the blood pool from the cardiac images. The indium excess represents the clot. Potential problems with this technique involve nonspecific uptake of red cells by the thrombus, the statistical significance of data derived by subtracting two large numbers with a small difference from each other, and patient movement during acquisition of the images. Stratton[50] recently demonstrated that ^{111}In-platelet scintigraphy is also an excellent predictor of embolic risk and further enhances the stratification of high-risk and low-risk patients and the selection of patients for therapy.

In conclusion, platelet imaging plays a complementary role with echocardiography for detecting thrombi.[9] Echocardiography reflects thrombus mass, whereas platelet scintigraphy reflects the activity on the thrombus surface. In general, echocardiography is a less cumbersome technique, but in those cases in which technical considerations preclude the acquisition of a technically satisfactory echocardiogram, platelet scintigraphy may be useful in identifying clot and directing therapy by predicting the risk of subsequent embolization.

Magnetic Resonance Imaging/X-ray Computed Tomography

State-of-the-art magnetic resonance imaging systems generate high-resolution images of the cardiovascular system. Thus, theoretically it is possible to image thrombi in the left ventricle. Studies have demonstrated the feasibility of this technique in identifying left ventricular masses,[57-61] and this technology is now widely available for clinical use. However, systematic studies during the acute phase of myocardial infarction have not been performed. This is likely due to the fact that the technique is costly and cumbersome and it is not feasible to transport sick patients to the imaging facilities. The same is true for computed tomography, which can accurately identify intraventricular masses or thrombi.[62-67]

Contrast Ventriculography

This technique[6,24,68-71] was the first utilized for the diagnosis of left ventricular clot. In general, it lacks both sensitivity and specificity. It is insensitive because clots are often laminated against the wall of the ventricle and cannot be seen. It is non-specific because thrombi form in large-volume ventricles that are incompletely opacified with contrast material, and, therefore, apparent filling defects due to incomplete mixing often lead to overdiagnosis.

TREATMENT

Treatment options for left ventricular thrombosis and for the prevention of systemic embolization fall into four categories. The first is anticoagulation, which is the most widely employed. Anticoagulation involves a combination of heparin followed by the chronic use of subcutaneous heparin or coumarin. Fibrinolytic agents and antiplatelet agents, as well as surgery, also have been employed.

ANTICOAGULATION

The possibility of preventing the development of mural thrombi in the presence of myocardial infarction by the use of anticoagulants was first suggested by Solandt and associates[72] in 1938. Although the prevention of thrombus formation by anticoagulation has not been consistently demonstrated, there is considerable evidence supporting a role for anticoagulation in the prevention of embolization.[7,8,28,41,42,73,74] Early trials of anticoagulation in a large number of patients with acute myocardial infarction provide the strongest evidence for the prevention of embolic events. In 1948, Wright and coworkers[75] treated 800 patients with acute myocardial infarction with heparin followed by dicumarol to maintain the pro-thrombin time at twice the normal value. They compared this group to an untreated group and found that 3.4 percent in the untreated group had cerebro-vascular accidents, compared with only 1.4 percent in the treated group. There was also a decrease in peripheral embolization from 3 percent in the control group to 1 percent in the treated group. Similar results were found in a British study published in 1969,[76] which showed a reduction in the frequency of clinically evident systemic embolic complications from 3.4 to 1.3 percent among 1427 patients randomized to either 36 hours of heparin administration with phenindione (mean dose 72 mg per day) to maintain the thrombotest at 15 percent or low-dose phenindione (1 mg per day) without heparin. Another study by Harvald and associates[77] published in 1962 further documented a reduction in strokes in a series of 315 patients. One of 45 (1 percent) of those treated with long-term dicumarol and 11 of 170 (6 percent) of those not anticoagulated suffered cerebrovascular accidents. Drapkin and Merskey's[78] study complicated the issue by demonstrating in over 1000 patients that a reduction in the incidence of cerebrovascular accidents was found only in women randomized to heparin and phenindione to maintain the prothrombin time at 2 to 2½ times control, or to placebo (1.5 percent versus 3.9 percent in controls), but not in men (1.5 percent versus 1.8 percent in controls). However, the absolute numbers in each subgroup, which ranged from 4 to 9, were small. In the Veterans Administration (VA) Cooperative Study of 999 patients,[79] there was also a decrease in emboli in patients treated with heparin and then coumarin to maintain the prothrombin time at twice normal, with a reduction of emboli from 3.8 percent in the placebo group to 0.8 percent in the treated group.

In the VA study, anticoagulated patients that went to autopsy had a decreased prevalence of mural thrombi as compared with controls, a finding also noted by Hilden and colleagues,[80] suggesting that the decreased incidence of emboli with anticoagulation might be due in part to a reduced incidence of ventricular clot. More recently, two small studies demonstrated by two-dimensional echocardiography a decreased incidence of left ventricular thrombus with anticoagulant therapy.[43,45] However, there are several other studies[6,8,28,29,41,42,73] in which no significant reduction in thrombus was encountered with anticoagulation. Interestingly, in three of these studies,[8,41,42] in spite of failing to show a reduction in ventricular clot, embolic complications were reduced nevertheless. In the study by Friedman and coworkers,[8] the incidence of left ventricular thrombi in patients who were anticoagulated was 9 of 45 (20 percent) and, similarly, thrombi occurred in 2 of 8 (25 percent) of those who did not receive anticoagulants. Nevertheless there appeared to be a trend toward reduction of emboli, with only one embolic event in the group of 44 anticoagulated patients and one embolic event occurring in one of only five patients not anticoagulated. In the study by Weinreich and associates[41] mural thrombi were noted in 44 of 130 (34 percent) of patients with anterior myocardial infarction. On follow-up of survivors at 6 months, there was no significant difference in the finding of persistent thrombus, with thrombi noted in 11 of 19 (58 percent) of patients receiving anticoagulants and similarly in 6 of 10 (60 percent) of those not receiving anticoagulants (p = NS). Nevertheless, there was a significant difference in embolic complications (p < 0.05), with no emboli in 25 anticoagulated patients and 7 emboli in 18 patients who did not receive anticoagulants. A similar finding was noted by Keating and colleagues.[42] In 54 patients with anterior myocardial infarction, 17 patients had mural thrombi—10 (18 percent) who were receiving anticoagulation and 7 (13 percent) who were not (p = NS). Nevertheless, there were no emboli in the anticoagulated group, but six cases (86 percent) were encountered in the group who were not anticoagulated (p < 0.001). In spite of the absence of a clear-cut effect on thrombi, these studies, in general, support the conclusion that anticoagulation prevents emboli in patients with left ventricular clot.

Stratton and Resnick[33] and Tramarin and associates[44] advanced our understanding by studying patients with chronic left ventricular thrombi, and they found benefit in terms of both emboli and clot using anticoagulation. Tramarin and associates[44] demonstrated the efficacy of long-term therapy with acenocoumarin on the resolution of left ventricular thrombi. In 19 treated patients compared with 19 control patients, there was significant (p < 0.001) improvement in the dimensions of mural thrombi at 15 days, at 3 months, and at 1 year. At the final follow-up evaluation at 1 year, 15 of 17 (88 percent) had resolution of thrombus in the treated group, whereas only 4 of 17 (24 percent) in the untreated group had complete resolution (p < 0.001). Stratton and Resnick[33] studied 85 patients with recent or remote myocardial infarction or cardiomyopathy who were found to have left ventricular thrombi by echocardiography. They noted that the presence of thrombus was associated with an increased risk of emboli, which occurred in 11 of 85 (13 percent) patients with thrombi. There were 11 emboli in 62 patients (18 percent) who received effective anticoagulation, and no emboli in 23 patients who had not been fully anticoagulated (p = 0.04.) These two studies demonstrate the efficacy of long-term anticoagulation both in the resolution of thrombi and in the prevention of emboli.

The timing of anticoagulation may influence the benefit. There is some suggestion that the earlier the anticoagulation is given, the more likely an effect is to be found. An animal study by Solandt and colleagues[72] as well as investigations in humans support this idea. When heparin was given early (4.6 ± 2.5 hours after the myocardial infarction),[46] a decreased incidence of thrombi was encountered, as opposed to slightly later therapy (6.5 ± 3.3 hours and 5.2 ± 4.6 hours after the myocardial infarction) in two other studies in which a decrease was not observed.[29,74] As discussed subsequently, early thrombolytic therapy as opposed to later therapy also resulted in a decreased frequency of thrombi. Although one study[29] demonstrated no difference between intravenous full-dose heparin therapy and lower-dose subcutaneous heparin, therapy was begun relatively late and the number of patients and the incidence of emboli were low, so that conclusions regarding low-dose compared with full-dose heparin are problematic.

THROMBOLYTIC THERAPY

Thrombolytic therapy has become standard therapy in the hyperacute phase of acute myocardial infarction; however, few studies have specifically evaluated the effect of thrombolysis on the formation, resolution, or embolization of ventricular thrombi, and, in addition, results have not been consistent (Table 6–2). In 1985, Stratton and coworkers[81] compared 45 patients treated with streptokinase for acute myocardial infarction with 38 concurrent controls receiving heparin. Only four patients had left ventricular thrombi on serial echocardiography, and all occurred in the streptokinase-treated group. Although this difference does not reach statistical significance, it does suggest that thrombolysis did not reduce the incidence of left ventricular thrombi; in fact, there was an increase, though not statistically significant. Sharma and associates[82] reported a 27 percent incidence of left ventricular thrombi after intracoronary streptokinase, and therefore they similarly concluded that thrombolysis did not reduce the incidence, although their study lacked a control group. Most recently, Held and coworkers[83] failed to find a statistically significant decrease in the incidence of left ventricular thrombi after lysis therapy with either tissue plasminogen activator or streptokinase (Thrombolysis in Myocardial Infarction Study), although there was a trend toward reduction, especially with streptokinase.[84] On the other hand, Eigler and associates[85] in one of the earliest studies, and Natarajan and coworkers[86] in a recent larger series of 40 patients with anterior myocardial infarction, did find statistically significant decrements in the incidence of left ventricular thrombi in patients treated early with thrombolytic therapy. In addition, Keren and colleagues[87] and Kremer and associates[88] have demonstrated efficacy in lysis of ventricular thrombi present in the postinfarction period.

The multiple effects of thrombolysis on mural thrombi may include prevention of thrombus formation, decreased infarct size with less substrate for thrombus formation, improved wall motion and ejection fraction, and lysis of preexisting thrombus. There is also the theoretic possibility, supported by isolated experimental observations (personal communication Funke-Kupper), that embolization may actually result from and occur during thrombolytic therapy, particularly in patients receiving thrombolytic therapy for a second myocardial infarction with a history of prior anterior myocardial infarction and preexisting thrombi. In large series of

Table 6–2. Thrombolytic Therapy and Left Ventricular Thrombus

Study	Anterior MI	Incidence of LVT		p Value	Therapy Treated
		Treated	Controls		
Eigler (1985)	22	(1) 1/12 = 8%	7/10 = 70%	p < .005	*Streptokinase 750,000 U < 3 hr after MI, then full anticoagulation with adjusted dose intravenous heparin, then Coumadin.
Stratton (1985)	29	(2) 5/19 = 26%	0/10 = 0%	p = NS	†IC streptokinase 1000 U/min up to 300,000 units, total 4.7 ± 2.5 hr after MI, then full anticoagulation with adjusted dose intravenous heparin, followed by Coumadin.
Sharma (1985)	30	(3) 8/30 = 27%	No controls		‡IC streptokinase 10,000 (1985) U/min up to 750,000 units 3.7 ± 2.0 hr after MI, then full anticoagulation with intravenous heparin.
Natarajan (1988)	40	(4) 0/22 = 0%	8/18 = 44%	p<.05	*Streptokinase 750,000 U < 6 hr after MI, then full anticoagulation with adjusted dose intravenous heparin for 3–4 days, followed by unspecified antiplatelet therapy.
Held (1988)	43	(5) 1/92 = 11%	6/14 = 43%	NS	§Streptokinase 1,500,000 U <7 hr after MI, then full anticoagulation with adjusted dose intravenous heparin
		(5) 7/20 = 35%	6/14 = 43%	NS	§t-PA, 80 mg over 3 hr, <7 hr after MI, then full anticoagulation with adjusted dose intravenous heparin.

Anterior MI = number of patients in the study with anterior myocardial infarction, LVT = left ventricular thrombus as determined echocardiographically, IC streptokinase = intracoronary streptokinase, t-PA = tissue plasminogen activator.

*Controls received no anticoagulation.

†Controls received adjusted dose heparin followed by oral Coumadin.

‡No control group.

§Controls received heparin 5000 U subcutaneously bid.

(1) Echocardiography performed <36 hours and 9 ± 2 days after infarction. (2) Echocardiogram performed at 8 ± 3 weeks after infarction. (3) Echocardiography performed <24 hr and 10 days after infarction. (4) Echocardiography performed at 8–10 days after infarction. (5) Echocardiography performed at 48–72 hrs.

patients receiving thrombolytic therapy, alterations in the incidence of strokes have been outweighed by the beneficial effects on mortality.[89] Thus, in the absence of consistent and strong evidence, the use of thrombolytic therapy specifically for ventricular thrombi remains experimental. In the setting of an acute myocardial infarction, thrombolytic therapy usage is indicated primarily for myocardial preservation, not thrombus prevention. Because of the danger of inducing an embolus, it may be contraindicating in situations in which a thrombus is demonstrated.

Thrombectomy/Aneurysmectomy/Infarctectomy

Whereas aneurysmectomy is indicated for recurrent thromboembolism,[90] surgical removal of thrombus in the setting of acute myocardial infarction has been undertaken only rarely.[91,92] As already discussed, the incidence of emboli is highest soon after infarction. This is also a period of high operative risk, and aneurysm resection is difficult and inexact because of the lack of definite margins or scar early after infarction. Nevertheless, if a subgroup of patients can be identified who are at sufficiently high risk of embolization and in whom operative removal poses less risk, surgery may be considered. However, this approach will require improved predictive capabilities. Therefore, surgery for this indication remains experimental.

Antiplatelet Drugs

Antiplatelet drugs have not been studied systematically. Whereas Ezekowitz and colleagues[54] demonstrated the lack of effect of aspirin on platelet scintigraphy, Stratton and Ritchie[51] found that platelet deposition as measured by ^{111}In-labeled platelets was inhibited by sulfinpyrazone as well as by aspirin and Persantine given together. Thrombus size by echocardiography was not significantly affected, however. Thus, although antiplatelet therapy may alter platelet activity or uptake by thrombus, there is no evidence of a clinically important effect.

CONCLUSION

The frequency of systemic emboli after myocardial infarction is only a few percent.[34,75–78] However, the reported incidence of emboli is markedly increased in certain subgroups. In patients with anterior myocardial infarctions, approximately one third will exhibit left ventricular thrombi.[5,8,21,22,31,42,44,48] The reported incidence of emboli in patients with detected left ventricular thrombus varies widely; in patients not treated with anticoagulants, the incidence varies from only a few percent in one large study[30] to 27 percent in another large study, and as high as 86 percent.[42] Improved selection of patients at risk may be enhanced by the finding of thrombus protrusion, thrombus mobility, positive platelet scintigraphy, advanced age, or Doppler evidence of low flow adjacent to poorly contracting myocardium. The best data to support the use of anticoagulation in acute infarction are found in the older literature. More recent studies have not been completely consistent but support the beneficial effect of anticoagulation. The role of thrombolytic agents is in the process of evolution. In the acute setting the importance of myocardial salvage overshadows consideration of embolic risk. The role of delayed thrombolysis, for example, for high-risk mobile thrombi has not been clarified and remains experimental. Antiplatelet agents have not been demonstrated to be useful. Surgery has been undertaken only rarely. Thrombectomy remains primarily an incidental procedure during surgery for other indications. The standard of therapy, therefore, remains full anticoagulation. There is evidence to guide the optimal timing of therapy. The occurrence of emboli early after infarction in concert with the delayed visualization of thrombi suggests that anticoagulation should be undertaken as soon as the risk of embolization is recognized, unless contraindications exist, and should not await visualization of thrombus (e.g., in all patients with anterior transmural myocardial infarction).

The optimal timing of echocardiography depends upon the peak occurrence of thrombus formation and the most cost-effective time to perform the study. In the case of anterior infarction, echocardiography is not necessary prior to starting anticoagulation. In the case of inferior infarction, involvement of the apex may confer similar risk and echocardiography is indicated to delineate apical involvement. The subsequent decisions after initial anticoagulation are less concrete. A reasonable approach would be to perform echocardiography after the first week— a time point that should detect 85 percent or more of thrombi and that also is a convenient time to start coumarin. If thrombus is present, then continued anticoagulation is indicated. The data from Stratton and Resnick[33] indicate that there is continued, albeit reduced, risk with chronic thrombi, and the benefit of long-term anticoagulation must be weighed against the bleeding risk. In patients without thrombus, anticoagulation may reasonably be discontinued. However, the late appearance of thrombi in longitudinal studies and the possibility that thrombus which had been prevented will develop on discontinuation of heparin suggest that a follow-up echocardiogram should be performed.

Echocardiography remains the imaging technique of choice. Alternative methods of imaging thrombi include platelet scintigraphy, magnetic resonance imaging, and computerized tomography—all of which may play a complementary role in cases with inadequate echocardiographic images.

ACKNOWLEDGMENT

The authors gratefully acknowledge the secretarial assistance of Paulette Trent.

REFERENCES

1. Ports, TA, Cogan, J, Schiller, NB, et al: Echocardiography of left ventricular masses. Circulation 58:528, 1978.
2. DeMaria, AN, Bommer, W, Neumann, A, et al: Left ventricular thrombi identified by cross-sectional echocardiography. Ann Intern Med 90:14, 1978.
3. Meltzer, RS, Guthaner, D, Rakowski, M, et al: Diagnosis of left ventricular thrombi by two-dimensional echocardiography. Br Heart J 42:261, 1979.
4. Come, PC, Mankis, JE, Vine, HS, et al: Echocardiographic diagnosis of left ventricular thombus. Am Heart J 100:523, 1980.
5. Asinger, RW, Mikell, FL, Elsperger, J, et al: Incidence of left ventricular thrombosis after acute transumural myocardial infarction: Serial evaluation by two-dimensional echocardiography. N Engl J Med 305:297, 1981.
6. Reeder, GS, Tajik, AJ, and Seward, JB: Left ventricular mural thrombus: Two dimensional echocardiographic diagnosis. Mayo Clin Proc 56:82, 1981.
7. Stratton, JR, Ritchie, JL, Hamilton, GW, et al: Left ventricular thombi: In vivo detection by indium-111 platelet imaging and two dimensional echocardiography. Am J Cardiol 47:874, 1981.
8. Friedman, MJ, Carlson, K, Marcus, FI, et al: Clinical correlations in patients with acute myocardial infarction and left ventricular thrombus detected by two-dimensional echocardiography. Am J Med 72:894, 1982.
9. Ezekowitz, MD, Wilson, DA, Smith, EO, et al: Comparison of indium-111 platelet scintigraphy and two-dimensional echocardiography in the diagnosis of left ventricular thrombi. N Engl J Med 306:1509, 1982.
10. Kloner, RA and Parisi, AS: Acute myocardial infarction: Diagnostic and prognostic applications of two-dimensional echocardiography. Circulation 75(3):521, 1987.
11. Horowitz, RS, Morganroth, J, Parrotto, C, et al: Immediate diagnosis of acute myocardial infarction by two dimensional echocardiography. Circulation 65:323, 1982.

12. Gibson, RS, Bishop, HL, Stamm, RB, et al: Value of early two dimensional echocardiography in patients with acute myocardial infarction. Am J Cardiol 49:1110, 1982.
13. Nishimura, RA, Tajik, AJ, Shub, C, et al: Role of two-dimensional echocardiography in the prediction of in-hospital complications after myocardial infarction. J Am Coll Cardiol 4:1080, 1984.
14. Horowitz, RS and Morganroth, J: Immediate detection of early high risk patients with acute myocardial infarction using two-dimensional echocardiographic evaluation of left ventricular regional wall motion abnormalities. Am Heart J 103:814, 1982.
15. Horgan, JH, O'M Shiel, F, and Goodman, AC: Demonstration of left ventricular thrombus by conventional echocardiography. J Clin Ultrasound 4:287, 1976.
16. Kramer, NE, Rathod, R, Chawla, KK, et al: Echocardiographic diagnosis of left ventricular mural thrombi occurring in cardiomyopathy. Am Heart J 96:381, 1978.
17. DeJoseph, RL, Shiroff, FA, Levenson, LW, et al: Echocardiograpic diagnosis of intraventricular clot. Chest 71:417, 1977.
18. van den Bos, AA, Bletter, WB, and Hagemeijer, F: Progressive development of a left ventricular thrombus: Detection and evolution studied with echocardiographic techniques. Chest 74:307, 1978.
19. Meltzer, RS, Visser, CA, Kan, G, et al: Two-dimensional echocardiographic appearance of left ventricular thombi with systemic emboli after myocardial infarction. Am J Cardiol 53:1511, 1984.
20. Haugland, JM, Asinger, RW, Mikell, FL, et al: Embolic potential of left ventricular thrombi detected by two-dimensional echocardiography. Circulation 70:588, 1984.
21. Visser, CA, Kan, G, Meltzer, RS, et al: Embolic potential of left ventricular thrombus after myocardial infarction: A two dimensional echocardiographic study of 119 patients. J Am Coll Cardiol 5:1276, 1985.
22. Visser, CA, et al: Two-dimensional echocardiography in the diagnosis of left ventricular thrombus. Chest 83:228, 1983.
23. Stratton, JR, Lighty, GW, Pearlman, AS, et al: Detection of left ventricular thrombus by two dimensional echocardiography: Sensitivity, specificity, and causes of uncertainty. Circulation 66:156, 1982.
24. Starling, MR, Crawford, MM, Sorenson, SG, et al: Comparative value of invasive and noninvasive techniques for identifying left ventricular mural thrombi. Am Heart J 106:1143, 1983.
25. Sheiban, I, Casarotto, D, Trevi, G, et al: Two dimensional echocardiography in the diagnosis of intracardiac masses: A prospective study with anatomic validation. Cardiovasc Intervent Radiol 10:157, 1987.
26. Maze, SS, Kotler, MA, and Pavy, WR: The contribution of color Doppler flow imaging to the assessment of left ventricular thrombus. Am Heart J 115:479, 1988.
27. Jordan, RA, Miller, RD, Edwards, JE, et al: Thromboembolism in acute and in healed myocardial infarction. I. Intracardiac mural thrombosis. Circulation 6:1, 1952.
28. Gueret, P, Duborg, O, Ferrier, A, et al: Effects of full-dose heparin anticoagulation on the development of left ventricular thrombosis in acute transmural myocardial infarction. J Am Coll Cardiol 8:419, 1986.
29. Davis, MJE and Ireland, MA: Effect of early anticoagulation on the frequency of left ventricular thrombi after anterior wall acute myocardial infarction. Am J Cardiol 57:1244, 1986.
30. Spirito, P, Bellotti, P, Chiarella, F, et al: Prognostic significance and natural history of left ventricular thrombi in patients with acute anterior myocardial infarction: A 2D echocardiographic study. Circulation 72:774, 1985.
31. Domenicucci, S, Bellotti, P, Chiarella, F, et al: Spontaneous morphologic changes in left ventricular thrombi: A prospective two-dimensional echocardiographic study. Circulation 75:737, 1987.
32. Komrad, MS, Coffey, CE, Coffey, KS, et al: Myocardial infarction and stroke. Neurology 34:1403, 1984.
33. Stratton, JR and Resnick, AD: Increased emboli risk in patients with left ventricular thrombi. Circulation 75:1004, 1987.
34. Drapkin, A and Merskey, C: Anticoagulant therapy after acute myocardial infarction: Relation of therapeutic benefit to patient's age, sex, and severity of infarction. JAMA 222:541, 1972.
35. Resnekov, L, Chediak, J, Hirsh, J, et al: Antithrombotic agents in coronary artery disease. Chest 89:54S, 1986.
36. Thompson, JE, Weston, AS, Signler, L, et al: Arterial embolectomy after myocardial infarction: A study of 31 patients. Ann Surg 171:979, 1970.
37. Darling, RC, Austen, G, and Linton, RR: Arterial embolism. Surg Gynecol Obstet 124:106, 1967.
38. Lary, BG and de Takats, G: Peripheral arterial embolism after myocardial infarction: Occurrence in unsuspected cases and ambulatory patients. JAMA 155:10, 1954.

39. Thompson, PL and Robinson, JS: Stroke after myocardial infarction: Relation to infarct size. Br Med J 2:457, 1978.
40. Bean, WB: Infarction of the heart. III. Clinical course and morphological findings. Ann Intern Med 12:71, 1938.
41. Weinreich, DJ, Burke, JF, and Pauletto, FJ: Left ventricular mural thombi complicating acute myocardial infarction: Long-term follow-up with serial echocardiography. Ann Intern Med 100:789, 1984.
42. Keating, EC, Gross, SA, Schlamowitz, RA, et al: Mural thrombi in myocardial infarctions: Prospective evaluation by two-dimensional echocardiography. Am J Med 74:989, 1983.
43. Johannessen, KA, Nordrehaug, JE, and Lippe, G: Left ventricular thombosis and cerebrovascular accident in acute myocardial infarction. Br Heart J 51:553, 1984.
44. Tramarin, R, Pozzoli, M, Feko, O, et al: Two-dimensional echocardiographic assessment of anticoagulant therapy in left ventricular thrombosis early after myocardial infarction. Eur Heart J 7:482, 1986.
45. Nordrehaug, JE, Johannessen, K, and von der Lippe, G: Usefulness of high-dose anticoagulants in preventing left ventricular thrombus in acute myocardial infarction. Am J Cardiol 55:1491, 1985.
46. Johannessen, K: Peripheral emboli from left ventricular thrombi of different echocardiographic appearance in acute myocardial infarction. Arch Intern Med 147:641, 1987.
47. Kinney, EL: The significance of left ventricular thrombi in patients with coronary heart disease: A retrospective analysis of pooled data. Am Heart J 109:191, 1985.
48. Johannessen, KA, Nordrehaug, JE, von der Lippe, G, et al: Risk factors for embolization in patients with left ventricular thrombi and acute myocardial infarction. Br Heart J 60:104, 1988.
49. Thakur, ML, Welch, MJ, Joist, JM, et al: Indium-111 labeled platelets: Studies on the preparation and evaluation of in vitro and in vivo functions. Thromb Res 9:345, 1976.
50. Stratton, JR: Indium-111 platelet imaging of left ventricular thrombi: Predictive value for systemic emboli. Presented at the International Meeting: Left Ventricular Thrombosis after Myocardial Infarction. Genoa, Italy, October 21, 1988.
51. Stratton, JR and Ritchie, JL: The effects of antithrombotic drugs in patients with left ventricular thrombi: Assessment with indium-111 platelet imaging and two-dimensional echocardiography. Circulation 69:561, 1984.
52. Ezekowitz, MD, Smith, EO, Rankin, R, et al: Left atrial mass: Diagnostic value of transesophageal two-dimensional echocardiography and indium-111 platelet scintigraphy. Am J Cardiol 51:1563, 1983.
53. Ezekowitz, MD, Smith, EO, and Streitz, TM: Identifying patients at risk for systemic emboli during the hospital phase of acute myocardial infarction—study using indium-11 labeled platelets. J Am Coll Cardiol 1:648, 1983 (abstr).
54. Ezekowitz, MD, Smith, EO, Cox, AC, et al: Failure of aspirin to prevent incorporation of indium 111 labeled platelets into cardiac thrombi in man. Lancet 1:440, 1981.
55. Powers, WJ and Siegel, BA: Thrombus imaging with indium-111 platelets. Seminars in Thrombosis and Hemostasis 9:115, 1983.
56. Bergman, SR, Lerch, RA, Mathias, CJ, et al: Noninvasive detection of coronary thrombi with indium-111 platelets: Concise communication. J Nucl Med 24:130, 1983.
57. Choyke, PL, Kressel, HY, Reichek, N, et al: Nongated cardiac magnetic resonance imaging: Preliminary experiences at 0.12 T. AJR 143:1143, 1984.
58. Higgins, CB, Lanzer, P, Stark, D, et al: Imaging by nuclear magnetic resonance in patients with chronic ischemic heart disease. Circulation 69:523, 1984.
59. Dooms, GC and Higgins, CB: MR Imaging of cardiac thrombi. J Comput Assist Tomogr 10:415, 1986.
60. Gomes, AS, Lois, JF, Child, JS, et al: Cardiac tumors and thrombus: Evaluation with MR imaging. AJR 149:895, 1987.
61. Council on Scientific Affairs: Magnetic resonance imaging of the cardiovascular system. Present state of the art and future potential. JAMA 259: 253, 1988.
62. Tomoda, H, Hoshai, M, Furuya, M, et al: Evaluation of left ventricular thrombus with computed tomography. Am J Cardiol 48:573, 1981.
63. Goldstein, JA, Schiller, NB, Lipton, MJ, et al: Evaluation of left ventricular thrombi by contrast enhanced computed tomography and two-dimensional echocardiography. Am J Cardiol 57:757, 1986.
64. Nair, CK, Sketch, MM, Mahoney, PD, et al: Detection of left ventricular thrombi by computerized tomography: A preliminary report. Br Heart J 45:535, 1981.

65. Goodwin, JD, Herykens, RJ, Skoldebrand, CG, et al: Detection of intraventricular thrombi by computed tomography. Radiology 138:717, 1981.
66. Tomora, H, Hoshia, M, Furuya, H, et al: Evaluation of intracardiac thrombus with computed tomography. Am J Cardiol 51:843, 1983.
67. Foster, CJ, Sekiya, T, Love, MG, et al: Identification of intracardiac thrombus: Comparison of computed tomography and cross sectional echocardiography. Br J Radiol 60:327, 1987.
68. Swan, HJC: Aneurysm of the cardiac ventricle: Its management by medical and surgical intervention. West J Med 129:26, 1978.
69. Raphael, MJ, Steiner, RC, Goodwin, JF, et al: Cineangiography of left ventricular aneurysm. Clin Radiol 23:129, 1972.
70. Cooley, DA: Surgical treatment of left ventricular aneurysm: Experience with excision of post infarction lesions in 80 patients. Prog Cardiovasc Dis 11:222, 1968.
71. Takamato, T, Kim, D, Uric, PM, et al: Comparative recognition of left ventricle thrombi by echocardiography and cineangiography. Br Heart J 53:36, 1985.
72. Solandt, DY, Nassim, R, and Best, CM: Production and prevention of cardiac mural thrombosis in dogs. Lancet 2:592, 1938.
73. Arvan, S: Mural thrombi in coronary artery disease: Recent advances in pathogenesis, diagnosis, and approaches to treatment. Arch Intern Med 144:113, 1984.
74. Simpson, MT, Oberman, A, Kouchoukos, NT, et al: Prevalence of mural thrombi and systemic embolization with left ventricular aneurysm: Effect of anticoagulation therapy. Chest 77:463, 1980.
75. Wright, IS, Marple, CD, and Beck, DF: Anticoagulant therapy of coronary thrombosis with myocardial infarction. JAMA 138:1074, 1948.
76. Arnott, WM, et al: Assessment of short-term anticoagulant administration after cardiac infarction. Br Med J 1:335, 1969.
77. Harvald, B, Hilden, T, and Lund, E: Long-term anticoagulant therapy after myocardial infarction. Lancet 2:626, 1962.
78. Drapkin, A and Merskey, C: Anticoagulant therapy after acute myocardial infarction: Relation of therapeutic benefit to patient's age, sex, and severity of infarction. JAMA 222:541, 1972.
79. VA Hospital Investigators: Anticoagulants in acute myocardial infarction. JAMA 225:724, 1973.
80. Hilden, T, Iversen, K, Raaschan, F, et al: Anticoagulation in acute myocardial infarction. Lancet 2:327, 1961.
81. Stratton, JR, Speck, SM, Caldwell, JM, et al: Late effects of intracoronary streptokinase on regional wall motion, ventricular aneurysm and left ventricular thrombus in myocardial infarction: Results from the western Washington randomized trial. J Am Coll Cardiol 5:1023, 1985.
82. Sharma, B, Carvalho, A, Wyeth, R, et al: Left ventricular thrombi diagnosed by echo in patients with acute myocardial infarction treated with intracoronary streptokinase followed by intravenous heparin. Am J Cardiol 56:422, 1985.
83. Held, AC, Gore, JM, Parasko, J, et al: Impact of thrombolytic therapy on left ventricular mural thrombi in acute myocardial infarction. Am J Cardiol 62:310, 1988.
84. The TIMI Study Group: The thrombolysis in myocardial infarction trial: Phase I finding. N Engl J Med 312:932, 1985.
85. Eigler, N, Maner, G, and Shah, PK: Effects of early systemic thrombolytic therapy on left ventricular mural thrombus formation in acute anterior myocardial infarction. Am J Cardiol 54:261, 1984.
86. Natarajan, D, Hotchandani, RK, and Nigan, PD: Reduced incidence of left ventricular thrombi with intravenous streptokinase in acute anterior myocardial infarction: Prospective evaluation by cross-sectional echocardiography, Int J Cardiol 20:201, 1988.
87. Keren, A, Medina, A, Gottleib, S, et al: Lysis of mobile left ventricular thrombi during acute myocardial infarction with urokinase. Am J Cardiol 60:1180, 1987.
88. Kremer, P, Fiebig, R, Tilsner, V, et al: Lysis of left ventricular thrombi with urokinase. Circulation 72:112, 1985.
89. ISIS-2 Collaborative Group: Randomized trial of intravenous streptokinase, oral aspirin, both or neither among 17,187 cases of suspected acute myocardial infarction: ISIS-1. Lancet 1:349, 1988.
90. Rutherford, JD, Braunwald, E, and Cohn, PF: In Braunwald, E (ed): Heart Disease: A Textbook of Cardiovascular Medicine. WB Saunders, Philadelphia, 1988, pp 1364–1366.
91. Lew, AS, Federman, J, Harper, RW, et al: Operative removal of mobile pedunculated left ventricular thrombus detected by 2-dimensional echocardiography. Am J Cardiol 52:48, 1983.
92. Fournial, G, Glock, Y, Berthoumieu, F, et al: Thrombus flottant du ventricule gauche apres infarctus du myocarde recent traite chirurgicalement. Arch Mal Coeur 73:1415,1980.

Commentary

Melvin D. Cheitlin, M.D.

Ezekowitz and Azrin have reviewed the literature on the development of mural thrombus and embolization in acute myocardial infarction and the role of anti-coagulation in preventing either the thrombus or the embolization. In most series the incidence of left ventricular thrombi in anterior wall myocardial infarction and inferior wall myocardial infarction with apical involvement is about 30 percent. The incidence of thrombus with localized inferior wall myocardial infarct and with non-Q-wave myocardial infarct is quite low. The overall incidence of embolization best obtained from the large controlled studies of anticoagulants in myocardial infarction done in the 1950s and 1960s suggests a low incidence of clinically recognized embolization, about 3 to 6 percent. One problem with the incidence of embolization in myocardial infarction is the definition of embolism. Certainly many emboli go unrecognized clinically. In studies that search for embolization, many transient symptoms that otherwise would be dismissed are attributed to emboli. This probably accounts for some of the wide variation in the literature in the incidence of embolization, inasmuch as it is reported that from 5 to 50 percent of patients with anterior wall myocardial infarction "have emboli." Unquestionably the incidence of clinically important cerebrovascular emboli with residua, coronary emboli with infarction, and peripheral emboli with residua, are much less frequent, and it is the incidence of these complications that must be balanced against the problems associated with long-term anti-coagulation.

From the data presented by Ezekowitz and Azrin, their conclusion is reasonable: because systemic emboli may occur early after infarction and detectable left ventricular thrombi may occur later, then emboli can occur before thrombus is detected by echocardiography. Therefore, in high-risk patients—that is, those with anterior wall myocardial infarction with akinesia or inferior wall infarct with apical involvement—heparin should be started. Also, because echocardiography is useful in risk stratification in myocardial infarction in estimating left ventricular function, it should be performed at the end of the first week after an anterior or apical myocardial infarction, and because the presence of a thrombus could indicate a potential late embolization, it is reasonable that anticoagulation is continued on those patients and discontinued in all others. Problems that remain unsettled are the time at which anticoagulation should be discontinued and the question of the recurrence of late thrombus formation and possibly the return of increased risk of embolization on discontinuing the anticoagulants. Until these problems are studied, any plan recommended will be tentative. It is our practice to restudy the patient after six weeks by echocardiography, and if the thrombus is either laminated or absent, to discontinue the anticoagulants. If the thrombus is vegetative or mobile, it is our practice to continue anticoagulants indefinitely.

CHAPTER 7

Has Multivessel Angioplasty Displaced Surgical Revascularization?

Spencer B. King III, M.D.
Russell J. Ivanhoe, M.D.

When Gruentzig developed coronary angioplasty in 1977, there was a broadly held view that it had a quite limited potential, and in fact most surgeons considered that patients having angioplasty would ultimately come to bypass surgery. Gruentzig limited the technique to single-lesion angioplasty in the beginning for two reasons. First, in order to ensure the safety of the procedure and to establish a record of favorable results, he selected patients in whom only one obstruction was causing the clinical syndrome, and, therefore, if relieved would lead to symptomatic and objective relief of ischemia. This approach would provide for safety of the procedure as well as clear documentation of its efficacy. As Gruentzig stated, if the technique would not work in single-vessel disease, it certainly could not be expanded beyond that. Documentation of the benefit of single-vessel angioplasty came early with reports of relief of angina and reversal of exercise test abnormalities. And, once long-term follow-up was available, it was obvious that the majority of the patients who had undergone single-vessel angioplasty could be managed chronically without the need for bypass surgery.

The second reason for selecting patients with single-vessel disease was the availablility of equipment in 1977. Lesions suitable for angioplasty were those that were quite proximal and discrete without intervening twists or turns in the coronary circulation, and, in fact, over 70 percent of the initial series were proximal anterior descending lesions.

The move to treating more complex disease, including multivessel angioplasty, has been a gradual one over the past 11 years, and it would not have been possible without technical developments that began in 1982 and are continuing. Improvements in guide catheters, guidewires, and balloons have brought distal and branch-vessel targets for angioplasty into easy range. Because safety is the most important principle to be considered, careful case selection has resulted in a respectable complication rate even for those patients with multivessel disease. Once these results were established, it was natural that more difficult cases would be attempted.

123

This chapter examines the experience with angioplasty to date, particularly in patients with various forms of multivessel disease, to examine how this development has had impact on surgical practice and to evaluate how far this technique is likely to go in displacing surgery as the primary therapy for patients with multivessel disease needing revascularization. There is current consensus regarding the selection for angioplasty or surgery in a large number of patients needing revascularization. The large cohort of patients in whom there is a continuing dilemma between selection for surgery and angioplasty are now undergoing prospective clinical testing. The results of these randomized trials will be important in further defining the value of angioplasty and surgery in patients with multivessel coronary artery disease.

PERCUTANEOUS TRANSLUMINAL CORONARY ANGIOPLASTY (PTCA)

Gruentzig's development of percutaneous transluminal coronary angioplasty (PTCA) was an extension of the work of Dotter and Judkins,[1] who first treated peripheral atherosclerosis with coaxial catheters. Gruentzig and colleagues[2] recognized early on and confirmed later that the procedure could yield a high primary success rate in well-selected patients; that emergency coronary artery bypass surgery (CABG) for failed angioplasty would limit infarct size; that restenosis would occur in about 30 percent; and that failure to attain clinical success may be related to the extent of undilated segments as much as to the success in dilating the primary segment.

EARLY RESULTS

Data that support the tenet that PTCA is not necessarily a prelude to coronary artery bypass surgery derive from long-term follow-up of the early experience in Zurich[3] and then at Emory.[4] In the early study, in which there was a 90 percent angiographic follow-up for single-vessel disease, the freedom from recurrence was 65 percent. Actuarial cardiac survival was 92 percent for multivessel disease and 98 percent for single-vessel disease at an average follow-up of 6 years. All patients undergoing PTCA at Emory University Hospital in 1981 have been followed prospectively. At five years, 82 percent were free from cardiac events (cardiac death, myocardial infarction, CABG). Furthermore, cardiac mortality in patients with proximal left anterior descending coronary artery (LAD) stenosis was 1.0 percent at 5 years, in stark contrast to that reported by Califf and colleagues,[5] who found a 10 percent mortality at 5 years in a similar cohort of patients treated medically.

COMPLICATIONS

The major complications of PTCA include emergency bypass surgery, acute infarction, and death. The rate of complications at Emory University Hospital is emergency bypass 2.5 percent, myocardial infarction (MI) 2.0 percent, and mortality 0.2 percent.[6] The usual cause of acute complications during PTCA is acute closure of the artery. This is typically the result of a dissection of the coronary artery, although it may be due also to acute thrombus formation. In the early years of angioplasty, abrupt closure was found to be related to female gender, unstable angina, right coronary artery PTCA, severe eccentric and long stenoses, multivessel disease, calcification, and thrombosis.[7] The Emory experience shows lesion length, female gender, tortuosity of the site, PTCA at a branch point, associated thrombus, and other stenoses in the same vessel to be related to acute closure.[8]

SURGICAL BACKUP

The importance of cardiac anesthesiology and surgical services in reducing the risk of failed PTCA is clear. Percutaneous transluminal coronary angioplasty should not be performed in centers incapable of providing appropriate surgical standby. Acute ischemic events during and after PTCA range from chest pain and electrocardiographic evidence of ischemia to transmural infarction and death. The effectiveness of emergency coronary bypass surgery in reducing mortality and infarction cannot be overemphasized and can be lifesaving.[10] In fact, it has been shown that early emergency surgery with establishment of extracorporeal circulation (within 30 minutes) can reduce the incidence of myocardial infarction.[11] During a four-year period at the Mid America Heart Institute, 286 patients underwent CABG following PTCA. Nearly 75 percent had multivessel disease. One hundred fifteen underwent surgery on an emergency basis. The 30-day mortality was 6.3 percent. Furthermore, the incidence of MI, low cardiac output syndrome, and operative death were far higher in patients requiring emergency surgery than in a nonemergency group. Early survivors of CABG after PTCA sustained a yearly mortality of 1.4 percent.[9]

At Emory University, the first 3500 patients to undergo PTCA had an emergency bypass rate of 2.7 percent. The mortality for the 96 emergency surgery patients was 2 percent.[12] Both groups of patients had multivessel disease, abnormal left ventricular function caused by previous myocardial infarction, underwent LAD angioplasty, and were hemodynamically unstable in the catheterization laboratory. There were no deaths among patients with single-vessel coronary artery disease or with normal left ventricular function undergoing emergency surgery for failed angioplasty in that series. Furthermore, there were no deaths in the five patients with a previous history of CABG who underwent emergency surgery for failed PTCA.

AHA/ACC GUIDELINES

In setting guidelines for PTCA, the American Heart Association (AHA)/ACC Task Force on PTCA has categorized the specific lesion morphology as an aid to determining which lesions carry a high risk of acute closure and a low rate of success (Table 7–1).[13] Those lesions which are short, concentric, discrete, and readily accessible in straight segments are most amenable to angioplasty. The absence of major branch involvement or intracoronary thrombus and location not in the ostium further enhance the likelihood of a successful procedure.

Furthermore, it is well known that diffuse lesions (more than 2 cm length), chronic occlusion (more than 3 months old), extremely tortuous or angulated segments, and inability to protect major side branches raise the risk of angioplasty considerably. These lesions should be attempted only in extenuating circumstances by operators who have considerable experience with these high-risk lesions. The patient should fully understand the low success rate and high risk inherent in dilating this type of lesion.

There is a group of lesions that fall between the aforementioned extremes of

Table 7–1. Lesion-specific Characteristics: Type A, B, and C
Lesions

Type A Lesions (High Success, >85%; Low Risk)	
• Discrete (<10 mm length)	• Little or no calcification
• Concentric	• Less than totally occlusive
• Readily accessible	• Not ostial in location
• Nonangulated segment, <45°	• No major branch involvement
• Smooth contour	• Absence of thrombus

Type B Lesions (Moderate Success, 60 to 85%; Moderate Risk)	
• Tubular (10 to 20 mm length)	• Moderate to heavy calcification
• Eccentric	• Total occlusions <3 months old
• Moderate tortuosity of proximal segment	• Ostial in location
• Moderately angulated segment, >45°, <90°	• Bifurcation lesions requiring double guide wires
• Irregular contour	• Some thrombus present

Type C Lesions (Low Success, <60%; High Risk)	
• Diffuse (>2 cm length)	• Total occlusion >3 months old
• Excessive tortuosity of proximal segment	• Inability to protect major side branches
• Extremely angulated segments >90°	• Degenerated vein grafts with friable lesions

Although the risk of abrupt vessel closure is moderate, in certain instances the likelihood of a major complication may be low as in dilation of total occlusions < months old or when abundant collateral channels supply the distal vessel.

AHA/ACC Task Force Report on Guidelines for Percutaneous Transluminal Coronary Angioplasty. JACC 12:538, 1988, with permission.

risk and difficulty. They are characterized by eccentricity, moderate tortuosity and angulation, some thrombus present, and irregular contours. These lesions may be total occlusions less than 3 months in duration, ostial lesions, or bifurcation lesions. These lesions carry a success rate of 60 to 85 percent and are of moderate risk. Percutaneous transluminal coronary angioplasty of this type of lesion should be performed by an experienced operator.

RESTENOSIS

In the years since PTCA has been applied, restenosis* has emerged as the primary factor limiting its application. Restenosis, particularly as it occurs in multivessel angioplasty, erodes the potential advantages PTCA holds over coronary bypass surgery. Each subsequent procedure adds to the cost and carries with it the risk of complication. Furthermore, when mildly stenotic lesions are dilated, restenosis may result in a more severe lesion than the primary one.[14] The incidence of restenosis has remained around 30 percent and typically presents within 6 months (although a small percentage occur after 6 months).[15] The evaluation of restenosis in large clinical trials that have assessed the progression to and extent of restenosis is complicated by data suggesting dependence of these factors on the definition and

---

*Restenosis can occur silently, and restenosis rates depend upon whether follow-up is clinical or angiographic.

quantitative method used.[16] At Emory University, restenosis is defined as greater than 50 percent luminal narrowing (measured by electronic calipers) at follow-up. Several risk factors have been identified, which may help determine those patients at risk for restenosis at the time of primary angioplasty and at repeat PTCA. These include the vessel dilated (LAD, right coronary artery [RCA], left circumflex [LCX]), the absence of an intimal dissection, a final translesional gradient greater than 15 mmHg, large residual stenosis (greater than 30 percent), and the presence of unstable angina.[14] The present management of restenosis is repeat PTCA, which has been shown to be effective and safe.[17]

There are a number of trials underway aimed at limiting the rate of restenosis. One initial report suggested that fish oil was effective in limiting restenosis.[18] However, a larger subsequent trial has shown a negative result.[19] A number of other pharmacologic approaches to limiting restenosis developed. Neither nifedipine[20] nor coumarin[21] have been effective in limiting restenosis. Various aspirin-dose programs and prolonged heparinization have not reduced the restenosis rate. Heparin subunits in combination with hydrocortisone have been shown to inhibit smooth muscle cell growth in cultures.[22] The role of platelets in the pathophysiology of restenosis of injured arteries[23] has led to the development of various antiplatelet antithrombosis approaches. Trapidil, an antianginal vasodilator, has been shown to limit restenosis in an *in vivo* animal model.[24]

Various mechanical approaches to inhibiting restenosis are also undergoing clinical trials. Atherectomy actually removes the plaque material. Laser balloon angioplasty induces permanent injury and fibrotic reformation at the site of angioplasty. Endovascular stents remodel the lumen and reduce elastic recoil.

Unfortunately, as yet no efforts aimed at reducing restenosis have proved efficacious. The frequently used approach, therefore, is to repeat PTCA, or to refer the patient for coronary bypass surgery.

PTCA IN MULTIVESSEL CORONARY ARTERY DISEASE

A specific definition of multivessel disease must be formulated in order to compare the results of multivessel PTCA with CABG properly. At Emory, we define multivessel disease as at least 50 percent diameter stenosis in two or more major vessels in either the LAD, LCX, or RCA systems. For example, a patient with critical stenosis in an obtuse marginal branch and a diagonal branch would be considered to have multivessel disease. However, a patient with disease in a marginal and the midcircumflex would not be considered to have multivessel disease. A further distinction should be made between multivessel and multilesion PTCA. The latter would, for example, include sequential LAD lesions.

It is not presently known whether such a grouping has any bearing on morbidity, mortality, restenosis, or crossover to CABG. It does allow us to compare patients who undergo multivessel angioplasty with those who receive surgical revascularization.

Gruentzig's first reported series included a significant percentage of patients with multivessel disease: 98 (58 percent) of those patients had single-vessel coronary artery disease (CAD) and 71 (42 percent) had multivessel disease.[2] In those patients with multivessel CAD, the artery considered to be responsible for the patients' symptoms was the only one dilated in all but two patients. Overall, in this initial group of patients, 73 percent had a technically successful angioplasty. There were six late deaths. A total of 35 patients with multivessel disease maintained patent vessels after dilatation. Four of these patients required bypass surgery because of progression of disease in a vessel that was not originally dilated. Overall, then, 31 of 71 patients (49 percent) have maintained a patent vessel after angioplasty and have not required coronary bypass surgery at 5 to 8 years of follow-up.[3]

The PTCA registry of the National Heart, Lung and Blood Institute (NHLBI) reopened in 1985 after having concentrated on follow-up of the first cohort from 1979 to 1981.[26] The later group was more anatomically complex, and the proportion of patients with multivessel disease was 53 percent, compared with only 25 percent in the earlier group. Despite the challenge of more difficult cases, the success rate improved dramatically. The angiographic success rate increased from 67 to 88 percent. The overall success rate increased from 61 to 78 percent. The shift in complexity, with the associated enhanced success, is likely the result of advancing technology as well as increasing operator experience.

There was also a sharp decrease in elective bypass surgery following angioplasty. Such surgery decreased in patients with two- and three-vessel CAD from 28 percent and 17 percent to 2 percent and 3 percent, respectively.[26]

The data from the Emory experience follow the same pattern as those observed in the NHLBI registry [Fig. 7-1 (A) and (B)]. From 1980 to 1987, there was a dramatic increase in the number of PTCA cases and a fall in the percent of cases with single-vessel disease from 80 to 85 percent to 50 percent. In the last five years the primary success rate has remained around 90 percent while the complication rate has not changed significantly. Only 11 percent of the cases in 1980 to 1981 had multivessel disease, and the rate of emergency coronary bypass surgery was 7.2 percent. By 1987, nearly 50 percent of angioplasties performed at Emory were for multivessel disease, whereas the rate of emergency surgery dropped to 2.2 percent. The incidence of Q-wave myocardial infarction also dropped from 2.5 percent to 0.9 percent in the same period. Death following PTCA rose gradually from 0.1 percent to 0.3 percent in the years 1980 to 1985. It has remained at that level for 1986 and 1987.

EXTENT OF REVASCULARIZATION

Concomitant with the trend toward more complex anatomy, the questions have arisen: To what extent should a patient be revascularized? Should all lesions present be dilated? Should only those vessels that have a very high-grade obstruction[27,28] or that correlate with a reperfusable defect on thallium scan be dilated?

The value of complete versus incomplete surgical revascularization has been studied. Reasons for not placing grafts are based on anatomic factors such as vessels less than 1 mm diameter, intramyocardial location, severe diffuse distal disease, or the vessel in question supplying a dyskinetic segment.[29,30] Therefore, there appears to be a selection bias that places patients who are not completely revascularized into a high-risk group. As surgical skills improved, the ability to bypass anatomically difficult arteries improved. This is reflected in the observation that the percent of patients who undergo complete revascularization is increasing. In one large series, the completeness of revascularization increased from 58.2 percent to 75.9 percent over a 13-year period.[30]

Complete revascularization, when possible, is, of course, favored in surgically

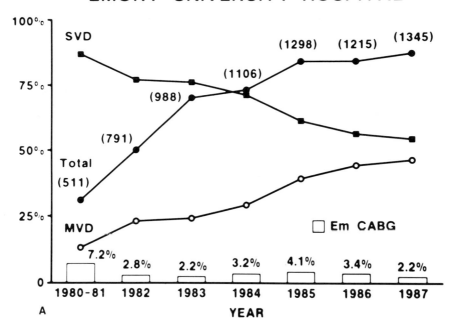

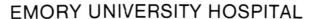

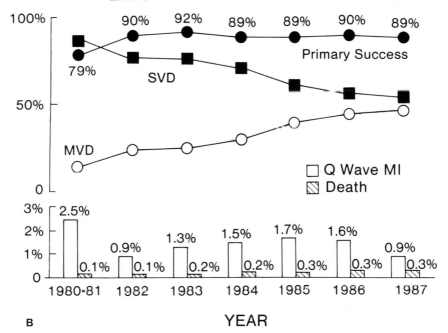

Figure 7–1. (*A*) Growth of PTCA at Emory University Hospital 1980–87. (*B*) Primary success and complication rate of coronary angioplasty at Emory University Hospital 1980–87.

Table 7–2. Multivessel Angioplasty—Primary Success, Restenosis

Author	N (#PT)	1° Success (%)	Angio F/U%	Complications Early (%)	Restenosis % PT (% Lesion)
Finci[32]	100	85	91	NR	51 (33)
Reeder[35]	286	NR	NR	NR	NR (NR)
Mata[37]	74	85	96	1.3	34 (23)
Cowley[38]	100	88	29	11	NR (NR)
Mabin[39]	66	77	37	NR	33 (32)
Roubin[40]	229	NR	67	NR	35 (20)
Hartzler[41]	312	92	NR	3.8	NR (NR)

NR = Not reported.

treated patients; and these patients have significantly better survival with fewer symptoms.[29–31] Jones and coworkers[31] showed that the improved clinical course with complete revascularization is due to the extent of revascularization. Differences in left ventricular (LV) function did not correlate with survival in their series. They concluded that as many grafts as possible should be constructed in order to achieve quality long-term survival.

The initial approach to evaluating PTCA in multivessel disease has been to analyze results and to divide patients into groups based on the degree of revascularization retrospectively.[32–41] The available data have been collected in Tables 7–2 and 7–3. Several points are evident. The primary success rate per patient—that is, successful dilatation with relief of symptoms—is slightly less than that reported for single-vessel PTCA. The reported rate of restenosis per vessel dilated hovers around 25 to 30 percent, but the rate of restenosis *per patient* is higher. The immediate, or acute, complications are no greater whether a patient undergoes complete or incomplete revascularization. However, there is an apparent difference in the long-term follow-up. Those patients undergoing incomplete revascularization were more symptomatic and had a higher rate of subsequent CABG. It must be kept in mind that these are trends and that there are insufficient data to draw firm conclusions, particularly with regard to late survival.

Table 7–3. Multivessel Angioplasty—Complete versus Incomplete Revascularization

Author	N (#PT)	No. PTS per Group		CABG(%)		Repeat PTCA (%)		Symptom Free (%)		Deaths (%)	
		CR	IR	CR	IR	CR	IR	CR	IR	CR	IR
Finci[32]	100	59	18	5	28	NR	NR	81	44	NR	NR
Thomas[33]	92	19	73	5	1	11	12	81	84	0	0
Deligonul[34]	470	128	342	7	16	14	13	NR	NR	5	5
Reeder[35]	286	127	159	9.4	17	19.7	8.8	69	68	3.1	5.0
Cowley[38]	100	NR	NR	6	6	NR	NR	NR	NR	NR	NR
Mabin[39]	66	31	35	13	23	NR	NR	71	37	NR	NR

NR = Not reported.

Breisblatt and associates[42] have attempted to identify those patients with multivessel disease who might benefit from incomplete revascularization by using exercise thallium scanning. They chose the primary stenosis to be dilated as that with the largest thallium perfusion defect prior to PTCA. At two to four weeks after PTCA, all patients had a repeat exercise thallium scan. The patients were then divided into two groups: those without (group I) and those with (group II) late thallium defects. At one year, 79 percent of the group II patients had required PTCA of a second vessel, whereas only 13 percent of group I had further PTCA. In this study, the positive thallium result may have influenced future therapy. Additional investigation is needed to discover whether the extent of revascularization influences long-term survival.

TRENDS IN SURGERY

During the PTCA era, patients selected for CABG have become more complex. The surgical experience at the Cleveland Clinic over the past 15 years shows that more patients have abnormal electrocardiograms, symptoms and signs of congestive heart failure (CHF), and documented preoperative myocardial infarction.[30] Furthermore, patients with triple-vessel disease now comprise more than half of the patients sent for CABG. The number of grafts per patient has risen as a consequence. In the 1970s, mortality rose with the number of grafts placed. This trend was reversed with the use of cold crystalloid cardioplegia. By the 1980s the predominant risk factors for mortality related to CABG had become emergency operation, preoperative CHF, age (especially the seventh and eighth decades), incomplete revascularization, and abnormal electrocardiograms.[30]

The risk of developing myocardial ischemia, and its consequences, following revascularization is primarily related to the frequency of graft occlusion and progression of atherosclerotic disease in native arterial segments.[43] In the Veterans Administration Cooperative study, initial improvement after CABG was followed by an increase in symptoms and a decrease in exercise tolerance to levels similar to those of medically treated patients 10 years after surgery.[44] Survival benefit also tends to diminish by 7 years after revascularization surgery in high-risk patients (three-vessel disease and depressed left ventricular function). At 5 years of follow-up, in patients who had previously undergone CABG and had an intercurrent MI, Wiseman and coworkers[45] found 42 percent of saphenous vein grafts were occluded, 12 percent were stenotic, and 45 percent were patent. All grafts were either occluded or stenosed in 30 percent of the patients. This is consistent with the annual attrition rate of grafts found previously to be 5.3 percent at 7 years of follow-up.[46]

The use of aspirin and dipyridamole may prolong graft patency when saphenous veins are used as the conduit.[47] More importantly, the use of the internal mammary artery (IMA) has improved long-term surgical results.[48–51] The CASS registry showed use of an IMA graft to be an independent predictor of survival with a reduced risk of 0.64.[49] The benefit of IMA use was not affected by the frequency of its use at a particular institution, the extent of impairment of ventricular function, sex, age, or the presence of left main coronary artery disease. The role of the IMA in CABG has been extended by use of both mammary arteries and sequential grafting.[51,52]

EFFECT OF PTCA ON REFERRAL PATTERNS TO SURGERY

Referral patterns for revascularization have changed at Emory. Referral patterns for treatment of CAD in patients undergoing their first angiogram in the Emory University Hospital system from 1981 to 1986 have been evaluated.[53] As expected, the percentage of patients revascularized by PTCA has risen considerably (from 6 to 22 percent over the years studied), while the percentage of patients referred for CABG has fallen (from 42 to 28 percent during the period 1981 to 1986). This shift has reflected not only an increase in PTCA at the expense of surgery but also the fact that the patients referred for surgery are now older and have worse ventricular function.

COSTS: PTCA VERSUS CABG

An important consideration in determining the degree to which PTCA has displaced or will displace CABG is that of cost. One of the earliest cost comparisons was completed in patients undergoing single-vessel PTCA or single-vessel CABG.[54] There was a large and significant difference between charges for angioplasty and for bypass grafting. This difference disappeared among patients with restenosis or failed PTCA. When surgical treatment was the result of restenosis, the average charge for PTCA nearly tripled ($7,508 to $20,036). It was calculated that to achieve a 30 percent reduction in expenditures for angioplasty compared with bypass, a 90 percent initial success rate and 20 percent restenosis rate and a 90 percent repeat-dilatation rate of those restenosed would be required. Another study of comparative costs of PTCA and CABG found a 43 percent cost advantage for PTCA after one year in patients with single-vessel disease.[55]

What are the costs for patients who have undergone multivessel PTCA or multivessel CABG in which at least one IMA graft has been constructed? Black and colleagues[56] carried out such an analysis at Emory in 100 consecutive patients undergoing elective PTCA to at least two vessels. Complete angiographic success was achieved in 81 percent, with a further 17 percent having at least one vessel dilated. During follow-up, repeat PTCA was required on 14 occasions (twice in one patient, once in 12 patients). Only six PTCA patients required CABG. The total one-year revascularization cost, including repeat procedures, was $11,100 for PTCA patients and $22,862 for the CABG patients.

In the present era of multivessel PTCA, the cost advantage will be diluted as long as the restenosis rate per vessel remains as high as it is. It should be kept in mind that the cost data presently available were not analyzed on a prospective randomized basis and that patients therefore may not be comparable. The true cost differential will become clear at the completion of the ongoing randomized PTCA versus surgery trials.

PRESENT INDICATIONS FOR MODE OF REVASCULARIZATION

There are certain patients for whom the preferred mode of revascularization is clear. Coronary bypass grafting is seldom undertaken for single-vessel disease. Although medical therapy for single-vessel disease is often effective, if symptoms are progressive and/or there is a large segment of myocardium at risk, PTCA is usually performed.

Patients with severe LV dysfunction and intractable angina, in whom the surgical risk exceeds that of PTCA, may undergo high-risk PTCA—accepting also the risks of not undergoing emergency bypass grafting should angioplasty fail.

Percutaneous transluminal coronary angioplasty has been shown to be very effective in dilating stenotic saphenous vein grafts. The success rate is high and the restenosis rate appears to be acceptable.[57] The risk can be minimized by proper case selection. A word of caution is necessary, as indicated by the AHA/ACC Task Force for PTCA; PTCA of old, friable saphenous vein grafts carries a high risk for distal embolization.

Surgery is unquestionably the treatment of choice for stenosis of an unprotected (i.e., no distal bypass grafts) left main coronary artery. The results of PTCA in that setting have been unfavorable and fall far short of surgical results.[58] Percutaneous transluminal coronary angioplasty of a vessel that supplies collaterals to a region of viable myocardium, such that acute closure in the former leads to ischemia in both segments, would constitute an extremely high-risk situation for PTCA. When the characteristics of the lesion are unfavorable (based on the classification system of the AHA/ACC Task Force, Table 7–1),[13] surgery is the treatment of choice.

Preservation of LV function should angioplasty fail underlies all strategies in multivessel angioplasty. For example, if a large RCA is occluded and receives collateral flow from the LAD, which has a proximal lesion, the RCA should be dilated first. This is needed in order to provide reversed collateral flow in the event the LAD angioplasty fails. Failure to revascularize the RCA would be an indication for elective surgery in this case.

Staging a multivessel procedure (dilating lesions on successive days) is indicated when a prolonged procedure is inevitable or acute closure of more than one vessel would lead to hemodynamic collapse. This is particularly true for patients with poor LV function, renal insufficiency, or diabetes or for patients who are unable to tolerate the additional time in the catheterization laboratory. One might approach a patient with disease in the RCA, LAD, and circumflex systems as a staged procedure by dilating the LAD at one sitting and approaching the RCA and circumflex arteries on another day in order to be assured of continued patency of the LAD. Any strategy must be designed to ensure preservation of LV function in the event of failed PTCA.

RANDOMIZED TRIALS

The preferred form of revascularization for patients with multivessel disease not involving the left main coronary artery is not yet established. There are several major studies underway designed to address this question. The Emory Angioplasty/ Surgery Trial (EAST), supported by the National Heart, Lung and Blood Institute (NHLBI), aims to recruit 500 to 600 patients. Those patients with multivessel CAD (as defined earlier) who are referred for PTCA or CABG are given the option of participating in the study. Should the patient decide to participate in the trial, he or she is randomized and then treated accordingly. Follow-up calls for angiography and exercise thallium scanning at one year and three years, unless indicated earlier. End points are mortality, MI, and objective ischemia as well as symptoms, economic and quality-of-life parameters, and angiographic degree of revascularization. Recruitment is about 70 percent completed in 1989.

The Bypass versus Angioplasty Revascularization Investigation (BARI) is another study designed to test whether angioplasty is a viable substitute for surgical revascularization for multivessel CAD. This 14-center trial, also funded by NHBLI, is in the early stages of recruitment. Two thousand eight hundred patients are to be enrolled and followed clinically for 5 years. Patients who have an established need for revascularization will be randomized to PTCA or CABG. At five-year follow-up, patients will be evaluated on the basis of mortality, rates of MI and repeat revascularization procedures, left ventricular status, and anatomic end points. Economic and quality-of-life parameters also will be analyzed.

A third randomized study of angioplasty versus surgery is the Randomized Interventional Treatment of Angina (RITA) being undertaken in the United Kingdom. Investigators ultimately will assign 1500 patients to either angioplasty or surgery. Once it is determined that a patient requires revascularization, a cardiac surgeon determines how many grafts should be placed. The cardiologist then determines whether it is possible to provide equivalent revascularization. The groups will be compared for mortality, new cardiac events, exercise tolerance by treadmill testing, LV function, and quality of life. Patients will undergo treadmill testing 6 months after randomization and again at 1 year, if the 6-month test is positive.

There are two other studies that will compare angioplasty to surgery on a randomized basis. The Coronary Angioplasty versus Bypass Revascularization Investigation (CABRI), a study to be conducted in Western Europe, and the German Angioplasty versus Bypass Investigation (GABI) are just getting underway.

It is expected that upon completion of these trials, firm guidelines for choosing multivessel revascularization strategies will evolve.

SUMMARY

Over the years, PTCA has been proved a safe and effective therapy for single-vessel CAD. Given the record of favorable results for single-vessel angioplasty, the extension of angioplasty to multivessel CAD soon followed. The successful application of PTCA to multivessel disease has been facilitated by developments in balloon, guidewire, and guide catheter technology. Success rates have been satisfactory, and complications have remained acceptable. Furthermore, as an outgrowth of an understanding of the mechanism and effect of PTCA, guidelines have been developed to aid case selection. As emphasized earlier, these guidelines should weigh heavily in deciding whether to select PTCA as a treatment modality.

Presently, in our opinion, PTCA has not yet completely displaced surgery for multivessel CAD. Surgical standby is required for safe PTCA, because emergency surgery can be lifesaving and limit myocardial infarction after failed angioplasty. It is doubtful that surgery will ever relinquish its position as the treatment of choice for left main coronary artery disease. Nor will elective surgery find wide application in single-vessel disease. Whether one mode of revascularization will emerge as the most efficacious for multivessel disease related to long-term survival, limitation of cardiac events, and cost will be addressed in the analysis of the ongoing randomized trials of surgery versus angioplasty.

Andreas Gruentzig established that it was possible to work within the coronary artery in an alert and comfortable patient. Interventional cardiology has experienced rapid technologic growth. Many patients formerly treated with bypass surgery can be managed effectively with angioplasty. If effective bail-out methods for acute closure are proven effective and restenosis is limited to a small percentage of patients, angioplasty in some form will further displace CABG. Until those ultimate goals are achieved, the value of angioplasty compared with bypass surgery must rest with current local experience and the eagerly awaited results of randomized trials.

REFERENCES

1. Dotter, CT and Judkins, MP: Tranluminal treatment of arteriosclerotic obstruction: Description of a new technique and a preliminary report of its application. Circulation 30:654, 1964.
2. Gruentzig, AR, Senning, A, and Siegenthaler, WE: Nonoperative dilatation of coronary artery stenosis. N Engl J Med 301:61, 1979.
3. Gruentzig, AR, King, SB, III, Schlumpf, M, et al: Long term follow-up after percutaneous transluminal coronary angioplasty: The early Zurich experience. N Engl J Med 316:1127, 1987.
4. Talley, JD, Hurst, JW, King, SB, III, et al: Clinical outcome 5 years after attempted percutaneous transluminal coronary angioplasty in 427 patients. Circulation 77:820, 1988.
5. Califf, RM, Tomabechi, Y, and Lee, KL: Outcome in one vessel coronary artery disease. Circulation 67:283, 1983.
6. King, SB, III: Current status of percutaneous transluminal coronary angioplasty. Cardiovasc Rev Reports 9:27, 1988.
7. Dorros, G, Cowley, MJ, Simpson, J, et al: Percutaneous transluminal coronary angioplasty: Report of complications from the National Heart, Lung and Blood Institute PTCA Registry. Circulation 67:723, 1983.
8. Ellis, S, Roubin, GS, Cox, W, et al: Angiographic and clinical predictors of acute closure after coronary angioplasty (abstr). Circulation 74 (Suppl IV):IV215, 1987.
9. Killen, DA, Hamaker, WR, and Reed, WA: Coronary artery bypass following percutaneous transluminal coronary angioplasty. Ann Thorac Surg 40:133, 1985.
10. Murphy, DA, Craver, JM, Jones, EL, et al: Surgical management of acute myocardial ischemia following percutaneous transluminal coronary angioplasty. J Thorac Cardiovasc Surg 87:332, 1984.
11. Reul, GJ, Cooley, DA, Hallman, GL, et al: Coronary artery bypass for unsuccessful percutaneous transluminal coronary angioplasty. J Thorac Cardiovasc Surg 88:685, 1984.
12. Bredlau, CC, Roubin, GS, Leimgruber, PP, et al: In-hospital morbidity and mortality in patients undergoing coronary angioplasty. Circulation 72:1044, 1985.
13. AHA/ACC Task Force Report on guidelines for percutaneous transluminal coronary angioplasty. J Am Coll Cardiol 12:529, 1988.
14. Leimgruber, PP, Roubin, GS, Hollman, J, et al: Restenosis after successful coronary angioplasty in patients with single vessel disease. Circulation 73:710, 1986.
15. Holmes, DR, Vlietstra, RE, Smith, HE, et al: Restenosis after percutaneous transluminal coronary angioplasty (PTCA): A report from the PTCA registry of the National Heart, Lung, and Blood Institute. Am J Cardiol 53:77C, 1984.
16. Serruys, PW, Luijten, HE, Beatt, KJ, et al: Incidence of restenosis after successful coronary angioplasty: A time related phenomenon. A quantitative angiographic study in 342 consecutive patients at 1,2,3, and 4 months. Circulation 77:361, 1988.
17. Meier, B, King, SB, III, Gruentzig, AR, et al: Repeat coronary angioplasty. J Am Coll Cardiol 4:463, 1984.
18. Dehmer, GJ, Popma, JJ, van der Berg, EK, et al: Reduction in the rate of early stenosis after coronary angioplasty by a diet supplemented with n-3 fatty acids. N Engl J Med 319:733, 1988.
19. Reis, GJ, Sipperly, ME, Boucher, TM, et al: Results of a randomized trial of fish oil for prevention of restenosis after PTCA. Circulation 78 (Suppl II):291, 1988.
20. Whitworth, HB, Roubin, GS, Hollman, J, et al: The effect of nifedipine on recurrent stenosis after percutaneous coronary angioplasty. J Am Coll Cardiol 8:1271, 1986.
21. Thornton, MA, Gruentzig, AR, Hollman, J, et al: Coumadin and aspirin in prevention of recurrence after transluminal coronary angioplasty: A randomized study. Circulation 69:721, 1984.
22. Gordon, JB, Berk, BC, Bittman, MA, et al: Vascular smooth muscle proliferation following balloon injury is synergistically inhibited by low molecular weight heparin and hydrocortisone. Circulation 76 (Suppl IV):213, 1987.

23. Adams, PC, Bodimon, JT, Bodimon, Z, et al: Role of platelets in atherogenesis: Relevance to coronary arterial restenosis after angioplasty. Cardiovasc Clin 18:49, 1987.
24. Liu, MW, Roubin, GS, Robinson, KA, et al: Trapidil (triazolopyrimidine) or platelet derived growth factors antagonist in preventing restenosis after balloon angioplasty in the atherosclerotic rabbit. Circulation 78 (Suppl II):II290, 1988.
25. Ischinger, T, Gruentzig, AR, Hollman, J, et al: Should coronary arteries with less than 60% diameter stenosis be treated by angioplasty (abstr)? Circulation 66 (Suppl II): II329, 1982.
26. Detre, K, Holubkov, R, Kelsey S, et al: Percutaneous transluminal coronary angioplasty in 1985–1986 and 1977–1981: The National Heart, Lung and Blood Institute Registry. N Engl J Med 318:265, 1988.
27. Ambrose, JA, Winters, SL, Stern, A, et al: Angiographic morphology and the pathogenesis of unstable angina pectoris. J Am Coll Cardiol 5:609, 1985.
28. Wohlgelernter, D, Cleman, M, Highman, HA, et al: Percutaneous transluminal coronary angioplasty of the "culprit" lesion for management of unstable angina pectoris in patients with multivessel coronary artery disease. Am J Cardiol 58:460, 1986.
29. Cukingnan, RA, Carey, JS, Wittig, JH, et al: Influence of complete coronary revascularization on relief of angina. J Thorac Cardiovasc Surg 79:188, 1980.
30. Cosgrove, DM, Loop, FD, Lythe, BW, et al: Primary myocardial revascularization: Trends in surgical mortality. J Thorac Cardiovasc Surg 88:673, 1984.
31. Jones, EL, Craver, JM, Goyton, RA, et al: Importance of complete revascularization in performance of the coronary bypass operation. Am J Cardiol 51:7, 1983.
32. Finci, L, Meier, B, DeBruyne, B, et al: Angiographic follow-up after multivessel percutaneous transluminal coronary angioplasty. Am J Cardiol 60:467, 1987.
33. Thomas, FS, Most, AS, and Williams, DO: Coronary angioplasty for patients with multivessel coronary artery disease: Follow-up clinical status. Am Heart J 115:8, 1988.
34. Deligonul, V, Vandormael, MG, Kern, MJ, et al: Coronary angioplasty: A therapeutic option for symptomatic patients with two and three vessel coronary disease. J Am Coll Cardiol 11:1173, 1988.
35. Reeder, GS, Holmes, DR, Detre, K, et al: Degree of revascularization in patients with multivessel coronary disease: A report from the National Heart, Lung, and Blood Institute Percutaneous Transluminal Coronary Angioplasty Registry. Circulation 77:638, 1988.
36. Vandormael, MB, Deligonul, V, Kern, MJ, et al: Multilesion coronary angioplasty: Clinical and angiographic follow-up. J Am Coll Cardiol 10:246, 1987.
37. Mata, LA, Bosch, X, David, PR, et al: Clinical and angiographic assessment 6 months after double vessel percutaneous coronary angioplasty. J Am Coll Cardiol 6:1239, 1985.
38. Cowley, MJ, Vetrovec, GW, DiSciacio, G, et al: Coronary angioplasty of multiple vessels: Short-term outcome and long-term results. Circulation 72:1314, 1985.
39. Mabin, TA, Holmes, DR, Jr, Smith, HE, et al: Follow-up clinical results in patients undergoing percutaneous transluminal coronary angioplasty. Circulation 71:754, 1985.
40. Roubin, GS, Redd, D, Leimgruber, P, et al: Restenosis after multilesion and multivessel coronary angioplasty (PTCA). J Am Coll Cardiol 7:22A, 1986.
41. Hartzler, GO: Percutaneous transluminal coronary angioplasty in multivessel disease. Cathet Cardiovasc Diag 9:537, 1983.
42. Breisblatt, WM, Barnes, JV, Weiland, F, et al: Incomplete revascularization in multivessel percutaneous transluminal coronary angioplasty: The role for stress thallium-201 imaging. J Am Coll Cardiol 11:1183, 1988.
43. Chatterjee, K: Is there any long-term benefit from coronary artery bypass surgery? J Am Coll Cardiol 12:881, 1988.
44. Peduzzi, P, Hultgren, H, Thomsen, J, et al: Ten year effect of medical and surgical therapy on quality of life: Veterans Administration Cooperative Study of Coronary Artery Surgery. Am J Cardiol 59:1017, 1987.
45. Wiseman, A, Walter, DD, Walling, A, et al: Long-term prognosis after myocardial infarction in patients with previous coronary artery bypass surgery. J Am Coll Cardiol 12:873, 1988.
46. Campeau, L, Eujalbert, M, Lesperance, J, et al: Atherosclerosis and late closure of aortacoronary saphenous vein grafts: Sequential angiographic studies at 2 weeks, 1 year, 5 to 7 years and 10 to 12 years after surgery. Circulation 68(Suppl II):II1, 1983.
47. Cheseboro, J, Fuster, V, et al: Effect of dipyridamole and aspirin on late vein graft patency after coronary bypass operations. N Engl J Med 310:209, 1984.
48. Loop, F, Lytle, B, Cosgrove, D, et al: Influence of the internal mammary artery graft on 10 year survival and other cardiac events. N Engl J Med 314:1, 1984.

49. Cameron, A, Davis, KB, Green, GE, et al: Clinical implications of internal mammary artery bypass grafts: The Coronary Artery Surgery Study Experience. Circulation 77:815, 1988.
50. Lytle, BW, Loop, FD, Cosgrove, DM, et al: Long-term (5 to 12 years) serial studies of internal mammary artery and saphenous vein coronary bypass grafts. J Thorac Cardiovasc Surg 89:248, 1985.
51. Lytle, BW, Cosgrove, DM, Saltus, GL, et al: Long-term results of bilateral internal mammary artery grafting. Ann Thorac Surg 36:540, 1983.
52. Jones, EL, Lutz, JF, King, SB, III, et al: Extended use of the internal mammary artery graft: Important anatomic and physiologic considerations. Circulation 74(Suppl III):42, 1986.
53. Weintraub, WS, Jones, EL, King, SB, III, et al: Changing utilization of coronary angioplasty and coronary bypass surgery in the treatment of chronic coronary artery disease (abstr). J Am Coll Cardiol.
54. Kelly, ME, Taylor, GJ, Moss, HW, et al: Comparative cost of myocardial revascularization: Percutaneous transluminal angioplasty and coronary artery bypass surgery. J Am Coll Cardiol 5:16, 1985.
55. Jang, GC, Block, PC, Cowley, MJ, et al: Relative cost of coronary angioplasty and bypass surgery in a one-vessel disease model. Am J Cardiol 53:52C, 1984.
56. Black, AJR, Roubin, GS, Sutor, C, et al: Comparative costs of percutantous transluminal coronary angioplasty and coronary artery bypass grafting in multivessel coronary artery disease. Am J Cardiol 62:809, 1988.
57. Douglas, JS, Jr, Gruentzig, AR, King, SB, III, et al: Percutaneous transluminal coronary angioplasty in patients with prior coronary bypass surgery. J Am Coll Cardiol 2:745, 1983.
58. Stertzer, SH, Myler, RK, Insel, H, et al: Percutaneous transluminal coronary angioplasty in left main stem coronary stenosis: A five year appraisal. Int J Cardiol 9:149, 1985.

Commentary

By Melvin D. Cheitlin, M.D.

This chapter deals with the mode of revascularization in patients with multi-vessel coronary artery disease when revascularization is deemed necessary. When comparing angioplasty with surgical revascularization, most of the studies cited are not randomized, making the population to which the study applies difficult to define and biased in results. For instance, given the variation in indications for angioplasty, it is possible, even probable, that many of the patients with single-vessel or even multivessel disease might have been very low-risk patients managed medically rather than by revascularization. In many institutions the indication for angioplasty is the presence of a significantly obstructed vessel, especially if some evidence of myocardial ischemia can be demonstrated, regardless of the symptomatic state of the patient or even the amount of myocardium subserved by the obstructed vessel. It is not certain that all angioplasty patients would have been considered for surgery, thus making the angioplasty and the surgical groups different populations.

The two groups also could be biased by indications within the institution for surgery or for angioplasty. It is apparent that in multivessel disease the ideal patients for angioplasty are those with severe, localized, proximal obstruction not associated with thrombus or heavy calcification; and not located in the areas of tortuosity or where significant branches are involved; and preferably those who do not have unstable angina. Furthermore, the more myocardium the involved vessel supplies, the greater the danger if the vessel is suddenly occluded during the angioplasty. The tendency is to perform multivessel angioplasty in the good-risk patients and to refer the higher-risk patients, especially those with decreased ventricular function, to surgery. This bias can go the other way in institutions in which the high-risk patient with intractable angina and poor ventricular function who is not a candidate for surgery is referred for *salvage* angioplasty.

All strategies are designed to preserve myocardial function maximally if PTCA fails. This includes performing angioplasty first in vessels protected by collaterals. If sudden obstruction occurs, immediate surgery can be done. Staged procedures also are recommended, for instance, dilating the left anterior descending coronary first and other lesions at a subsequent procedure on another day after patency of the left anterior descending coronary is assured. With multistaged procedures the expense of angioplasty increases, and this must be taken into account.

The ultimate comparison of PTCA with bypass surgery in multivessel coronary artery disease awaits the outcome of the multiple randomized trials men-

138

tioned, the EAST, BARI, RITA, GABI, and CAPRI trials. From these trials clear advantages should be evident in comparable groups of patients for angioplasty and for surgical revascularization, and firm recommendations as to the form of revascularization in a given patient should be possible.

It is obvious from the patients' point of view that PTCA is the preferable procedure. Even with the high incidence of restenosis and especially the return of symptoms, with proper indications, repeat PTCA would be preferable to sending the patient to surgery; however, the cost advantages that PTCA affords depend upon how many times PTCA is needed, because with each procedure the cost and the total incidence of complications also increases. Depending upon the incidence of restenosis and the rate of progression of coronary atherosclerosis in the native vessels, a single bypass procedure might very well be more economical and better for the patient in the long run than multiple angioplasties.

With the use of the internal mammary artery as a bypass conduit already extending the excellent results of bypass surgery, and the widespread changes in diet and life style that can decrease the progression of coronary artery disease in the native and bypass vessels, even with the presently ongoing controlled trials, which have a limited follow-up period of 1 to 5 years, it may be difficult to prove which revascularization technique is better.

The problem with long-term controlled trials continues to be changing technology. The results of the trial are applicable to the patients selected and to the technical methods used in the trial. While the bypass surgery-versus-medical management trials have been proceeding, the type of patients, the types of surgical procedures, and the methods of myocardial preservation during surgery have changed, so that by the time the trials are reported, the claims that *that's not what we do now* and *the results do not apply to our present techniques of revascularization* have elements of truth. As has been known for a long time, it is difficult to hit a moving target.

Ultimately the results of these trials will pit technical advances in surgery against those in angioplasty. To be fair, the groups randomized must be comparable. The patients choosing not to be randomized must be characterized and followed in order to know the patient characterizations to which the results of the study apply. Finally, the follow-up must be long enough to really test the probably excellent, long-term results of a single bypass operation against the probability for the requirement of multiple angioplasties with their accompanying complications.

PART 2

Valvular Heart Disease

CHAPTER 8

Is the Mitral Valve Prolapse Patient at High Risk of Sudden Death Identifiable?

Paul Kligfield, M.D.
Richard B. Devereux, M.D.

The frequent occurrence of atrial and ventricular arrhythmias and the sporadic occurrence of sudden death have been associated with mitral valve prolapse since its early description.[1-6] Although it is intuitive that arrhythmias are the most likely immediate cause of sudden death in mitral valve prolapse, the relative prevalence and clinical correlates of arrhythmias in these subjects have been controversial, and their ability to predict mortality remains unknown. At the same time, other clinical features that have been suggested to predict sudden death in subjects with mitral prolapse have been found inconstantly in fatal cases.[7-9]

Inasmuch as mitral valve prolapse has been estimated to occur in up to four percent of the general adult population, seven million affected subjects may be found in the United States alone.[10,11] Although it is recognized that complications of mitral prolapse are uncommon, even a rare event in such a large population can affect a substantial number of people. Until accurate predictors of mortality are available for the general population of patients with mitral valve prolapse, uncertainty will remain a major feature of their management. This problem, of course, accounts for much of the controversy that surrounds clinical management of asymptomatic subjects with mitral prolapse. At the same time, a number of recent observations suggest that some patients with mitral valve prolapse at higher risk for sudden death can indeed be identified.[8]

Accordingly, this chapter will assess and integrate observations bearing on identification of sudden death risk in mitral valve prolapse:

1. What evidence suggests that sudden death is indeed a feature of mitral valve prolapse?
2. Can the incidence of sudden death in the general prolapse population be estimated?

143

3. What is the prevalence of complex atrial and ventricular arrhythmias in affected subjects?
4. What evidence is available to suggest that arrhythmias detected during routine evaluation are actually predictive of subsequent mortality in patients with mitral valve prolapse?
5. Can other findings consistently identify a subgroup of patients with mitral valve prolapse at high risk of sudden death?
6. Is there a rationale for antiarrhythmic therapy to reduce mortality in asymptomatic or minimally symptomatic patients with mitral valve prolapse?

WHAT EVIDENCE SUGGESTS THAT SUDDEN DEATH AND MALIGNANT ARRHYTHMIAS ARE FEATURES OF MITRAL VALVE PROLAPSE?

Mitral valve prolapse has been reported as the only autopsy finding in cases of sudden death[12,13] and the only detectable abnormality among survivors of cardiac arrest.[14-16] Wei and associates[14] found 10 patients with mitral prolapse and 10 otherwise normal subjects among 60 consecutive patients who were referred for electrophysiologic study of refractory, potentially fatal ventricular arrhythmias; and Somberg[15] has found 15 patients with isolated mitral prolapse and 72 otherwise normal subjects among approximately 900 patients referred for similar indications. The proportion of subjects with mitral valve prolapse in each series is significantly higher, relative to affected normals, than would be expected by chance alone.[11]

Despite such reports of occasional sudden death in patients with mitral valve prolapse, it is also quite clear that the actual occurrence of sudden death is rare.[1,17] Estimated mortality has ranged from 0 to as high as 0.5 percent per year,[8,17-19] but it must be appreciated that these populations are often highly selected by virtue of referral to cardiologists interested in the complications of mitral prolapse, and therefore these groups may be at higher risk than the general prolapse population.[20]

Duren and coworkers[19] found three cases of sudden death among 300 patients with mitral prolapse followed prospectively for a mean period of six years, from which yearly risk in this selected population can be estimated at approximately 0.2 percent. Of note, two of the three patients who died had evidence of important mitral regurgitation and were over 50 years of age, so that actual risk in hemodynamically uncomplicated cases may be even lower. Two younger men in this group, including the remaining case with subsequent sudden death, were successfully resuscitated from ventricular fibrillation. Interestingly, ventricular tachycardia was detected and suppressed in a surprisingly high 19 percent of this population. It is possible that this treatment might have contributed to the low mortality in these patients with advanced arrhythmias, but without control data this assumption is speculative.

Nishimura and colleagues[18] reported six cases of sudden death over six years among 237 subjects with mitral prolapse who were minimally symptomatic, in whom no clinical or echocardiographic findings suggestive of severe mitral regurgitation were present. This approximates an annual risk of just under 0.5 percent, which is twice the risk found in the general population in the Albany-Framingham studies.[21] However, most of these deaths occurred in older men with mitral prolapse, and autopsy exlcusion of coronary artery disease or other possible etiologies of these deaths is not available.

WHAT RISK FACTORS FOR SUDDEN DEATH HAVE BEEN SUGGESTED IN MITRAL VALVE PROLAPSE?

A number of potential risk factors have been proposed for the identification of subjects with mitral valve prolapse who are at risk for sudden death (Table 8–1). Because sudden death is most often an arrhythmic event, it has long been suspected that complex ventricular arrhythmias might play a role in mortality. Evidence supporting a role for repetitive ventricular arrhythmias is found among survivors of out-of-hospital cardiac arrest who have episodes of spontaneous nonsustained or inducible ventricular tachycardia.[14–16,22,23] However, although complex arrhythmias certainly occur among subjects with mitral valve prolapse,[24–26] the excess prevalence of these arrhythmias may not be as great as has been previously suspected in the general prolapse population.[27,28] It should be emphasized also that it remains to be demonstrated that these arrhythmias indeed are present prior to sudden death in a prognostically useful manner.

Recent evidence suggests that hemodynamically important mitral regurgitation, a complication affecting a small proportion of the general prolapse population, markedly increases the risk of sudden death in patients with mitral valve prolapse.[8,29–31] Inasmuch as it has been recognized that mitral regurgitation occurs more commonly in older men with mitral valve prolapse,[32–34] and inasmuch as it is also recognized independently that complex ventricular arrhythmias in the general population are more common in the older age groups,[35–38] it might be speculated that age, and perhaps also sex, might prove to be additional risk factors for sudden death in mitral valve prolapse. At the same time, it remains clear that occasional instances of sudden death occur in otherwise healthy young subjects with mitral valve prolapse.

Electrocardiographic findings, such as prolongation of the QT interval and inferior repolarization abnormalities, also have been suggested as potential markers for sudden death risk among subjects with mitral valve prolapse.[4–6,39,40] Although it has been demonstrated recently that QT prolongation may be no more common among the prolapse population than in the general population,[11,41] this observation does not exclude its potential contribution to the occurrence of arrhythmic death in some individuals. However, the demonstration of repolarization changes in only a rather small proportion of patients who have suffered sudden death and in a comparably small proportion of survivors of out-of-hospital cardiac arrest with mitral valve prolapse argues against a strong predictive value for these findings.[12,16]

Redundant, or thickened, mitral valve leaflets detected at echocardiography have been suggested by Nishimura and coworkers[18] to be highly sensitive for pre-

Table 8–1. Potential Risk Factors for Sudden Death in Mitral Valve Prolapse

Complex or repetitive ventricular arrhythmias
Mitral regurgitation
Prolonged QT interval
Inferolateral repolarization abnormalities
Redundant or thickened mitral leaflets
History of syncope, presyncope, palpitations
Older age; male gender

dicting subsequent complications, including sudden death, among a prospectively
followed mitral valve prolapse population. However, the sensitivity of this finding
for stratifying risk of sudden death has been questioned by its low prevalence
among resuscitated survivors of out-of-hospital cardiac arrest in whom mitral valve
prolapse is the only detectable abnormality.[16]

Finally, it has been suggested that syncope, presyncope, and symptomatic palpitations may identify a subset of the general prolapse population at increased risk
for sudden death. When related to sustained ventricular tachycardia, and certainly
in resuscitated survivors of cardiac arrest, these symptoms and signs may identify
individuals who need treatment, perhaps guided by electrophysiologic testing.[42-45] However, the sensitivity and specificity of these symptomatic findings
for identification of prolapse subjects at risk of sudden death remain unknown.

WHAT IS THE PREVALENCE OF ARRHYTHMIAS IN MITRAL VALVE PROLAPSE?

Arrhythmias are common in mitral valve prolapse.[7,24-28] Ventricular premature complexes have been reported in 58 to 89 percent of study populations, and
complex ventricular arrhythmias have been reported in 43 to 56 percent of the
subjects. Although the definition of ventricular arrhythmia complexity has varied
among studies, ventricular couplets have been reported in from 6 to 50 percent of
patients and nonsustained ventricular tachycardia has been found in 5 to 21 percent of these subjects (Table 8-2).

A number of problems affect these observations. First, it must be appreciated
that similar arrhythmias also occur in the general population,[38,46-49] so that disorders of impulse formation cannot necessarily be attributed to the presence of mitral
valve prolapse without appropriate control group studies. Second, selection bias
can increase arrhythmia prevalence in populations with mitral prolapse referred for
further study because of highly symptomatic palpitation or previous detection of

Table 8-2. Prevalence of Arrhythmias in Adult
Populations with Mitral Valve Prolapse, Detected by
Ambulatory Electrocardiography

		Arrhythmia Prevalence (%)			
	n	APCs	PAT	VPCs	Complex VPCs
Kramer et al[28]	63	81	32	63	43
Savage et al[27]	61	90	24	89	56
De Maria et al[24]	31	35	3	58	52
Campbell et al[25]	20	—	10	80	50
Winkle et al[26]	24	63	29	75	50

Adapted from Kramer et al.[28]

n = number of patients with mitral valve prolapse, APCs = atrial premature complexes, PAT = paroxysmal atrial tachycardia, VPCs = ventricular premature complexes; complex VPCs include VPC couplets and ventricular tachycardia with additional arrhythmias as defined in specific studies.

these arrhythmias themselves.[20,28,50] Finally, evidence is now available that complex arrhythmias are substantially more common in the small segment of the mitral prolapse population with associated significant mitral regurgitation,[29] the prevalence of which has varied in previously reported study groups.

The prevalence of ventricular arrhythmias detected by ambulatory electrocardiography in patients with mitral valve prolapse but no important mitral regurgitation, from the work of Kramer and associates,[28] is shown in Figure 8–1. Ventricular premature complexes occurred in nearly two thirds of 63 such subjects but were generally infrequent (with a mean density greater than 10 per 1000 total beats in only two subjects). Multiform ventricular premature complexes were found in more than one third of the total population, and three of 63 subjects had nonsustained ventricular tachycardia. However, in a similarly selected control population with comparable symptoms, the frequency and complexity of ventricular arrhythmias were quite similar. No significant differences in group prevalence of multiform ventricular ectopy, ventricular couplets, or nonsustained ventricular tachycardia were found.[28]

The similar prevalence of complex arrhythmias in unselected subjects with and without mitral valve prolapse was also observed by Savage and coworkers[27] among a cohort of offspring of the original Framingham population. Thus, when compared with similarly selected symptomatic control subjects, or with similarly asymptomatic randomly selected controls, patients with mitral valve prolapse do not appear to have the substantial excess of complex ventricular arrhythmias suggested in early reports.

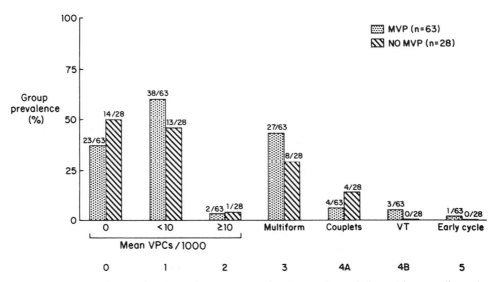

Figure 8–1. Group prevalence of ventricular arrhythmias detected by ambulatory electrocardiography in subjects with mitral valve prolapse and in similarly symptomatic controls. Each subject is represented once in the appropriate mean ventricular premature complex (VPC) density group, and once in each complexity category when multiform VPCs, VPC couplets, ventricular tachycardia, or early cycle forms occurred. Thus, each bar represents the proportion of subjects having the arrhythmia frequency or complexity indicated below. No significant differences were found between prolapse and control subjects. (From Kramer, et al,[28] with permission.)

HOW OFTEN CAN SUDDEN DEATH BE ATTRIBUTED TO MITRAL VALVE PROLAPSE IN UNSELECTED POPULATIONS?

Epidemiologic data regarding mortality among unselected subjects with mitral valve prolapse are scarce.[8,9] Among forensic necropsies in London, Davies and colleagues[13] found 13 cases of unexpected death associated only with mitral valve prolapse during a five-year search. Of note, more than two thirds of these cases (9 of 13) were associated with evidence of significant mitral regurgitation, a finding that provides our best insight into the relative risk of mortality in this important subgroup. Interestingly, a similar proportion of sudden deaths was associated with important mitral regurgitation in the prospective follow-up by Duren and associates.[19]

Unfortunately, Davies and colleagues[13] did not report the total number of deaths during the period of their study or the size of the total population in which these deaths occurred. However, it was noted that during the same period approximately 1250 cases of sudden death due to underlying coronary artery disease were found at autopsy. From this observation it can be inferred that approximately 10 cases of sudden death associated with mitral valve prolapse might be found for every 1000 deaths due to coronary artery disease in the general population. Based on the observations of Davies and colleagues,[13] supported by those of Duren and associates,[19] perhaps two thirds of the mitral prolapse sudden deaths might occur in patients who also have hemodynamically significant mitral regurgitation, whereas one third might occur in prolapse patients without evidence of mitral insufficiency.

These approximations can be used to estimate the risk of sudden death in unselected populations of prolapse patients with and without mitral regurgitation.[8] Although considerable error is likely to exist in these calculations, useful conclusions can be drawn regarding the relative risk of mortality among subsets of patients with mitral valve prolapse.

WHAT IS THE RISK OF SUDDEN DEATH IN UNSELECTED POPULATIONS OF MITRAL VALVE PROLAPSE PATIENTS WITHOUT IMPORTANT MITRAL REGURGITATION?

It has been estimated that there are 400,000 sudden deaths due to coronary artery disease each year in the United States.[23] Based on the approximations provided by the findings of Davies and coworkers,[13] if slightly more than three sudden deaths were to occur in patients with mitral valve prolapse and no mitral regurgitation for every 1000 deaths due to coronary disease, we would expect approximately 1300 sudden deaths in patients with mitral valve prolapse who have no important mitral regurgitation to occur each year in the United States.

Based on a 4 percent prevalence of mitral valve prolapse among the 180 million adults in the United States,[10,11,51] the adult population of mitral prolapse subjects approaches seven million. Inasmuch as 4 percent or fewer of these subjects with mitral prolapse have prognostically important mitral regurgitation,[10,11] the estimated 1300 sudden deaths within this population would translate to an annual risk of sudden death among mitral valve prolapse subjects who do not have significant mitral regurgitation of 1.9 per 10,000 (approximately 0.02 percent per year).[8]

For the purpose of comparison, the annual risk of sudden death among the entire adult US population can be estimated at approximately 22 per 10,000 (0.22 percent per year), an overall mortality that is predominantly due to coronary artery disease in the United States.[23] For further comparison, the annual risk of sudden death among 45- to 54-year-old subjects with no clinical evidence of coronary artery disease in the combined Albany-Framingham population[21] has been reported as 7 per 10,000 (0.07 percent per year). Thus, the estimated risk of sudden death potentially attributable to uncomplicated mitral valve prolapse appears to be far less than the risk attributable to known or unsuspected coronary disease in the general adult population, and even less than the annual sudden death risk reported in otherwise apparently normal middle-aged adults.

The low estimated sudden death risk among patients with mitral valve prolapse who have no important mitral regurgitation is certainly compatible with the general impression in clinical practice that uncomplicated mitral valve prolapse is inherently a rather benign finding. Thus, for example, based on this estimated risk, a physician caring for 100 unselected subjects with mitral valve prolapse and no mitral regurgitation would be unlikely to see a case of unexpected sudden death in this group during a 25-year period. This is consistent with the absence of apparent primary arrhythmic death found by Allen and associates[17] during a 14-year retrospective follow-up of 62 patients with isolated late systolic murmurs compatible with underlying mitral prolapse and minimal regurgitation.

Although it might be argued from these estimates that the risk of sudden death in uncomplicated mitral valve prolapse might indeed be unrelated to the presence of prolapse itself, other arguments noted previously support the reality of attributable risk in this situation. The apparent excess prevalence of subjects with even uncomplicated mitral valve prolapse among survivors of out-of-hospital cardiac arrest and among patients referred for electrophysiologic study of refractory, potentially life-threatening cardiac arrhythmias cannot be explained easily as coincidence.

Furthermore, a low risk is not inconsistent with substantial epidemiologic importance of this problem among the general prolapse population, inasmuch as the same estimates may still account for 1300 total deaths yearly in the United States, even in this rather prognostically benign group.[8] These seemingly discordant impressions are entirely compatible, of course, because of the high prevalence of mitral valve prolapse itself in the general populaton.[1,11]

IMPLICATIONS OF TREATMENT OF COMPLEX ARRHYTHMIAS IN PATIENTS WITH MITRAL VALVE PROLAPSE WHO DO NOT HAVE IMPORTANT MITRAL REGURGITATION

Estimated mortality due to sudden death in mitral valve prolapse can be combined with data regarding prevalence of arrhythmias in these subjects to examine the logistics and consequences of any attempt to prevent sudden death by antiarrhythmic drug treatment in patients with mitral valve prolapse.[8] Based on 1300 cases of sudden death each year in the United States occurring among 7 million adults with mitral valve prolapse, together with a 50 percent group prevalence of complex ventricular ectopy (defined as either multiform or repetitive ventricular premature complexes), it can be estimated that approximately 2500 prolapse subjects with complex ventricular ectopy would require treatment for one year to prevent one episode of sudden death.

If treatment were restricted to the 8 to 9 percent of subjects with more complex repetitive forms (ventricular couplets, ventricular salvos, or ventricular tachycardia), then approximately 300 people with these repetitive forms would require treatment to prevent one episode of sudden death each year. In this context, it is speculative to conclude that the low incidence of sudden death found by Duren and associates[19] among prolapse subjects with treated ventricular tachycardia is the result of arrhythmia suppression. It is also apparent from these estimates that the potential role of antiarrhythmic therapy for reducing the occurrence of sudden death in mitral valve prolapse can be answerable only by means of a prospective, controlled study of large, multicenter proportion.

Of course, these estimates also are based on the assumption that complex arrhythmias in fatal cases are indeed present prior to death, that antiarrhythmic drug therapy is completely effective to prevent sudden death, and that, importantly, there is no offsetting proarrhythmic drug effect or other side effects that might make treatment more dangerous than no treatment in this population. Unfortunately, each of these assumptions can be seriously questioned.

No long-term data exist to demonstrate that complex arrhythmias are highly sensitive or predictive for subsequent mortality among patients with mitral valve prolapse who do not have mitral regurgitation. Mortality in these subjects might alternatively result from a unique and perhaps random clustering of other pathophysiologic events leading to fatal arrhythmogenesis.[7,12,52–54] In addition, there is no conclusive evidence that antiarrhythmic drug therapy is effective for the prevention of sudden death, as distinguished from the suppression of arrhythmias, in mitral prolapse. Finally, the estimated 5 to 15 percent proarrhythmic effect[55] of many currently used drugs might, in theory, do more harm in otherwise uncomplicated subjects with mitral prolapse who have complex arrhythmias than their projected benefits would justify.

Available data suggest that the prognostic value of electrophysiologic testing in patients with mitral valve prolapse who do not have sustained ventricular tachycardia is limited.[42–45] Combined with the low incidence of sudden death in this group, these findings suggest that these methods alone are unlikely to provide a general solution to the problem of identifying prolapse patients at risk of arrhythmic mortality.

WHAT IS THE RISK OF SUDDEN DEATH IN MITRAL VALVE PROLAPSE PATIENTS WITH IMPORTANT MITRAL REGURGITATION?

Based on available evidence, it appears that the risk of sudden death in patients with mitral valve prolapse is significantly higher when hemodynamically severe mitral regurgitation develops as a complication.[8,29–31] The data of Davies and colleagues[13] suggest that slightly fewer than seven cases of sudden death due to mitral valve prolapse associated with severe mitral regurgitation might occur for every 1000 sudden deaths due to coronary artery disease. Concentration of sudden death risk among prolapse patients with mitral regurgitation is supported by the observations of Duren and associates.[19] Accordingly, based on the 400,000 deaths due to coronary artery disease reported each year in the United States, approximately 2700 sudden deaths might be expected each year in this country among mitral valve prolapse patients who have hemodynamically important mitral regurgitation.

This is a fairly large number of deaths, concentrated in a rather small proportion of the general prolapse population. Based on a 2 to 4 percent prevalence of significant mitral regurgitation among subjects with mitral valve prolapse,[10,11] the annual risk of sudden death in this subset can be estimated at 94 to 188 per 10,000 (in the range of 1 to 2 percent per year). Therefore, compared with the estimated risk of sudden death in uncomplicated mitral prolapse subjects of 1.9 per 10,000 per year, the risk of sudden death when mitral regurgitation complicates mitral valve prolapse may be 50 to 100 times greater.[8]

This striking concentration of risk for sudden death suggests that more than half of the mortality associated with mitral valve prolapse may occur in a subset comprising less than five percent of the total prolapse population. Although mitral regurgitation as a complication of mitral valve prolapse is more common in older men,[32-34] and it is generally appreciated that the frequency and complexity of ventricular arrhythmias also tend to increase with age,[38] the relationship of age and sex to risk of sudden death among subjects with mitral valve prolapse remains to be established. In this context, it is relevant to note that two-thirds of the cases of sudden death reported by Nishimura and coworkers[18] during a longitudinal follow-up of a large prolapse population occurred in men over the age of 50 years, even though no clinical evidence of hemodynamically severe mitral regurgitation was reported in this group.

ARE COMPLEX ARRHYTHMIAS IN MITRAL PROLAPSE MORE PREVALENT WHEN SEVERE MITRAL REGURGITATION IS PRESENT?

Group prevalence of the frequency and complexity of ventricular arrhythmias in patients with mitral valve prolapse, with and without mitral regurgitation, and in patients with mitral regurgitation of other etiologies, is shown in Figure 8-2.[29] In contrast to mitral prolapse subjects with no important mitral regurgitation, all patients with mitral prolapse complicated by severe mitral regurgitation had ventricular premature complexes, and the ventricular ectopy was significantly more likely to be frequent than rare. Approximately 80 percent of prolapse subjects with complicating mitral regurgitation had multiform ventricular premature complexes, more than two thirds had ventricular couplets, and nearly one third had ventricular salvos or brief bursts of nonsustained ventricular tachycardia detected by ambulatory electrocardiography. Each of these complex forms was significantly more prevalent among patients with mitral valve prolapse when mitral regurgitation was present (Table 8-3).

However, the frequency and complexity of ventricular arrhythmias in mitral prolapse patients with mitral regurgitation were nearly identical to those in a group of patients with comparably severe mitral regurgitation that was unassociated with mitral valve prolapse.[29] These findings suggest that the complex arrhythmias found among prolapse patients with mitral regurgitation are more directly related to the hemodynamic load imposed by valvular insufficiency than to the presence of mitral valve prolapse itself.

Taken together, the concentration of risk for sudden death among prolapse

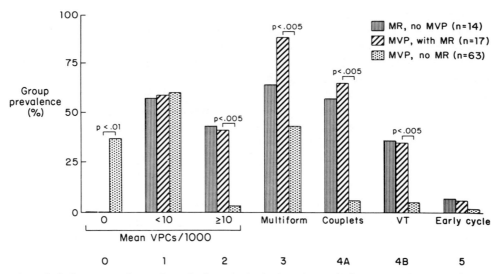

Figure 8–2. Group prevalence of ventricular arrhythmias in patients with important mitral regurgitation, with and without underlying mitral prolapse, contrasted with arrhythmias in prolapse subjects without mitral regurgitation. Definitions as in Figure 8–1. Arrhythmia frequency and complexity is greater when mitral regurgitation complicates mitral prolapse, but these features are independent of the etiology of mitral regurgitation. (From Kligfield, et al,[29] with permission.)

Table 8–3. Prevalence of Ventricular Arrhythmias in Mitral Valve Prolapse, with and without Mitral Regurgitation

	MVP Subgroups		
	MVP − MR (n = 63)	MVP + MR (n = 17)	P
VPC Frequency			
No VPCs	37% (23/63)	0% (0/17)	<0.01
Mean > 10/1000	3% (2/63)	41% (7/17)	<0.005
VPC Complexity			
Multiform VPCs	43% (27/63)	88% (15/17)	<0.005
VPC couplets	6% (4/63)	65% (11/17)	<0.005
VPC salvos/VT	5% (3/63)	35% (6/17)	<0.005
Peak Lown Grade			
0–2	58% (36/63)	6% (1/17)	<0.001
3	33% (21/63)	24% (4/17)	ns
4A	3% (2/63)	35% (6/17)	<0.005
4B	5% (3/63)	29% (5/17)	<0.005
5	2% (1/63)	6% (1/17)	ns

Adapted from Kligfield et al.[29]

MR = mitral regurgitation, MVP = mitral valve prolapse, VPC = ventricular premature complex, VT = ventricular tachycardia.

patients with mitral regurgitation and the higher prevalence of complex ventricular arrhythmias provide suggestive evidence for arrhythmic mortality in this population.[8] Although the sensitivity, specificity, and predictive value of complex arrhythmias for subsequent sudden death have not been established in a pure population of patients with severe mitral regurgitation due to mitral valve prolapse, recent data have addressed this issue in patients with mitral regurgitation of diverse etiologies.[30,31]

HOW DO ARRHYTHMIA COMPLEXITY AND VENTRICULAR FUNCTION RELATE TO MORTALITY IN MITRAL REGURGITATION?

Selected observations among patients with coronary artery disease,[56–59] particularly those after myocardial infarction, and in patients with ischemic and non-ischemic dilated cardiomyopathy,[60–62] have suggested that both ventricular dysfunction and complex ventricular arrhythmias may be independent risk factors for mortality and, in particular, for sudden death. This model for risk stratification has been applied recently to patients with hemodynamically important mitral regurgitation of diverse etiologies.[31] Although mitral valve prolapse is currently emerging as the most common cause of severe pure mitral regurgitation among adults in the United States,[63,64] the relatively small number of prolapse patients with marked ventricular dysfunction in any single series has so far precluded meaningful analysis of similar data in prolapse subjects alone.

Two-year mortality in medically treated patients with hemodynamically severe mitral regurgitation[31] is shown in relation to etiology, arrhythmia complexity, and ventricular function in Table 8–4. Arrhythmia complexity was defined by serial ambulatory electrocardiography, and any frequency of single ventricular premature complexes, including multiform ventricular ectopy, was considered to represent a simple arrhythmia. Complex ventricular arrhythmias in these patients were defined as repetitive ventricular forms, comprising only ventricular couplets, ventricular salvos, or brief bursts of nonsustained ventricular tachycardia. Ventricular function in these patients was considered abnormal when either left ventricular ejection fraction was less than 45 percent or right ventricular ejection fraction was less than 30 percent.[30]

Two-year mortality in these patients was strikingly related to the presence of abnormal ventricular function and occurred in 4 of the 6 patients with subnormal ejection fraction but in none of the 25 patients with normal ventricular function.[31] Because of the high prevalence of repetitive ventricular arrhythmias in this population, the predictive value of arrhythmias alone for mortality was low. Furthermore, the single patient with subnormal ventricular function who had only simple arrhythmias precludes even speculation regarding the possible role of rhythm stability in survival. However, such speculation would be consistent with the observation in patients with dilated cardiomyopathy that absence of repetitive ventricular arrhythmias is associated with a more favorable short-term prognosis even when ventricular function is poor.[60,62]

Of note, three of the four deaths in this population were either witnessed or inferred sudden cardiac arrest, including the one patient in this group with underlying mitral valve prolapse who died a witnessed sudden death while playing tennis. Therefore, although these data do not demonstrate a high predictive value of repet-

Table 8–4. Mortality in Patients with Mitral Regurgitation, with
and without Mitral Valve Prolapse, according to Ventricular
Function and Ventricular Arrhythmia

	MR with MVP (n = 15)		MR with Other Etiology (n = 16)	
	Simple Ventricular Arrhythmias	Repetitive Ventricular Arrhythmias	Simple Ventricular Arrhythmias	Repetitive Ventricular Arrhythmias
Normal or not importantly depressed RVEF and LVEF	0/3	0/11	0/5	0/6
Importantly depressed RVEF or LVEF	0/0	1/1*	0/1	3/4†

*Witnessed sudden death.

†Sudden death (witnessed and inferred) in two of three deaths.

MR = mitral regurgitation, MVP = mitral valve prolapse, RVEF = right ventricular ejection fraction, LVEF = left ventricular ejection fraction.

From Kligfield et al,[31] with permission of the publisher.

itive ventricular arrhythmias for subsequent sudden death in mitral regurgitation, they do demonstrate that these complex arrhythmias were indeed present prior to mortality in all patients who died. These findings also suggest the fascinating possibility that repetitive ventricular arrhythmias alone, in the absence of ventricular dysfunction, are not strongly predictive of death in mitral prolapse even when complicated by mitral regurgitation (see Table 8–4).

SUDDEN DEATH AND ARRHYTHMIAS IN MITRAL VALVE PROLAPSE: AN OVERVIEW

Available evidence suggests that sudden death does occur, but quite uncommonly, in patients with mitral valve prolapse who do not have significant mitral regurgitation. In contrast, the risk of sudden death appears to be highly concentrated, by perhaps 50- to 100-fold, in patients with mitral valve prolapse complicated by severe mitral regurgitation. These patients also can be shown to have a high prevalence of complex ventricular arrhythmias.

When complex ventricular arrhythmias are associated with important ventricular dysfunction in patients with mitral prolapse who have mitral regurgitation, the risk of sudden arrhythmic death appears to be high. At the same time, complex ventricular arrhythmias alone, in the absence of ventricular dysfunction, may not in and of themselves be highly predictive for sudden death in prolapse patients who have mitral regurgitation. Surgical management of patients with prolapse who have severe mitral regurgitation with ventricular dysfunction may be more effective for prevention of sudden death than antiarrhythmic therapy.[30]

Although sudden death is ultimately an arrhythmic event, complex arrhythmias have not been shown to predict mortality in unselected populations of subjects with mitral valve prolapse who have no associated mitral regurgitation. Other associated findings of potential predictive value for sudden death in mitral valve prolapse—such as QT interval prolongation, inferior repolarization changes, and thickened mitral leaflets—are only inconstantly present in subjects with mitral valve prolapse who have died suddenly or who have been resuscitated from otherwise fatal cardiac arrest. Large, multicenter prospective studies will be required to identify which patients with uncomplicated mitral valve prolapse are at risk for sudden death, if this is indeed possible prior to the fatal event.

It is evident, therefore, that until accurate predictors of sudden death are available, antiarrhythmic intervention designed to reduce mortality cannot be accurately targeted in a large proportion of prolapse subjects. As a result, the risk of drug treatment of arrhythmias may exceed the estimated mortality in asymptomatic subjects with uncomplicated mitral prolapse.

REFERENCES

1. Devereux, RB, Perloff, JK, Reichek, N, et al: Mitral valve prolapse. Circulation 54:3, 1976.
2. Hancock, EW and Cohn, K: The syndrome associated with midsystolic click and late systolic murmur. Am J Med 41:183, 1966.
3. Pocock, WA and Barlow, JB: Etiology and electrocardiographic features of the billowing posterior mitral leaflet syndrome. Am J Med 51:731, 1971.
4. Shappell, SD, Marshall, CE, Brown, RE, et al: Sudden death and the familial occurrence of midsystolic click, late systolic murmur syndrome. Circulation 48:1128, 1973.
5. Winkle, RA, Lopes, MG, Popp, RL, et al: Life-threatening arrhythmias in the mitral valve prolapse syndrome. Am J Med 60:961, 1976.
6. Jeresaty, RM: Sudden death in the mitral valve prolapse-click syndrome (editorial). Am J Cardiol 37:317, 1976.
7. Kligfield, P and Devereux, RB: Arrhythmias in mitral valve prolapse. Clin Prog Electrophysiol Pacing 3:403, 1985.
8. Kligfield, P, Levy, D, Devereux, RB, et al: Arrhythmias and sudden death in mitral valve prolapse. Am Heart J 113:1298, 1987.
9. Boudoulas, H, Kligfield, P, and Wooley, CF: Mitral valve prolapse: Sudden death. In Boudoulas, H and Wooley, CF: Mitral Valve Prolapse and the Mitral Valve Prolapse Syndrome. Futura Publishing, Mt Kisco, NY, 1988, pp 591–605.
10. Devereux, RB, Kramer-Fox, R, Shear, MK, et al: Diagnosis and classification of severity of mitral valve prolapse: Methodologic, biologic, and prognostic considerations. Am Heart J 113:1265, 1987.
11. Levy, D and Savage, D: Prevalence and clinical features of mitral valve prolapse. Am Heart J 113:1281, 1987.
12. Chesler, E, King, RA, and Edwards, JE: The myxomatous mitral valve and sudden death. Circulation 67:632, 1983.
13. Davies, MJ, Moore, BP, and Braimbridge, MV: The floppy mitral valve: Study of incidence, pathology, and complications in surgical, necropsy, and forensic material. Br Heart J 40:468, 1978.
14. Wei, JY, Bulkley, BH, Schaeffer, AH, et al: Mitral-valve prolapse syndrome and recurrent ventricular tachyarrhythmias: A malignant variant refractory to conventional drug therapy. Ann Intern Med 89:6, 1978.
15. Somberg, JC: Personal communication, 1987.
16. Boudoulas, H, Schaal, SF, Stang, JM, et al: Mitral valve prolapse-sudden death with long term survival (abstr). J Am Coll Cardiol 7:29A, 1986.
17. Allen, H, Harris, A, and Leatham, A: Significance and prognosis of an isolated late systolic murmur. Br Heart J 36:525, 1974.
18. Nishimura, RA, McGoon, MD, Shub, C, et al: Echocardiographically documented mitral-valve prolapse. N Engl J Med 313:1305, 1985.
19. Duren, DR, Becker, AE, and Dunning, AJ: Long-term follow-up of idiopathic mitral valve prolapse in 300 patients: A prospective study. J Am Coll Cardiol 11:42, 1988.

20. Motulsky, AG: Biased ascertainment and the natural history of diseases. N Engl J Med 298:1196, 1978.
21. Kannel, WB, Doyle, JT, McNamara, PM, et al: Precursors of sudden coronary death: Factors related to the incidence of sudden death. Circulation 51:606, 1975.
22. Myerburg, RJ, Conde, CA, Sung, RJ, et al: Clinical, electrophysiologic and hemodynamic profile of patients resuscitated from prehospital cardiac arrest. Am J Med 68:568, 1980.
23. Ruskin, JN, DiMarco, JP, and Garan, H: Out-of-hospital cardiac arrest. Electrophysiologic observations and selection of long-term antiarrhythmic therapy. N Engl J Med 303:607, 1980.
24. DeMaria, AN, Amsterdam, EA, Vismara, LA, et al: Arrhythmias in the mitral valve prolapse syndrome: Prevalence, nature, and frequency. Ann Intern Med 84:656, 1976.
25. Campbell, RWF, Godman, MG, Fiddler, GI, et al: Ventricular arrhythmias in syndrome of balloon deformity of mitral valve: Definition of possible high risk group. Br Heart J 38:1053, 1976.
26. Winkle, RA, Lopes, MG, Fitzgerald, JW, et al: Arrhythmias in patients with mitral valve prolapse. Circulation 52:73, 1975.
27. Savage, DD, Levy, DL, Garrison, RJ, et al: Mitral valve prolapse in the general population, part 3: Dysrhythmias. The Framingham Study. Am Heart J 106:582, 1983.
28. Kramer, HM, Kligfield, P, Devereux, RB, et al: Arrhythmias in mitral valve prolapse: Effect of selection bias. Arch Intern Med 144:2360, 1984.
29. Kligfield, P, Hochreiter, C, Kramer, H, et al: Complex arrhythmias in mitral regurgitation with and without mitral valve prolapse: Contrast to arrhythmias in mitral valve prolapse without mitral regurgitation. Am J Cardiol 55:1545, 1985.
30. Hochreiter, C, Niles, N, Devereux, RB, et al: Mitral regurgitation: Relationship of noninvasive descriptors of right and left ventricular performance to clinical and hemodynamic findings and to prognosis in medically and surgically treated patients. Circulation 73:900, 1986.
31. Kligfield, P, Hochreiter, C, Niles, N, et al: Relation of sudden death in pure mitral regurgitation, with and without mitral valve prolapse, to repetitive ventricular arrhythmias and right and left ventricular ejection fractions. Am J Cardiol 60:397, 1987.
32. Devereux, RB, Hawkins, I, Kramer-Fox, R, et al: Complications of mitral valve prolapse: Disproportionate occurrence in men and older patients. Am J Med 81:751, 1986.
33. Wilcken, DEL and Hickey, AJ: Lifetime risk for patients with mitral valve prolapse of developing severe valve regurgitation requiring surgery. Circulation 78:10, 1988.
34. Devereux, RB: Mitral valve prolapse and severe mitral regurgitation (editorial). Circulation 78:234, 1988.
35. Glasser, SP, Clark, PI, and Applebaum, HJ: Occurrence of frequent complex arrhythmias detected by ambulatory monitoring: Findings in an apparently healthy asymptomatic elderly population. Chest 75:565, 1979.
36. Camm, AJ, Evans, KE, Ward, ED, et al: The rhythm of the heart in active elderly subjects. Am Heart J 99:598, 1980.
37. Kantelip, J-P, Sage, E, and Duchene-Marullaz, P: Findings on ambulatory electrocardiographic monitoring in subjects older than 80 years. Am J Cardiol 57:398, 1986.
38. Kligfield, P: Clinical applications of ambulatory electrocardiography. Cardiology 71:69, 1984.
39. Bekheit, SG, Ali, AA, Deglin, SM, et al: Analysis of QT interval in patients with idiopathic mitral valve prolapse. Chest 81:620, 1982.
40. Puddu, PE, Pasternac, A, Tubau, JF, et al: QT intérval prolongation and increased plasma catecholamine levels in patients with mitral valve prolapse. Am Heart J 105:422, 1983.
41. Cowan, MD and Fye, WB: Prevalence of QTc prolongation in women with mitral valve prolapse. Am J Cardiol 63:133, 1989.
42. Engel, TR, Meister, SG, and Frankl, WS: Ventricular extrastimulation in the mitral valve prolapse syndrome: Evidence for ventricular reentry. J Electrocardiol 11:137, 1978.
43. Morady, F, Shen, E, Bhandari, A, et al: Programmed ventricular stimulation in mitral valve prolapse: Analysis of 36 patients. Am J Cardiol 53:135, 1984.
44. Rosenthal, ME, Hamer, A, Gang, ES, et al: The yield of programmed ventricular stimulation in mitral valve prolapse patients with ventricular arrhythmias. Am Heart J 110:970, 1985.
45. Naccarelli, GV, Prystowsky, EN, Jackman, WM, et al: Role of electrophysiologic testing in managing patients who have ventricular tachycardia unrelated to coronary artery disease. Am J Cardiol 50:165, 1982.
46. Southall, DP, Johnston, F, Shinebourne, EA, et al: 24-hour electrocardiographic study of heart rate and rhythm patterns in population of healthy children. Br Heart J 45:281, 1981.

47. Brodsky, M, Wu, D, Denes, P, et al: Arrhythmias documented by 24 hour continuous electrocardiographic monitoring in 50 male medical students without apparent heart disease. Am J Cardiol 39:390, 1977.
48. Sobotka, PA, Mayer, JH, Bauernfeind, RA, et al: Arrhythmias documented by 24-hour continuous ambulatory electrocardiographic monitoring in young women without apparent heart disease. Am Heart J 101:753, 1981.
49. Hinkle, LE, Carver, ST, and Stevens, M: The frequency of asymptomatic disturbances of cardiac rhythm and conduction in middle-aged men. Am J Cardiol 24:629, 1969.
50. Alpert, JS: Association between arrhythmias and mitral valve prolapse (editorial). Arch Intern Med 144:2333, 1984.
51. Savage, DD, Garrison, RJ, Devereux, RB, et al: Mitral valve prolapse in the general population. I. Epidemiologic features: The Framingham Study. Am Heart J 106:571, 1983.
52. Wit, AL and Cranefield, PF: Triggered activity in cardiac muscle fibers of the simian mitral valve. Circ Res 38:85, 1976.
53. Ware, JA, Magro, SA, Luck, JC, et al: Conduction system abnormalities in symptomatic mitral valve prolapse: An electrophysiologic analysis of 60 patients. Am J Cardiol 53:1075, 1984.
54. Mason, JW, Kock, FH, Billingham, ME, et al: Cardiac biopsy evidence of a cardiomyopathy associated with symptomatic mitral valve prolapse. Am J Cardiol 42:557, 1978.
55. Velebit, V, Podrid, P, Lown, B, et al: Aggravation and provocation of ventricular arrhythmias by antiarrhythmic drugs. Circulation 65:886, 1982.
56. Schulze, RA, Strauss, HW, and Pitt, B: Sudden death in the year following myocardial infarction: Relation to ventricular premature contractions in the late hospital phase and left ventricular ejection fraction. Am J Med 62:192, 1977.
57. Ruberman, W, Weinblatt, E, Goldberg, JD, et al: Ventricular premature beats and mortality after myocardial infarction. N Engl J Med 14:750, 1977.
58. Bigger, JT, Heller, CA, Wenger, TL, et al: Risk stratification after acute myocardial infarction. Am J Cardiol 42:202, 1978.
59. Ruberman, W, Weinblatt, E, Goldberg, JD, et al: Ventricular premature complexes and sudden death after myocardial infarction. Circulation 64:297, 1981.
60. Holmes, JR, Kubo, SH, Cody, RJ, et al: Arrhythmias in ischemic and nonischemic dilated cardiomyopathy: Prediction of mortality by ambulatory electrocardiography. Am J Cardiol 55:146, 1985.
61. Meinertz, T, Hofmann, T, Kasper, W, et al: Significance of ventricular arrhythmias in idiopathic dilated cardiomyopathy. Am J Cardiol 53:902, 1984.
62. Romeo, F, Pelliccia, F, Cianfrocca, C, et al: Predictors of sudden death in idiopathic dilated cardiomyopathy. Am J Cardiol 63:138, 1989.
63. Waller, BF, Morrow, AG, Maron, BJ, et al: Etiology of clinically isolated severe, chronic, pure mitral regurgitation: Analysis of 97 patients over 30 yeras of age having mitral valve replacement. Am Heart J 104:276, 1982.
64. Olson, LJ, Subramanian, R, Ackermann, DM, et al: Surgical pathology of the mitral valve: A study of 712 cases spanning 21 years. Mayo Clin Proc 62:22, 1987.

Commentary

By Melvin D. Cheitlin, M.D.

Mitral valve prolapse continues to be a challenging problem to the practicing physician. Unlike other disease, it is identified frequently by physical examination or perhaps too frequently—given the uncertain criteria for diagnosis—by echocardiography. Of the complications of mitral valve prolapse, that of progression to severe mitral regurgitation is most important, and mitral valve prolapse is now recognized as the most common etiology for severe isolated mitral regurgitation requiring mitral valve surgery. Other complications, such as the development of infective endocarditis and thromboemboli, are less frquent, and evidence is accumulating that those patients most susceptible to these complications are those with thickened myxomatous valves as seen by echocardiography.[1-3] It is generally agreed that patients with mitral regurgitation should receive prophylactic antibiotics at the time of bacteremia and that patients with transient cerebral ischemic episodes should receive antiplatelet drugs or anticoagulants.

The major complication that still perplexes the physician is that of asymptomatic ventricular arrhythmias, especially frequent early premature ventricular contractions or runs of nonsustained ventricular tachycardia, because it is generally believed that these arrhythmias may be precursors to the much rarer catastrophe of sudden death.

It is generally agreed that unpleasant symptomatic ventricular arrhythmias should be suppressed, and patients with sustained ventricular tachycardia or with arrhythmia-related syncope or arrhythmia requiring resuscitation should be evaluated by electrophysiologic studies and appropriate antiarrhythmic drugs should be instituted. The patient with asymptomatic, high-grade ventricular ectopy remains a problem. To believe that these arrhythmias predict the patient is at risk of sudden death, and that suppression of these arrhythmias will prevent this tragedy is tempting; however, these complex ventricular beats are extremely frequent, occurring in about 50 percent of patients, and sudden death is very uncommon. With the known proarrhythmic effect of antiarrhythmic drugs in 10 to 20 percent of cases, more harm that good would probably come from treating these complex arrhythmias in all patients.

In this chapter Kligfield and Devereux review other factors that have been implicated as risk factors for high-grade arrhythmias or sudden death. They have shown that patients with severe mitral regurgitation with and without mitral valve prolapse have high-grade ectopy, and they suggest that perhaps it is the patient with both high-grade ectopy and severe mitral regurgitation who is at risk. They refer to the study of Davies and colleagues,[4] in which 8 of 13 of the sudden-death patients with mitral valve prolapse had evidence of probable severe mitral regurgitation. However, in the reported cases of patients with mitral valve prolapse resuscitated from sudden arrest, mitral regurgitation is not always or even frequently a prominent factor.

A more interesting observation is that of the association of poor left ventricular function and high-grade ectopy as a risk factor for sudden death. This is consistent with what is known of high-grade ectopy in coronary artery disease and cardiomyopathy; that is, those patients after myocardial infarct with high-grade ectopy and poor left ventricular function are at the greatest risk of sudden death. In the study quoted in this chapter by Kligfield and colleagues[5] that related decreased ventricular function and sudden death in patients with mitral regurgitation, all but one patient who died suddenly had a diagnosis other than mitral valve prolapse. The problem is how to differentiate the patient with mitral regurgitation causing poor left ventricular function from the patient with poor left ventricular function causing mitral regurgitation.

In identifying the group of patients with mitral valve prolapse at highest risk of complications, perhaps including sudden death, most compelling is the evidence by Nishimura and colleagues[2] of the myxomatous thickened valve as the marker of significant disease. A study reported by Marks and colleagues[3] substantiates the observation that the thickened leaflet is the best marker of risk for complications. In this paper, no sudden deaths were reported, but endocarditis, severe mitral regurgitation, and requirement for mitral valve replacement occurred in 62 of 319 patients with thickened valves, compared with 1 of 137 patients with thin valves. The incidence of stroke was the same whether the valve was thickened or not.

In hearts that I have examined of patients who have died with the complications of mitral valve prolapse, including several with sudden death, I have been impressed with the thickened myxomatous valve as being present most of the time. Jeresaty[6] also has mentioned the thickened myxomatous valves he has seen in most hearts of patients with mitral valve prolapse who have died suddenly.

In the sudden-death literature, mitral valve prolapse is not a prominent diagnosis. In young people the common etiology is hypertrophic cardiomyopathy and, to a lesser extent, coronary artery anomalies. In older patients it is overwhelmingly coronary artery disease. Given the prevalence of mitral valve prolapse in the population, the risk of sudden death in any patient must be extremely small. In any sudden death population, 10 percent are found to have no gross anatomic abnormality and presumably have had an electrophysiologic basis for the fatal arrhythmia. Certainly, as Kligfield and Devereux point out, mitral valve prolapse has been found in patients dying suddenly; however, as shown by the studies of Davies[4] and Lucas[7] and their colleagues the incidence in consecutive autopsies of mitral valve prolapse is 4 to 7 percent. Therefore, even if there were no etiologic association between the sudden death and the mitral valve prolapse, we would expect to find mitral valve prolapse coincidentally in 4 to 7 percent of patients dying suddenly. Only if the incidence of mitral valve prolapse exceeded this could we say that the mitral valve prolapse is probably not coincidental.

From the elegant analysis presented in this chapter using rates of mitral valve prolapse in the population, rates of sudden death associated with mitral valve prolapse, the incidence of proarrhythmic effects of antiarrhythmic drugs, and other figures, it is apparent to me that at present there is no indication that patients with asymptomatic complex arrhythmias will benefit from treatment with antiarrhythmic drugs. For me at least, what to do about arrhythmias in the asymptomatic patient with mitral valve prolapse is clear: We observe and reassure the patient. It is much more likely that one can make an asymptomatic patient concerned to the point of symptoms and neurosis by focusing on the potential danger of arrhythmias than it is that any benefit can be derived from treating asymptomatic arrhythmias with drugs. Until better information is available, this conservative reassuring attitude will provide the patient with the greatest benefit.

REFERENCES

1. Chandraratna, PA, Nimalasuriya, A, Kawanishi, D, et al: Identification of the increased frequency of cardiovascular abnormalities associated with mitral valve prolapse by two-dimensional echocardiography. Am J Cardiol 54:1283, 1984.
2. Nishimura, RA, McGoon, MD, Shub, C, et al: Echocardiographically documented mitral valve prolapse. Long-term follow-up of 237 patients. N Engl J Med 313:1305, 1985.
3. Marks, AR, Choong, CY, San Filippo, AJ, et al: Identification of high-risk and low-risk subgroups of patients with mitral valve prolapse. N Engl J Med 320:1031, 1989.
4. Davies, MJ, Moore, BP, and Braimbridge, MV: The floppy mitral valve: Study of incidence, pathology, and complications in surgical, necropsy, and forensic material. Br Heart J 40:468, 1978.
5. Kligfield, P, Hochreiter, C, Niles, N, et al: Relation of sudden death in pure mitral regurgitation, with and without mitral valve prolapse to repetitive ventricular arrhythmias and right and left ventricular ejection fractions. Am J Cardiol 60:397, 1987.
6. Jeresaty, RN: Sudden death due to mitral valve prolapse click syndrome (editorial). Am J Cardiol 37:317, 1976.
7. Lucas, RV, Jr and Edwards, JE: The floppy mitral valve. Curr Probl Cardiol 7:1, 1982.

CHAPTER 9

Is Valve Surgery Indicated in Patients with Severe Mitral Regurgitation Even If They Are Asymptomatic?

Herbert J. Levine, M.D.

Deciding whether to operate on patients with chronic volume overload is more difficult when it involves patients with mitral regurgitation (MR) than it is among patients with chronic aortic regurgitation (AR). The reasons for this difficulty are several. First, the etiology of chronic AR can be traced, for the most part, to either primary disease of the aortic valve itself or disease of the aortic root, and the consequence of the disease is generally manifest as a pure volume overload of the left ventricle. Any functional impairment of the left ventricle (LV), therefore, is the result of either volume overload or a second disease process, for example, coronary artery disease. However, the etiology of chronic mitral regurgitation is much more varied, and frequently the volume overload may be secondary to LV dysfunction that in turn is due to primary disease of the coronary arteries. Second, the size of the regurgitant orifice in chronic AR is generally constant, whereas in some forms of chronic MR the mitral regurgitant valve orifice is dynamic and critically dependent upon ventricular dimensions (as in papillary muscle dysfunction, mitral valve prolapse, or idiopathic hypertrophic subaortic stenosis).

As a consequence of these important differences, it is not surprising that in recent years a large portion of the literature has been devoted to an analysis of the natural history of patients before and after aortic valve replacement for chronic AR, and guidelines for determining the response to corrective surgery and the optimal time for surgery have evolved. However, the complexities of etiology, the dynamic aspects of the magnitude of regurgitant flow, and the importance of primary disease of the LV have made a comparable analysis of patients with chronic MR a challenging task. To compound the problem further, assessment of LV function in MR has been difficult because of the special loading conditions of a ventricle faced with a low pressure runoff into the left atrium. The necessity to pay close attention to these issues when we analyze data in studies of the natural history and response to surgery in patients with chronic MR is clear.

Four major issues need to be addressed in answering the question: Is valve surgery indicated in patients with severe MR, even if they are asymptomatic?

1. The natural history of patients with severe asymptomatic MR treated medically
2. The risk of surgery in this group of patients
3. The natural history of patients with severe asymptomatic MR treated surgically
4. The consequences of waiting until symptoms develop in asymptomatic patients with MR.

To begin, we should establish a few ground rules. For the purpose of discussion, assume that severe MR includes those patients whose MR, as assessed by Doppler study, radionuclide ventriculography, or contrast ventriculography, is 3–4 plus. However, because estimation of the severity of MR in some older studies of this lesion was frequently made on the basis of clinical data, the contour of the pulmonary capillary or left atrial pressure pulse, or the Korner-Schillingford analysis of indicator dilution curves, the validity of the assessment of the severity of MR must at times remain in question. Second, before routine coronary angiography was performed during diagnostic cardiac catheterization, it was not always possible to establish how much of the hemodynamic consequences of MR could be attributed to valvular disease and how much to associated coronary heart disease. Thus, it should be apparent that historical data on the etiology of LV dysfunction in patients with chronic MR often may be less firm than those from comparable studies of chronic AR.

THE NATURAL HISTORY OF PATIENTS WITH SEVERE ASYMPTOMATIC MITRAL REGURGITATION

The natural history of asymptomatic severe MR remains unknown. Published information on the course of patients with chronic MR treated medically is meager and generally refers to patient groups dominated by symptomatic patients. Dr. Paul Wood's[1] classic review of rheumatic valve disease included 300 patients, 82 of whom had either pure MR or mitral stenosis (MS) with *serious incompetence.* Although coronary anatomy was not investigated in these patients, it is likely that the great majority had rheumatic MR, inasmuch as their average age was 37.6 years and in 72 percent of the MR group a clear history of rheumatism was elicited. Wood[1] reported that the interval between initial rheumatic inflammation and death was the same in MS and in MR patients, but the symptom-free period was slightly longer in the MR patients, whereas the period from the onset of symptoms to death was slightly shorter in MR patients. An analysis of the life history of these rheumatic MR patients is summarized in Table 9–1. Of those patients with chronic MR who were asymptomatic, the interval between the subsequent onset of symptoms and total disability averaged 5.4 years.

Hochreiter and associates[2] reported that among 20 patients with severe asymptomatic MR treated medically, one died during an average follow-up of 28 months. During the same period of observation, 12 patients with class II symptoms were followed on medical therapy, and 2 of these died.

The natural history of patients with mitral and aortic valve disease treated medically at the University of California in San Francisco was reported by Rapa-

Table 9–1. Natural History of Rheumatic Mitral Valve Disease

	Latent Period			Duration of Symptoms (Years)				From Onset of Symptoms to Total Incapacity (Years)
	Age of Initial Attack (Year)	Latent Period (Years)	Age Onset of Sx (Years)	Grade I	Grade II	Grade III	Grade IV	
Mitral stenosis	12	19	31	2.7 (0–17)	2.7 (0–18)	1.9 (0.5–11)	2 (0.5–4)	7.3
Mitral regurgitation	12.5	20	32.5	2 (0–9)	1.1 (0–5)	2.3 (0–7)	> 1 (0.3–3)	5.4

(From Wood, P,[1] with permission.)

port[3] in 1975. Among patients with pure chronic MR, approximately 80 percent were alive at 5 years and almost 60 percent survived 10 years following diagnosis. When the group with combined mitral stenosis and regurgitation was examined, the prognosis was less favorable, with 65 percent alive at 5 years and only 33.3 percent alive at 10 years. Unfortunately, the symptomatic classification of these patients was not given, and we must assume that the majority were symptomatic at the time of initial evaluation. Munoz and coworkers[4] reported that the survival of patients with MR or combined MS and MR treated medically was 89 percent at 3 years and only 46 percent at 5 years.

These sparse data suggest that among medically treated patients with chronic MR (most of whom were symptomatic), approximately 20 to 54 percent were either dead or totally disabled within 5 years of initial evaluation. Although the clinical course of asymptomatic patients with substantial MR is not known, the data provided by Wood suggest that the interval between initial evaluation and total disability averages approximately 7½ years. We also must consider that much of the aforementioned data was collected before the introduction of potent diuretics and vasodilator therapy, and it is likely that modern medical therapy for chronic MR would improve these estimates somewhat.

THE EARLY AND LATE RISKS OF SURGERY IN ASYMPTOMATIC PATIENTS WITH CHRONIC MITRAL REGURGITATION

Cohn and associates[5] reported that the operative mortality of 363 symptomatic patients with MR who underwent valve replacement (MVR) between 1972 and 1984 was 11.5 percent, and the long-term survival rate was significantly better in those who had a bioprosthesis than in those with a prosthetic disk valve. Among 105 patients with isolated MR who underwent MVR at Massachusetts General Hospital between 1974 and 1979, Phillips and associates[6] observed an operative mortality of 4 percent. Carpentier and colleagues[7] reported a 4 percent operative mortality among 377 patients with isolated MR who underwent reconstructive surgery of the mitral valve. Actuarial data revealed that 82 percent survived 9 years, and the thromboembolic rate was only 0.6 percent per patient year, although almost half of the patients were not given anticoagulants. Cosgrove and associates[8] reported their results of mitral valve reconstruction in 117 consecutive cases of MR.

Operative mortality was 4.3 percent, and one-third of the patients underwent simultaneous myocardial revascularization. Only two patients sustained embolic events, and the two-year actuarial survival was 90.6 percent. In ischemic MR, too, mitral valve repair has provided better short- and long-term results than has MVR. Kay and coworkers[9] observed that 62 percent of patients who underwent mitral repair were alive at five years following surgery compared with 37 percent of those who had MVR. Among mitral valve repair patients with ejection fractions of 40 percent or more, 87 percent were alive five years following surgery.

An important surgical trend during the past decade has been the growing enthusiasm for reconstructive surgery of incompetent mitral valves. A number of reviews support the view that the early and late results of mitral valve repair compare favorably with the results of MVR in chronic MR, particularly in patients with myxomatous degeneration of the valve, ruptured chordae tendineae, or ischemic MR[10–12] and in young patients with rheumatic MR.[13,14] Not only does the operative mortality appear to be less with reconstructive procedures, but the incidence of postoperative thromboembolism and endocarditis is markedly reduced and, in the absence of atrial fibrillation, most patients are spared the risks of long-term anticoagulant therapy. It is generally considered that the incidence of endocarditis following repair of the mitral valve is similar to that of the native lesion and clearly less than that among patients with MVR. Even more convincing are the data demonstrating a lower incidence of thromboembolism in mitral repair patients compared with valve replacement patients. Cohn and associates[12] found that the actuarial freedom from emboli 36 months following surgery was 86 percent for MVR patients and 100 percent for the repair group. In ischemic MR, Kay and colleagues[9] reported that the incidence of thromboembolism was 5 percent and 10 percent per patient year for the repair group and MVR group, respectively, and other comparative studies indicate thromboembolic incidence rates of 8.0 percent versus 1.8 percent[15] and 4.1 percent versus 2.4 percent[11] per patient year in the MVR and repair groups, respectively.

The major determinants of the short- and long-term results of corrective surgery for patients with chronic MR are the functional classification of the patient, the etiology of the MR, the contractile state of the left ventricle, and the type of repair or replacement of the mitral valve. Although for many patients the results of mitral repair appear to be better than those of valve replacement, the success of mitral repair is dependent on the experience of the surgeon, and a learning curve is an important part of this procedure. Furthermore, one cannot always be assured preoperatively that repair of the mitral lesion will be possible, and the decision to repair or to replace the valve frequently will be made at the time of surgery. Thus, a clinician may need to make a recommendation for surgery without full knowledge of whether the downstream risks will be those associated with repair or replacement.

The literature does not provide a clear estimation of the short- and long-term results of corrective surgery for asymptomatic MR. However, on the basis of the data available, it is estimated that the operative risk of mitral valve repair in an asymptomatic patient with severe MR and normal systolic function is likely to be no greater than 1 to 2 percent. Although the clinical classification of the patient with MR is probably the most potent predictor of the short- and long-term risks of corrective surgery of MR, this factor may be closely rivaled by the functional state of the left ventricle.

THE ROLE OF VENTRICULAR FUNCTION IN THE NATURAL HISTORY OF CHRONIC MITRAL REGURGITATION

It should come as no surprise that a major determinant of the natural history of chronic MR is the functional state of the left ventricle. Borrowing from the extensive literature devoted to the natural history of patients with coronary heart disease and of patients with chronic aortic regurgitation, we would predict a critical and dominant role for left ventricular function in determining the course of medically and surgically treated patients with MR.

There are, however, several peculiarities of the hemodynamic abnormalities in chronic MR that frustrate conventional assessment of the functional state of the left ventricle in this condition. Systolic pump function is determined by preload, afterload, and the contractile state of the ventricular myocardium. In acute MR, left ventricular filling pressure (a measure of preload) is increased by the augmented filling volume, and afterload is reduced as a consequence of the low pressure runoff into the left atrium.[16] These loading conditions combine to increase ejection fraction in acute MR.[16,17]

In chronic compensated MR, dilatation and hypertrophy of the left ventricle proceeds, and chamber compliance of the ventricle increases, permitting a larger stroke volume to be ejected with a decrease (or at least without a further increase) in preload. Several studies indicate that, at this stage of the disease, systolic stress is generally within the normal range.[18-20] According to Carabello,[21] this chronic, compensated phase of MR is characterized by increased preload, normal contractile function, and an afterload that has increased from subnormal to normal levels as a consequence of an increased ratio of chamber radius to wall thickness.

Elimination of the mitral leak results in a further increase in left ventricular afterload. When a chronic shunt from the left ventricle to the left atrium in dogs was eliminated, LV wall stress increased acutely[22] and a similar finding was observed by Wong and Spotnitz[23] in six patients with MR studied intraoperatively immediately following valve replacement. In acute experimental MR, Berko and coworkers[24] found that when LV elastance was normalized for heart size, contractile state remained unchanged and the increase in systolic ejection fraction (SEF) observed was due to an increase in ventricular preload. However, numerous studies indicate that MVR in patients with chronic MR results in a fall in SEF regardless of the preoperative state of LV function. In a recent review of the response to surgical correction of chronic AR and MR, Gaasch and coworkers[25] reported that in chronic MR an average decrease in SEF was found following MVR in each of 10 separate reports, with an overall reduction in SEF among the 10 studies from 0.59 to 0.49. Logic would suggest that the explanation for this fall in SEF is the combined decrease in preload and increase in afterload observed following MVR. There are, however, several reasons to question this conclusion. First, although LV wall stress increases immediately following MVR, when regression of hypertrophy and remodeling of the ventricle has occurred months later, this may not be the case. Zile and associates[20] reported no change in systolic wall stress one year following MVR for chronic MR. Second, whereas SEF predictably falls following MVR, this does not appear to be the case when surgical correction of MR is accomplished by mitral valve repair. Of three studies of systolic function following repair of MR, SEF rose in two, and the overall SEF for the three groups increased from 0.59 to 0.62.[11,26,27] It has been suggested that loss of the integrity of papillary muscles and chordae tendineae following MVR is an important factor responsible for postoperative reduction in systolic function and that valve repair with preservation of the continuity between mitral annulus and the LV wall plays a critical role in sustaining LV function.[11,25–28] Although a fall in SEF is uniformly observed following MVR in chronic MR, this phenomenon cannot be attributed to elimination of the MR per se.

ASSESSMENT OF VENTRICULAR FUNCTION IN MITRAL REGURGITATION

Systolic ejection fraction and fractional shortening are the most commonly used indices of LV pump function. Both indices, however, are influenced importantly by acute changes in preload and afterload, and the unique loading conditions imposed by severe MR preclude the use of these indices to estimate reliably the contractile state of the ventricle in this condition. This dilemma has prompted some investigators to look for alternative indices of systolic performance that are less susceptible to the vagaries of variable loading conditions in MR.

Accordingly, Borow and colleagues[29] examined the utility of end-systolic volume (ESV), an index that is independent of preload, in patients with AR and in those with MR. Postoperative LV function in MR correlated well with preoperative ESV and did so substantially better than with preoperative SEF, end-diastolic volume (EDV), or LV end-diastolic pressure. Carabello and associates[30] carried this approach a step further in search of an index that was relatively insensitive to both preload and afterload. They examined the end-systolic wall stress (ESWS) to end-systolic volume index (ESVI) ratio in patients with MR and found that among the preoperative variables of age, pulmonary wedge pressure, end-diastolic volume index (EDVI), ESVI, SEF, and the ESWS/ESVI ratio, only the ESWS/ESVI ratio proved to be an independent predictor of the clinical outcome of surgical correction of MR. In a recent review of the proper timing of surgical correction of MR, Carabello and associates[30] suggested that the preoperative markers of a probably good outcome are: (1) an SEF of greater than 0.70, (2) an end-systolic dimension index of less than 2.4 cm/M^2, (3) an ESVI of less than 60 ml/M^2, and (4) an ESWS/ESVI ratio of greater than 2.6. The predictors of a probable poor outcome are: (1) an SEF of less than 0.55, (2) an end-systolic dimension index of greater than 2.6 cm/M^2, (3) an ESVI of more than 75 ml/M^2, and (4) an ESWS/ESVI ratio of less than 2.4.

THE ASYMPTOMATIC PATIENT WITH SEVERE MITRAL REGURGITATION

The first question might be: Is the patient truly asymptomatic? Many patients with volume or pressure overload of the ventricle gradually and imperceptibly adjust their life-style in such a way that precludes easy detection of an effort syndrome. They may limit their activities to an extent that they are free from clinical symptoms of pulmonary congestion or ischemia and indeed are asymptomatic. Others may be limited by musculoskeletal disease, or by what might be conveniently interpreted as signs of early aging. In some instances, observing their performance on a treadmill will bring to light undetected cardiorespiratory symptoms. Exercise testing may be particularly rewarding in patients with asymptomatic ischemic MR, especially those with dynamic papillary muscle dysfunction, in which severe MR occurs as as result of regional or global myocardial ischemia. Indeed, an exercise study at the time of diagnostic cardiac catheterization may be useful in determining the impact of MR upon right heart pressures, especially in those who demonstrate normal pulmonary pressures at rest. The importance of examining right ventricular (RV) function in patients with MR has been emphasized by Hochreiter and associates.[2] These investigators have shown that RV dysfunction, generally associated with LV dysfunction, identifies a high-risk group of patients with MR.

In addition to an aggressive search for an effort syndrome in patients with asymptomatic MR, a special effort must be made to detect the earliest signs of LV dysfunction in these patients. In patients with an SEF of less than 0.55, one must assume the presence of LV dysfunction, and an examination of LV chamber dimensions, stress-shortening relations, and systolic elastance at this point may further help characterize the extent of underlying myocardial failure.

This stage of the analysis is particularly important because the detection of early LV dysfunction in a truly asymptomatic patient with severe MR may be sufficient reason to proceed with corrective surgery. There is also good reason to believe that the duration as well as the extent of LV dysfunction will have an important bearing on the results of surgery. Although a proper study of this issue has not yet been carried out in patients with chronic MR, lessons learned from experience with another form of chronic volume overload of the LV may be applicable here. Bonow and associates[31] have examined the results of aortic valve replacement in a large series of patients with chronic AR and found that the long-term surgical results in patients with LV dysfunction of short duration (i.e., less than 14 months) were as good as those in patients with severe AR who had normal LV function. On the other hand, if LV dysfunction had been long-standing (i.e., greater than 18 months), the long-term prognosis was clearly less good. Should these observations apply to patients with chronic MR as well, there would be good reason to identify the onset of LV dysfunction promptly and to proceed with corrective surgery without delay and with the expectation of a good clinical outcome.

INDICATIONS FOR SURGERY IN ASYMPTOMATIC MITRAL REGURGITATION

Once it has been established that a patient with severe MR is truly asymptomatic, the first priority is an accurate assessment of LV function. As outlined in Table 9–2, if the SEF is greater than 0.70, one can safey assume that LV function is within normal limits, and it is prudent at this point to recommend continued medical therapy. In those patients in whom the etiology remains in doubt, the finding of an

Table 9–2. Asymptomatic Severe Mitral Regurgitation

Pump Function	Ventricular Function	Recommendation
SEF > 0.70	Presumed normal	Medical treatment
SEF = 0.55–0.70	Probably normal	Serial echo or RVG every 4–6 months
SEF < 0.55	LV dysfunction	Consider corrective surgery

SEF = systolic ejection fraction.
RVG = radionuclide ventriculography.

unusually high SEF should, however, raise the possibility of obstructive hypertrophic cardiomyopathy.

In those patients whose SEF is between 0.55 and 0.70, one may suspect that LV function is likely to be normal, but it behooves the clinician to examine LV chamber volumes carefully, particularly ESV, and to proceed with an analysis of stress-shortening relations in an effort to characterize myocardial function better. Serial examinations using echocardiography or radionuclide ventriculography at 4 to 6 month intervals should be helpful in identifying a trend in the patient's hemodynamic profile.

If the SEF is less than 0.55, one must assume that there is some LV dysfunction, and both the extent and duration of this dysfunction should be documented as accurately as possible. Should an asymptomatic patient with convincing LV dysfunction be identified, one can make a strong case for proceeding promptly with surgery.

The decision to recommend surgery will, of course, be influenced by the estimated operative risk. In circumstances in which the clinical and echocardiographic data strongly suggest a relatively normal mitral valve anatomy (i.e., ruptured chordae, mitral valve prolapse, or ischemic MR), and when the patient has access to a surgical service experienced in mitral valve repair, the threshold for proceeding with surgery will be less, knowing that the long-term risks of MVR probably can be avoided. On the other hand, a heavily calcified valve due to either rheumatic disease or mitral annular calcification is almost certain to require replacement, and the clinician should weigh the decision for surgery with the short-term and long-term risks of valve replacement. It is estimated that the operative risk of mitral valve repair in asymptomatic MR will be no greater than 1 to 2 percent, whereas the risk of MVR is probably 2 to 4 percent.

Although it is unlikely that a patient with severe MR and advanced LV dysfunction would be asymptomatic, finding a moderately depressed SEF (i.e., 0.40 to 0.50) does not preclude a satisfactory surgical result even if contractile function is found to be subnormal.[18] An additional factor in the long-term results of surgery for MR is the role of loss of the atrial transport mechanism. In many patients with volume or pressure overload of the LV, clinical decompensation may coincide with the onset of atrial fibrillation. As emphasized by Cohn,[32] the long-term results of surgery for MR are better among those in sinus rhythm than in those with atrial fibrillation, and there may be reason to preempt the development of atrial fibrillation, especially in those with progressive enlargement of the left atrium who remain in normal sinus rhythm.

SUMMARY

There is a natural reluctance among clinicians to recommend surgery in asymptomatic patients with cardiac disease and in patients with stenotic disease of the mitral and aortic valves; this instinct will mislead us very rarely. However, among patients with chronic volume overload of the LV, this rule-of-thumb does not always apply. For truly asymptomatic patients with severe MR who clearly have normal LV function, continued medical therapy with serial monitoring of LV dynamics is a prudent alternative to the small risk of corrective surgery. However, the major challenge in addressing this problem is the definition and detection of LV dysfunction in chronic MR. Thus, for MR patients with questionable impairment of myocardial function (generally those with an SEF between 0.55 and 0.70), an examination of chamber dimensions and particularly stress-shortening relations may be necessary to detect early LV dysfunction. Should LV dysfunction be identified or should serial studies indicate an adverse trend in LV performance, a strong case can be made for proceeding with surgery. Patients with an SEF of less than 0.55 must be assumed to have LV dysfunction and analogous data from patients with chronic AR suggest that a satisfactory surgical result may be achieved if the duration of LV dysfunction is brief. Those patients with chronic MR whose disease is likely to be amenable to mitral valve repair rather than valve replacement deserve a lower threshold for corrective surgery.

REFERENCES

1. Wood, P: An appreciation of mitral stenosis. Part 1: Clinical features. Br Med J 1:1051, 1954.
2. Hochreiter, C, Niles, N, Devereux, RB, et al: Mitral regurgitation: Relation of non-invasive descriptors of right and left ventricular performance to clinical and hemodynamic findings in medically and surgically treated patients. Circulation 73:900, 1986.
3. Rapaport, E: Natural history of aortic and mitral valve disease. Am J Cardiol 35:221, 1975.
4. Munoz, S, Gallardo, J, Diaz-Gorrin, JR, et al: Influence of surgery on the natural history of rheumatic mitral and aortic valve disease. Am J Cardiol 35:234, 1975.
5. Cohn, LH, Allred, EN, Cohn, LA, et al: Early and late risk of mitral valve replacement. J Thorac Cardiovasc Surg 90:872, 1985.
6. Phillips, HR, Levine, FH, Carter, JE, et al: Mitral valve replacement for isolated mitral regurgitation: Analysis of clinical course and late post-operative left ventricular ejection fraction. Am J Cardiol 48:647, 1981.
7. Carpentier, A, Fabiani, JN, Relland, J, et al: Reconstructive surgery of mitral valve incompetence. J Thorac Cardiovasc Surg 79:338, 1980.
8. Cosgrove, DM, Chavez, AM, Lytle, BW, et al: Results of mitral valve reconstruction. Circulation 74:I82, 1986.
9. Kay, GL, Kay, JH, Zubiate, P, et al: Mitral valve repair for mitral regurgitation secondary to coronary artery disease. Circulation 74:I88, 1986.
10. Sand, ME, Naftel, DC, Blackstone, EH, et al: A comparison of repair and replacement for mitral valve incompetence. J Thorac Cardiovasc Surg 94:208, 1987.
11. Duran, CG, Pomar, JL, Revuelta, JM, et al: Conservative operation for mitral insufficiency. J Thorac Cardiovasc Surg 79:326, 1980.
12. Cohn, LH, Kowalker, W, Bhatia, S, et al: Comparative morbidity of mitral valve repair versus replacement for mitral regurgitation with and without coronary artery disease. Ann Thorac Surg 45:284, 1988.
13. Antunes, MJ, Magalhaes, MP, Colsen, PR, et al: Valvuloplasty for rheumatic mitral valve disease. J Thorac Cardiovasc Surg 94:44, 1987.
14. Lessana, A, Viet, TT, Ades, F, et al: Mitral reconstructive operations: A series of 130 consecutive cases. J Thorac Cardiovasc Surg 86:553, 1983.
15. Orszulak, TA, Schaff, HV, Danielson, GK, et al: Mitral regurgitation due to ruptured chordae tendinae. J Thorac Cardiovasc Surg 89:491, 1985.
16. Kleaveland, JP, Kussmaul, WG, and Carabello, B: Left ventricular hemodynamics in a new experimental model of mitral regurgitation (abstr). J Am Coll Cardiol 5:486, 1985.
17. Urschel, CW, Covell, JW, Sonnenblick, EH, et al: Myocardial mechanics in aortic and mitral valvular regurgitation: The concept of instantaneous impedance as a determinant of the performance of the intact heart. J Clin Invest 47:867, 1968.
18. Wisenbaugh, T: Does normal pump function belie muscle dysfunction in patients with chronic severe mitral regurgitation? Circulation 77:515, 1988.
19. Corrin, WJ, Monrad, ES, Murakami, T, et al: The relation of afterload to ejection performance in chronic mitral regurgitation. Circulation 76:59, 1987.
20. Zile, MR, Gaasch, WH, and Levine, HJ: Left ventricular stress-dimension-shortening relations before and after correction of chronic aortic and mitral regurgitation. Am J Cardiol 56:99, 1985.

21. Carabello, B: Mitral regurgitation. Part 2: Proper timing of mitral valve replacement. Mod Concepts Cardiovasc Dis 57:59, 1988.
22. Rankin, JS, Nicholas, LM, and Kouchoukos, NT: Experimental mitral regurgitation: Effect on left ventricular function before and after elimination of chronic regurgitation in the dog. J Thorac Cardiovasc Surg 70:478, 1975.
23. Wong, CYH and Spotnitz, HM: Systolic and diastolic properties of the human left ventricle during valve replacement for chronic mitral regurgitation. Am J Cardiol 47:40, 1981.
24. Berko, B, Gaasch, WH, Tanigawa, N, et al: Disparity between ejection and end-systolic indexes of left ventricular contractility in mitral regurgitation. Circulation 75:1310, 1987.
25. Gaasch, WH, Levine, HJ, and Zile, MR: Chronic aortic and mitral regurgitation: Mechanical consequences of the lesion and the results of surgical correction. In Levine, HJ and Gaasch, WH (eds): The Ventricle. Martinus Nijhoff, Boston, 1985.
26. Bonchek, L, Siegel, R, Olinger, G, et al: Left ventricular function is better after mitral repair than after valve replacement. Am J Cardiol 49:922, 1982.
27. David, TE, Uden, DE, and Strauss, HD: The importance of the mitral apparatus in left ventricular function after correction of mitral regurgitation. Circulation 68:II76, 1983.
28. Hansen, DE, Cahill, PD, DeCampli, WM, et al: Valvular-ventricular interaction: Importance of the mitral apparatus in canine left ventricular systolic performance. Circulation 73:1310, 1986.
29. Borow, KM, Green, LH, Mann, T, et al: End-systolic volume as a predictor of post-operative left ventricular performance in volume overload from valvular regurgitation. Am J Med 68:655, 1980.
30. Carabello, B, Nolan, SP, and McGuire, LB: Assessment of pre-operative left ventricular function in patients with mitral regurgitation: Value of the end-systolic wall stress–end-systolic volume ratio. Circulation 64:1212, 1981.
31. Bonow, RO, Picone, AL, McIntosh, CL, et al: Survival and functional results after valve replacement for aortic regurgitation from 1976 to 1983: Impact of pre-operative left ventricular function. Circulation 72:1244, 1985.
32. Cohn, LH: Surgery for mitral regurgitation. JAMA 260:2883, 1988.

Commentary

Melvin D. Cheitlin, M.D.

A decision to undertake surgical intervention in valve disease must be based on knowledge of the natural history of the disease treated medically compared with the risks at surgery and later risks, some of which are secondary to the surgery and artificial valve. Currently at most centers in the United States, surgery for mitral regurgitation almost always means valve replacement, which carries a risk of perioperative mortality of 3 to 10 percent and of late mortality after successful valve replacement of 2 to 3 percent per year. In addition, the problems of thromboembolism, bleeding on anticoagulants, valve disruption with the bioprosthetic valves, and infective endocarditis all result in a pattern of disease—*prosthetic valve disease*—which has a substantial mortality and morbidity. Certainly this fact must weigh heavily in making a decision to recommend surgery, especially to an asymptomatic patient.

Unfortunately, the loading conditions of the left ventricle, both preload and afterload, encountered in patients with mitral regurgitation encourage the concept that myocardial dysfunction may occur and be masked by the increased preload and possibly decreased afterload found in these patients. Obviously, some means of following myocardial function as distinct from global left ventricular function is necessary. If myocardial dysfunction is allowed to occur, it may be irreversible and might be an indication for surgery even if the patient remains asymptomatic.

In this chapter Dr. Levine reviews the problem of following myocardial function and concludes that the most sensitive index of myocardial function, which is closest to being independent of loading conditions, is the end-systolic volume or, even better, the relationship of end-systolic stress to end-systolic volume. As shown recently by Wisenbaugh,[1] patients with mitral regurgitation who have ejection fractions greater than 60 percent probably have normal left ventricular myocardial contractility, and these patients can be followed safely with periodic measurements of left ventricular ejection fraction. The reason for concern is the implication that some patients will have significant deterioriation of myocardial function while remaining truly asymptomatic, but one must realize that symptoms are subjective and that some patients rationalize symptoms or reduce activity to the point at which they no longer have the symptoms. These patients can appear *asymptomatic* when questioned superficially. When taking the history, it is necessary to evaluate the patient's activity against the activity that the patient *should* be able to do, given the patient's age, sex, and personality. If a judgment cannot be made of the patient's true level of activity, then a meaningful evaluation of the patient's symptoms or lack thereof cannot be made. It is in this situation that objective measurements, such as exercising along with the patient or walking upstairs together, or more formal standardized exercise testing is valuable.

In my opinion, it is unusual for patients with mitral regurgitation due to a primary valve problem such as rheumatic heart disease or mitral valve prolapse to have markedly abnormal myocardial function while remaining truly asymptomatic. More frequently, the question arises in the patient with myocardial dysfunction and mitral regurgitation as to which came first. Did the mitral regurgitation cause the myocardial dysfunction, or are we seeing a patient with underlying myocardial disease—for instance, coronary heart disease or cardiomyopathy—who has dilated the left ventricle and developed mitral regurgitation?

Valuable insight into the problem of how often left ventricular dysfunction occurs in relatively asymptomatic patients with mitral regurgitation can be obtained by examining a surgical series of patients after mitral valve replacement. Salomon and colleagues[2] reported almost 900 patients with isolated mitral valve replacement. About one third had mitral stenosis, one third had mitral stenosis and mitral regurgitation, and one third had mitral regurgitation. Ninety percent of the patients were very symptomatic, that is, New York Heart Association class III or IV, and only a few were class II. Furthermore, 90 percent of the survivors became class I or II, so the surgery was successful in relieving symptoms. Although the patients with mitral stenosis or mitral stenosis plus mitral regurgitation had a better late survival than patients with mitral regurgitation alone, the difference in late mortality was found exclusively in the patients with mitral regurgitation due to ischemic heart disease. After the removal of those patients with coronary artery disease, class III and IV mitral regurgitation patients with mitral valve replacement had a similar good result and late prognosis as did those with mitral valve replacement due to mitral stenosis, in which the left ventricular muscle function is probably normal no matter how symptomatic the patient. It is probable that those patients with mitral regurgitation who were class III or IV, therefore, had little deterioration of left ventricular myocardial function. However, patients with mitral regurgitation and decreased myocardial function possibly were less likely to be operated upon and therefore were less likely to appear in such a series. Poor left ventricular function leading to late mortality after valve replacement in the absence of coronary artery disease most likely was unusual, even in these very symptomatic patients.

Because the development of severe mitral regurgitation leads to dilatation of the left ventricle and left atrium and a further increase in mitral insufficiency and atrial fibrillation, eliminating mitral regurgitation by valve surgery once it becomes severe would be desirable. The major problem with this approach still is that the patient with mitral regurgitation must be sent to surgery with the expectation that a prosthetic valve replacement will be necessary. This remains true at the great majority of centers in the United States except in the case of mitral prolapse confined to the mural leaflet or ruptured chordae of the mural leaflet, either of which can be repaired by most surgeons. With increasing experience based on the excellent results obtained by Carpentier, Duran, Yacoub, and others, more surgeons will become proficient in the techniques of valve repair for mitral regurgitation. At present, 90 percent of mitral valve prolapse causing mitral regurgitation can be repaired. The success rate of repair is lower with the scarred and retracted leaflet of rheumatic heart disease. Although echocardiography and, more recently, transesophageal two-dimensional echo-Doppler study have been very helpful in assessing the mitral apparatus and the pathophysiologic reasons for mitral regurgitation preoperatively, the decision for repair versus replacement must be made at the time of surgery.

No matter how asymptomatic a patient with severe mitral regurgitation is, mitral valve surgery is certainly indicated if myocardial function is deteriorating as shown by a sustained decrease in ejection fraction below 55 percent with progressive increase in left ventricular end-systolic volume. Preferably, the patient should be sent to a surgeon experienced in mitral valve repair. However, until we are able to predict repair of the valve before the patient goes to surgery with the certainty that we now predict repair in the patient with mitral stenosis, choosing to send the asymptomatic patient with mitral regurgitation to surgery remains a difficult decision.

REFERENCES

1. Wisenbaugh, T: Does normal pump function belie muscle dysfunction in patients with chronic severe mitral regurgitation? Circulation 77:515, 1988.
2. Salomon, NW, Stinson, EB, Griepp, RB, et al: Patient-related risk factors as predictors of results following isolated mitral valve replacement. Ann Thorac Surg 24:519, 1977.

CHAPTER 10

Should Patients with Mitral Stenosis Who Are Acceptable Surgical Commissurotomy Candidates Now Have Balloon Valvuloplasty Treatment?

Charles R. McKay, M.D.

> *Mitral stenosis is not only one of the most distressing forms of cardiac disease, but in its severe forms it resists all treatment by medicine. On looking at the contracted mitral orifice in a severe case of this disease . . . the wish unconsciously arises that one could divide the constriction as easily during life as one can after death. The risk that such an operation would entail naturally makes one shrink from it.*

—Sir Lauder Brunton, 1902[1]

Several surgeons worked over the four decades[2,3] after Brunton's initial challenge in 1902 to develop the technique of closed mitral commissurotomy.[4,5] Relief of mitral stenosis by closed mitral commissurotomy has, since 1949, dramatically altered the prognosis of patients with severe symptomatic mitral stenosis and is still practiced throughout the world. Even in the early experiences with closed mitral commissurotomy the dramatic clinical results, with decreased symptoms and the increased survival in these patients, warranted the use of surgical treatment despite procedure-related short- and long-term risks.[6]

The development of mechanical heart-lung bypass and mitral annuloplasty[7] offered increased surgical control and the possibility of performing open mitral valve commissurotomy,[8] or optional valve replacement,[9] in cases deemed at surgery to be unsuitable for commissurotomy.[10] The open technique with optional valve replacement has therefore been adopted by surgeons as the current standard of treatment for mitral stenosis patients in the United States and Europe. However,

175

the data supporting the currently held beliefs regarding the superiority of open commissurotomy, with optional valve replacement, over closed commissurotomy are not based on direct comparisons of these techniques. The case selection for these techniques differed greatly in different institutions and in different surgical eras.

Percutaneous balloon valvuloplasty treatment of mitral stenosis was developed only recently.[11] This technique now offers the possibility of achieving clinical and hemodynamic results similar to surgical commissurotomy in pediatric[12,13] and younger adult[14,15] patients. Early in the experience with balloon valvuloplasty, it was hoped that these results also could be achieved in some elderly patients without the associated risks of surgery.[16-18] Although mitral balloon valvuloplasty remains investigational, clinical experience in many centers has accumulated rapidly. Encouraging immediate results and midterm follow-up results of balloon valvuloplasty[19-24] have been demonstrated.

The use of catheter procedures rather than thoracotomy is especially appealing to the patients.

However, the procedure remains technically difficult and carries its own acute and long-term risks, which are being documented carefully by a long-term cooperative multicenter Balloon Valvuloplasty Registry sponsored by the National Heart, Lung and Blood Institute.[25,26] The clinician caring for patients with symptomatic mitral stenosis now must decide whether to refer patients with symptomatic mitral stenosis (especially those patients who are good surgical candidates) for balloon valvuloplasty treatment or to continue to recommend surgical therapy by open commissurotomy with optional mitral valve replacement. This review, which explores these issues and compares currently available surgical and balloon valvuloplasty data, supports the thesis that balloon valvuloplasty performed in an experienced setting should now be considered the preferred treatment for many patients with symptomatic mitral stenosis.

NATURAL HISTORY AND MORPHOLOGY OF RHEUMATIC MITRAL STENOSIS

Despite descriptions by early anatomists of fused and calcified mitral commissures, the observations and proposals of Brunton were surprisingly controversial. They challenged the view that prevailed early in this century that the primary problem of *rheumatoid heart* was a persistent carditis and myopathy.[27]

Despite this limited understanding of pathophysiology and hemodynamics, clinicians followed patients with auscultatory findings of mitral stenosis over many years and carefully documented their prognosis without surgery. These studies are listed in Table 10–1 in order of increasing mean age of the patient populations. Many younger patients had asymptomatic murmurs diagnosed two years after the episode of acute rheumatic fever. They presented after 7 to 10 years with mild symptoms that were usually stable for up to ten years. Patients without symptoms and without cardiomegaly had a good prognosis with a 95 percent 5-year survival,[28,30,33] and mild symptoms progressed in 10 to 38 percent of these patients. They had an 84 to 96 percent 10-year survival and a 35 to 84 percent 20-year survival.[28-30] Decreased survival occurred in patients who on initial evaluation were older,[30-32] had cardiomegaly,[29] or had more severe symptoms at presentation. Patients with functional class III symptoms had a 15 to 62 percent 10-year survival.[31,32] Patients with mixed mitral stenosis and regurgitation or with cardiomeg-

Table 10–1. Natural History of Patients with Mitral Stenosis without Surgical Treatment

Author (Ref #)	# of Pts	Mean Age at Entry	% With Atrial Fib.	Comparison Groups	Follow-Up Data Survival			Sx %	SBE %	Comments
					5 yr	10 yr	20 yr			
Bland (28)	653	8	0	RHD pts	—	69	54	80	4.4	653 of 1000 ARF pts with RHD
	117	8	0	MS only	—	96	84	10	—	117 of 653 with pure MS
Wilson (29)	269	<20	5	All MS	—	92	84	10	2.0	MS murmur heard 1–2 years after ARF
				Mild CM	—	96	92			
				Severe CM	—	72	44			
Rowe (30)	250	30	29	All MS	75	61	21	20	4.5	26% with emboli at 20 years
				FC I	95	84	35			
				FC II	55	42	10			
				FC III	25	15	0			
Grant (31)	238	31	9.4		65	50	—	33	5.5	All males
Bannister (33)	105	37	28	All FC I	95	—	—	38	1	22 pts with emboli
Olesen (32)	271	42	57	All MS	58	34	14	12	—	
				FC III		62	38			
				FC IV		15	0			

Atrial fib. = atrial fibrillation, Sx % = percent of patients with progressive symptoms over the follow-up period, SBE % = percent of patients with bacterial endocarditis over the follow-up period, RHD = rheumatic heart disease, ARF = acute rheumatic fever, MS = mitral stenosis, CM = cardiomegaly on chest x-ray, FC = New York Heart Association functional class.

aly on chest x-ray examination[29] or with severe pulmonary hypertension[34] also had reduced survival.

Early morphologic observations of stenotic mitral valves in patients[1] and in laboratory models[2] led to early attempts to sever fused commissures in order to improve mitral valve function.[2,3] During this time, Rusted and colleagues[35] demonstrated the frequency and importance of commissural fusion in a large autopsy series of hearts with rheumatic mitral valves. In 22 of 70 valves, commissural fusion was the primary cause of stenosis. Commissural fusion contributed to the stenosis, along with thickening of the leaflets, and shortening and fusion of the chordae tendineae, in 31 other valves. Appreciation of the importance of changes in the mitral valve morphology led to the classic description of the clinical presentations in these patients.[36] After the technical improvements in surgery and in blood banking that were developed during World War II, it was possible for surgeons to develop effective closed commissurotomy techniques in the late 1940s.

RESULTS OF TRANSATRIAL CLOSED MITRAL COMMISSUROTOMY

After the initial reports[4–6] documented the technical possibility and success of closed transatrial *finger fracture* of the mitral valve commissures, the technique was practiced widely. Hemodynamic studies[37] documented in detail the improvements in intracardiac hemodynamics and respiratory function at rest and at exercise. Within three weeks after operation, the pulmonary arterial wedge pressures, mean pulmonary artery pressures, and pulmonary arterial resistances decreased. Increases in cardiac output at maximum exercise were associated with relatively lower pulmonary arterial wedge pressures. These beneficial hemodynamic changes persisted in patients 2 to 3 years after transatrial commissurotomy.[38]

The perioperative results and long-term clinical follow-up after transatrial mitral commissurotomy were documented in two large series of cases. Harken and colleagues[39] continued long-term follow-up in over 1800 cases, with many cases followed up to 20 years. Glenn and colleagues[40] followed over 400 cases for 12 years. The mean age at operation of the patient groups was 29 and 45 years. From 90 to 95 percent of these patients were in functional class III or IV. From 30 to 54 percent were in atrial fibrillation; 19 to 32 percent had a history of previous systemic embolization; 15 to 23 percent had moderate mitral regurgitation preoperatively; and 13 to 30 percent had clinically documented associated valvular diseases. At operation, assessment of the valve by palpation demonstrated mitral valve calcification in 32 to 40 percent of the patients. Calcification was more common in younger males. Mitral regurgitation was palpated in 30 to 44 percent of the patients.

By sequentially applying direct pressure to the anterior and posterior commissures, it was possible in over 80 percent of patients to open one commissure, and in approximately one third of patients it was also possible to open two commissures. Approximately 20 percent of patients had significant thrombus in the left atrial appendage, which was removed, and the atrial appendage was amputated or oversewn. Mitral regurgitation was noted to increase slightly in approximately one third of the patients. Severe increase in mitral regurgitation occurred rarely and indicated a poor prognosis. Perioperative emboli were noted in 2 to 8 percent of the patients, and the overall perioperative 30-day mortality was from 3.8 to 8 percent. In addition, those patients who presented in functional class IV had increased risks of operative mortality from 10 to 20 percent compared with patients in class II or III with a 2 to 6 percent risk. The perioperative mortality was also lower in the later experience of these surgeons. In the series reported by Ellis's group, there was a 2 percent overall mortality in the last 500 of 1500 patients reported; and in the late 1950s, after 8 years of experience, Glenn's group reported a zero operative mortality.

At five-year follow-up, Ellis and associates[41] analyzed the results of transatrial commissurotomy in various patient subsets based on preoperative criteria. In patients less than 40 years of age at operation, 76 to 100 percent reported persistent improvement 5 years after surgery. In patients greater than 40 years of age, 63 percent reported persistent improvement. In patients who had no mitral regurgitation or mild mitral regurgitation either before the operation or induced immediately after the operation, 78 percent reported persistently improved symptoms, whereas in patients who had greater degrees of mitral regurgitation, only 48 percent reported persistently improved symptoms. Whereas 76 percent of patients with pliable valves reported persistent improvement, only 58 percent of those with thickened fibrotic valves reported persistent improvement. Of those patients with no calcium palpated on the valve at the time of surgery, 63 percent noted persistent improvement, whereas of those patients with palpable calcium on the mitral valve, only 44 percent noted persistent improvement. At this 5-year follow-up and at later follow-up, neither the sex of the patient nor the presence of atrial fibrillation influenced the persistence of a good clinical result.

Ten years after commissurotomy,[42,43] 69 percent of the patients who had been in functional class III preoperatively had persistently improved symptoms, whereas 55 percent of the patients in functional class IV preoperatively remained improved. The annual risk of systemic embolization was 0.25 to 0.59 percent. The risk of late embolization increased in patients with atrial fibrillation. Repeat mitral commissurotomy, performed in 10 percent of patients by 10-year follow-up, carried a 5.8 percent operative mortality. Patients who were in functional class III preoperatively had an actuarial 10-year survival of 79 percent, and those in functional class IV had a 64 percent survival. Those who had been in sinus rhythm had a 90 percent survival, whereas those in atrial fibrillation had a 79 percent survival. Those with no calcification or mitral regurgitation had an 84 percent survival; those with mild calcification or regurgitation had 60 percent survival; and those with heavy calcification or significant mitral regurgitation had a 47 percent 10-year survival.

Two other important studies reviewed results of transatrial mitral commissurotomy in special patient subgroups. Black and Harken[44] reviewed the results of surgical mitral valvuloplasty performed in 148 patients who were over 50 years of age at time of operation. All patients were in functional class III or IV. From 68 to 84 percent of the patients had atrial fibrillation. At least 42 percent of the patients had histories of previous arterial embolic events, and 14 percent had associated aortic valve disease, coronary disease, or hypertensive disease. At operation, 48 to 65 percent of these patients had palpable mitral valve calcification, and 35 to 70 percent had thrombus in the left atrium. The perioperative embolic rate was high at 10 to 16 percent. For patients in functional class III, regardless of their age, the perioperative mortality from all causes was 3.1 percent, and for those in class IV it was 27 percent. At follow-up 2 years after surgery, 80 percent of the patients in preoperative functional class III remained improved and 50 percent of the patients in functional class IV remained improved. The cardiac mortality was 8 percent at 2 years. Thus, despite severe symptoms and stiff calcified valves, these patients had satisfactory clinical improvement after commissurotomy.

Fraser[45] reviewed the late results 7 to 13 years after transatrial mitral commissurotomy in 68 patients who had received *inadequate opening* of the mitral valve. The mitral valve opening was defined as inadequate when it was palpated after fracture to be less than 2.5 cm². There were 21 patients who initially improved but had recurrent symptoms and successful reoperation by the transventricular technique. Late mortality occurred in 11 patients owing to heart failure or embolic events. There were 35 other patients who had excellent results and did not have reoperation at least 6 years after initial surgery; 20 patients had persistently good results and 15 patients had late recurrent symptoms. Those patients with (1) shorter symptomatic duration (less than 6 years) prior to the commissurotomy, (2) no mitral valve calcification, and (3) no cardiomegaly on chest x-ray examination were more likely to have persistently good symptomatic results despite *inadequate opening* of the valve at surgery.

These studies show that the advantages of the transatrial closed commissurotomy included (1) ease of access through a lateral thoracotomy, (2) the ability to assess mitral valve calcification and mitral regurgitation, and the extent of commissural opening by digital palpation in the beating heart, and (3) the ability to open the mitral valve without using cardiopulmonary bypass. The disadvantages of transatrial commissurotomy include (1) the small but definite risk of atrial tears, especially in the early experience with this technique, (2) the inability to repair mitral regurgitation that increased due to the procedure, and (3) a 2 to 8 percent perioperative embolic rate. There also were persistent technical difficulties. Sequentially applying digital pressure unilaterally to each commissure could only partially open the commissures in some patients. Surgeons attempted to improve the commissural opening using various digital knives and valvulotomes. Logan and Turner[46] then proposed the use of the Tubbs transventricular mitral dilator, which has become the standard technique for closed mitral valvulotomy and is still used in many institutions.

RESULTS OF TRANSVENTRICULAR CLOSED MITRAL COMMISSUROTOMY

The immediate and long-term results of closed commissurotomy using the transventricular Tubbs dilator have been the subject of many surgical reports over the last three decades. Perioperative results from several large series of patients are shown in Table 10-2. The table is organized with the clinical findings before surgery on the left side of the table, and the intraoperative results in the center and the postoperative findings at the right of the table. The studies have reviewed cases operated from 1952 to 1967, and are arranged in order of increasing age of the patient populations at the time of operation. This arrangement was chosen because the proportions of patients with atrial fibrillation or calcified mitral valve, two important determinants of clinical outcome, also increase with increasing patient age in these studies.

Before surgery, most patients had severe symptoms and were in New York Heart Association functional class III or IV. Even in the studies of younger patients,[47] all patients were severely symptomatic. In studies with the mean patient age of less than 40 years of age, atrial fibrillation occurred in 13 to 45 percent, and in older patients it occurred in 60 to 75 percent. The previous history of embolization also increased with age. From 3 to 21 percent of the younger patients and 22 to 27 percent of older patients reported previous embolic episodes. Moderate mitral regurgitation, assessed preoperatively by physical examination, occurred in 10 to 27 percent. Associated valvular disease occurred in 10 to 19 percent of cases.

The perioperative findings were assessed by the surgeon by palpating the valve in the operating room. Calcified mitral valves occurred in 15 to 36 percent of younger patients, and in 37 to 52 percent of older patients. In other studies published later, severely calcified valves were found in 16 to 28 percent of eligible patients and were treated by *converting* the procedure to mitral valve replacement using standby heart-lung bypass.[56,57] The incidence of mild to moderate mitral regurgitation immediately after commissurotomy varied from 18 to 38 percent in younger patient groups and from 5 to 53 percent in older patients. Although mild mitral regurgitation was induced in 10 to 30 percent of patients, the incidence of severe mitral regurgitation was 0.3 to 3 percent and did not increase with increasing patient age or valve calcification. Induction of moderate to severe mitral regurgitation was associated with poor long-term prognosis.[48] A *good valve opening* was assessed by surgical palpation in 60 to 90 percent of patients in these studies and was strongly associated with the clinical and surgical assessment of valve mobility.[49] Embolic events at operation or in the perioperative period occurred in 1 to 12 per-

Table 10–2. Perioperative Results of Transventricular Mitral Commissurotomy

Author	Ref #	Total # of Pts	Mean Age (Yr)	Preoperative*				Intraoperative Period*			Postoperative*		
				FC II and IV	At. Fib.	Hx Emboli	Mod. MR	Calcified Valve	MR Post CMC	Good Valve Opening	Embolic Event	FC III and IV	30-Day Mortality
John	47	3724	27	99	13	3	13	15	18	98	1–6	—	3.8
Manteuffel	48	1700	30	79	35	16	27	25	38	81	3	14	4.5
Commerford	49	654	33	91	21	—	—	26	—	79	—	—	3
Hoeksema	50	291	35	59	—	18	10	16	19	86	12.4	4	3.4
Logan	46	521	35	—	—	—	—	—	19	61	1.4	—	6.4
Otto	51	555	37	82	36	6.3	8	25	26	60	3	—	4.9
Turina	52	137	38	69	45	21	25	28	35	—	—	—	1.5
Lowther	53	500	39	—	39	—	27	36	19	84	3	16	6.2
Fraser	54	287	35	95	—	—	—	7	—	79	—	—	4.2
Austen	55	100	40	—	60	23	—	37	38	51	2	—	3.2
Salerno	56	139	46	100	—	—	6	—	14	—	3	10	2
Grantham	57	273	47	77	63	25	6	52	—	90	2.7	3	3,7
Kulbertus	58	77	55	67	75	27	21	49	53	84	—	—	6.7
Skagen	59	90	56	71	74	22	—	—	5	—	3.3	19	7.8

*Percent of patients (Pts) in each category. At. Fib. = atrial fibrillation, Hx Emboli = history of embolic events, Mod. MR = auscultatory mild to moderate mitral regurgitation, MR Post CMC = surgeon's assessment by palpation of mitral regurgitation after closed mitral commissurotomy, Good Valve Opening as assessed by surgeon at commissurotomy, Embolic Event = peripheral emboli.

cent of patients. Patients in sinus rhythm had a lower embolic rate (1 to 3 percent) compared with those with atrial fibrillation (6 to 12 percent). Usually in the perioperative period there was a remarkable decrease in symptoms, only 3 to 19 percent of patients remaining in functional class III or IV. The 30-day operative mortality in these studies, which were reported during 20 years of operative experience with the technique, was 3 to 5 percent for patients under the age of 50 years. Operative mortality was increased for patients over the age of 50 and for those patients in functional class IV. *Operative mortality was not increased in those patients with mildly calcified valves or with associated mild to moderate mitral regurgitation not requiring valve replacement.*

These surgeons followed their patients for 2 to 24 years and documented the late clinical results (Table 10–3). Persistently good clinical results were noted at follow-up in 57 to 86 percent of younger patient groups and in 41 to 90 percent of older patients. Late embolic events ranged from 0.5 to 2.4 percent for younger groups of patients, and up to 14 percent for patients who were above 60 years of age at operation. Many of these latter patients were already in functional class IV or in atrial fibrillation at the time of operation. Younger patients, even in functional class III or IV, had a long-term incidence of late embolization of only 0.16 percent per year. Patients who developed atrial fibrillation also had progressive symptoms. Follow-up from 3 to 9 years showed that the prevalence of atrial fibrillation progressed in older and more symptomatic patients. Patient groups with mean ages above 50 at operation had an 83 to 95 percent incidence of atrial fibrillation at 3- to 5-year follow-up.

Open heart surgery early after closed mitral commissurotomy was necessary in 1 to 3 percent of patients who had markedly increased mitral regurgitation, or incomplete commissurotomy. *The surgical impression was that the distribution of*

Table 10–3. Follow-Up Results After Transventricular Mitral Commissurotomy*

Author	Ref #	F/U Length (Yr)	Good Results at F/U	FC III or IV	Late Emboli	Late Atrial Fib.	Repeat Mitral Comm.	Mitral Valve Replace.	Late Survival
John	47	24	78	20	0.5	—	3.5	—	85
Manteuffel	48	6	66	—	—	25	3	—	95
Commerford	49	12	—	—	—	—	31	—	78
Hoeksema	50	2.5	86	—	2.4	—	—	4	93
Logan	46	—	—	—	—	—	—	—	—
Otto	51	2	85	—	—	—	6	5	—
Turina	52	3	73	9	2	31	4	1	95
Lowther	53	9	57	56	9	27	17	—	88
Fraser	54	11	79	21	—	—	5	7	86
Austen	55	—	—	—	4	—	—	—	—
Salerno	56	11	—	—	4	—	17	15	90
Grantham	57	4.4	90	—	4	—	8	8	87
Kulbertus	58	3	41	50	8	95	13	13	85
Skagen	59	5	—	32	14	83	—	18	77

*Percent of patients in each category. F/U = follow-up. Other abbreviations same as Table 10–2.

calcium in these valves was more important than the total amount of calcification in relation to induced mitral regurgitation. Tears of the posterior leaflet of the mitral valves occurred in those valves with calcium nodules in the leaflets and in commissures. Repeat mitral commissurotomy, either by a transventricular closed technique or by open technique, was necessary after 4 to 24 years in 3 to 31 percent of the patients. The need for repeat commissurotomy was very small for the first 5 to 6 years after the surgical procedure and was related to the mean age at operation. For young selected patients, repeat mitral commissurotomy was necessary in 3.5 percent of patients over a 24-year follow-up period. For unselected patients 30 to 40 years of age, the need for repeat commissurotomy was 4 to 17 percent.[52,54] In older patient groups, with mean ages at operation from 47 to 56 years, the incidence was 13 to 17 percent at 3- to 5-year follow-up.

The long-term survival after transventricular closed mitral commissurotomy is excellent. The 3- to 24-year survival ranges from 77 to 95 percent. Younger patients demonstrated an 85 percent 24-year survival. In patients having commissurotomy at 40 to 50 years of age, there was a 77 to 87 percent 3- to 5-year survival.

Review of these experiences with transventricular commissurotomy showed the following:

1. In younger patients with shorter duration of symptoms, it is uncommon to find atrial fibrillation and calcified mitral valves. Pliable mitral valves may be assessed by auscultation.
2. These patients are likely to have good to excellent results from closed transventricular commissurotomy. Good clinical results may persist from 12 to 24 years in 80 percent of these patients.
3. Older patients are more likely to have atrial fibrillation, longer history of symptoms, and a higher probability of calcified mitral valve, but they can

also have excellent clinical results with commissurotomy if they are in functional class II or III.

4. Older patients with more severe symptoms often have associated atrial fibrillation before surgery and more heavily calcified valves palpated at surgery. They have increased incidence of atrial thrombus and have higher incidences of perioperative embolization.

5. The incidence of increased mitral regurgitation after a transventricular commissurotomy may be related to the *distribution* of calcium on the valve rather than the total amount of calcium seen on fluoroscopy.

6. In patients with advanced age, atrial fibrillation, or valve calcification, there is an initial good clinical result in 77 to 90 percent, which may last from 3 to 7 years. Thereafter, there is progressive symptomatic deterioration.

RESULTS OF OPEN MITRAL COMMISSUROTOMY

With the development of the pump-oxygenator, Lillehei,[60] Kay,[61] and Nichols[62] pioneered the surgical treatment of mitral stenosis under direct visualization with the heart open on cardiopulmonary bypass. Despite the early technical difficulties with cardiopulmonary bypass, the perceived advantages of open commissurotomy were (1) surgical control of the heart during cardiopulmonary bypass; (2) direct visual evaluation of the mitral valve and the subvalvular apparatus with the possibility of precise dissection of the commissures and fused chordae; and (3) after valve inspection or an attempted valve repair, the surgeon could immediately proceed to mitral valve replacement as a back-up procedure. These options resulted in improved results of open commissurotomy, both as a result of improved surgical technique and as a result of case selection by the surgeon based on valve morphology at the time of operation. Less calcified valves with simple commissural fusion were subjected to open commissurotomy, whereas heavily calcified or regurgitant valves, or valves that were regurgitant or persistently stenotic after an attempted repair, were replaced. Because of the varying techniques and approaches to repair or replacement in various institutions, it is difficult to compare closed commissurotomy with open commissurotomy directly. However, several centers have reviewed their long-term experience with open mitral commissurotomy and have reported on 8- to 10-year follow-up on series of 100 to 200 patients who were operated over an 8- to 20-year period.[63–66]

In comparing the preoperative characteristics of these patient groups with those listed for patients undergoing closed mitral commissurotomy, there are several differences. First, the patients having open commissurotomy tend to be older; the mean ages ranged from 39 to 49 years. Second, there was a tendency to select patients with earlier symptoms; only 45 to 86 percent of these patients were in functional class III or IV. Third, atrial fibrillation was present in only approximately one third of these patients despite their increased age. Fourth, only 9 to 20 percent of patients reported previous episodes of systemic emboli. In approximately 90 percent of these selected patients, open mitral commissurotomy alone was performed. In up to 10 percent, tricuspid repair was also performed.

In several studies, the authors have carefully documented their case selection process. For example, in the study by Laschinger and colleagues[64] over the 12-year period in which 150 open mitral commissurotomies were performed, there were at the same time many patients in whom open commissurotomy was planned but who went on to mitral valve replacement. Porcine valves were placed in 74 patients and Starr-Edwards valves in 187 patients. The operative morbidity and mortality were greater in both valve replacement groups. In the study of Kay and coworkers,[63] one quarter of the valves were *decalcified,* and approximately 22 percent of the valves had moderate to severe mitral valve regurgitation induced by attempting to open the commissures down to the annulus. These valves therefore were immediately treated with mitral valve replacement. In other long-term studies, the incidence of mitral valve replacement in patients in whom open commissurotomy was planned varied from 2 to 20 percent.[67–69]

This patient selection process resulted in notable differences in perioperative results. For example, 83 to 95 percent of patients in these studies achieved *excellent or good valve opening* with the open commissurotomy. Moderate to severe mitral regurgitation was induced more often, in 2 to 22 percent of the patients who then required mitral valve replacement at the same sitting. The perioperative embolic rate was reduced to 0.6 to 1 percent with the use of cardiopulmonary bypass. Immediately postoperatively, only 8 to 10 percent of the patients remained in functional class III or IV. Most important, the 30-day mortality in some studies ranged from 0.6 to 2 percent.[64,66,67] Operative mortality also decreased with increasing surgical experience. Finnegan and associates[70] demonstrated that in 314 patients operated over a 10-year period of time, the patients who were operated in the first 5 years of the series had a 10 percent operative mortality, whereas those operated in the last 5 years of the series had a 0.7 percent mortality. The variability in operative mortality was attributed to a *learning curve* in using the cardiopulmonary bypass systems, the early lack of appreciation of avoiding air emboli, and the early attempts at extensive decalcification and debridement of calcified mitral valves (associated with perioperative emboli 2 to 15 days after the surgery). In contrast, the patients who had valve replacement rather than open commissurotomy consistently had a 7 to 11 percent perioperative mortality.

These studies also reported follow-up data in series of 105 to 212 patients over 8 to 10 years. Most patients remained stable for 3 to 5 years after the operation. Only 2 to 16 percent required intervention in this early follow-up period. The incidence of late embolization was dramatically reduced to approximately 0.7 to 1 percent. Some patients had a relatively short duration of atrial fibrillation before operative intervention, or they developed atrial fibrillation only postoperatively and therefore they were able to be converted to sinus rhythm after recovery from the surgery.

Despite these differences in perioperative results, the late follow-up results after open commissurotomy in these patients are similar to the late results reported after closed commissurotomy by Ellis[41] and Glenn[40]. Late survival ranged from 85 to 100 percent at 8 to 10 years. However, only 38 to 79 percent of the patients survived free of a second operation. This second operation was usually mitral valve replacement.

There is no study that directly compares open versus closed mitral commissurotomy. The foregoing discussion demonstrates that there are wide variations between institutions and over time within an institution in selecting patients for commissurotomy versus valve replacement. It is unlikely therefore that a direct comparison study will be possible in the future. Case-controlled studies from a single large institution, even if chosen from different surgical eras, might afford better direct comparisons of the comparative risks and benefits of closed versus open operative techniques.

CURRENT TECHNIQUES OF MITRAL BALLOON
VALVULOPLASTY

The first cases treated by percutaneous mitral balloon valvuloplasty in adults[11] reported the transseptal placement of a special latex balloon, 25 mm in diameter, fixed on the distal end of a preformed curved catheter shaft. Later reports of mitral balloon valvuloplasty in adolescents and elderly patients also utilized an antero-grade transseptal approach and a single 25-mm diameter commercially available balloon catheter.[13,16,17] Although procedures were performed with catheters that underdilated the mitral valve, these achieved partial opening of the commissures, which decreased left atrial pressures and pulmonary artery pressures and increased cardiac output. During the early experiences with mitral balloon valvuloplasty in both pediatric and adult laboratories,[12] several difficulties were identified with the use of this single large balloon catheter: (1) The small vessel diameters in pediatric patients precluded the routine use of larger balloons to achieve further opening of the mitral valve orifice. (2) Placing large balloons into the femoral vein and across the atrial septum was difficult and traumatic. (3) The larger-diameter balloon was globular in shape and was difficult to hold in position across the stenotic mitral valve orifice. (4) The large fluid volume required to inflate and to deflate the balloon caused prolonged occlusion of the mitral orifice and hypotension. (5) After the valve was opened, pulling these large deflated balloons back across the atrial septum caused persistent atrial septal defects in some patients.

Using a double balloon technique overcame these problems and, in addition, achieved wider opening of the mitral valve. In adult patients, areas of 2 to 3 cm^2 and residual valve gradients of 4 to 6 mmHg were obtained immediately after the procedure.[14,19] Most investigators now routinely use a double balloon technique. Although it is more demanding technically, it usually achieves superior hemodynamic results.

In performing double balloon mitral valvuloplasty,[19] one or two transseptal catheter-sheath systems are placed across the atrial septum. A small balloon catheter can be advanced through the sheaths to the left ventricle. Long, stiff guide-wires with preshaped curled ends are then advanced into the left ventricular apex. After dilatation of the venous entry site at the groin and the interatrial septum, the large balloon valvuloplasty catheters are introduced across the septum and across the mitral valve orifice. They are inflated simultaneously to put stress directly on the fibrosed mitral commissures. Newer catheters have dual inflation ports, *pigtail* distal ends, and use thinner polyethylene catheter shafts and balloon materials. These new catheters may help to protect the left ventricular apex from trauma or perforation and may reduce the size of the entry hole across the interatrial septum. The selection of balloon sizes tends to vary. For younger patients the overdilatation of the mitral annulus seems to be well tolerated, and often two 20-mm diameter balloons are used. In older patients with a calcified mitral annulus, overdilatation of the annulus may contribute to acute annulus tears or to mitral regurgitation.

IMMEDIATE RESULTS OF MITRAL BALLOON
VALVULOPLASTY

Studies documenting the immediate hemodynamic results of single and double balloon mitral balloon valvuloplasty are listed in Table 10–4. These studies demonstrate that the mitral valve gradient can be reduced from the 15- to 21-

Table 10–4. Immediate Results of Mitral Balloon Valvuloplasty

Author	Ref #	# of Pts	Mean Age (Yr)	Gradient (LA-LV) mmHg		Cardiac Output (Liters/Min)		Mitral Valve Area (cm²)		Comments
				Pre	Post	Pre	Post	Pre	Post	
Lock	13	8	15	21	10	3.8	4.9	0.7	1.3	1–25 mm balloon used; 2 of 8 pts were adults
Palacios	20	100	55	15	5	3.9	4.3	0.9	1.8	1 balloon, 22 pts; 2 balloons, 20 + 20 mm
Al Zaibag	21	41	26	—	—	—	—	0.8	1.6	15 + 18 mm balloons
McKay CR	19	27	43	17	6	4.2	4.8	1.1	2.2	18 + 20 mm balloons
Mullins	12	5	17	21	4	—	—	—	—	2 balloon diam. = 1.2 × annulus
McKay RG	22	18	49	15	9	4.3	5.1	0.9	1.6	14 pts 1–25 mm balloon
Vahanian	23	100	43	16	6	2.6	3.1	1.1	2.2	23 pts w/1 balloon
Babic	24	76	39	19	8	—	—	1.1	2.4	33 pts single balloon
Chen	72	23	31	19	5	4.0	5.2	0.8	1.9	All double balloon
Nobuyoshi	73	64	—	12	7	—	—	1.4	2.0	Inoue balloon
Block (NHLBI-BVR)	74	72	56	15	6	—	—	0.9	2.0	73% w/2 balloons

mmHg range down to 4 to 7 mmHg immediately after the procedure. In series where single balloons were used, the residual gradients may be higher.[13] Usually the cardiac output increases by 10 to 30 percent and the mitral valve area increases by about 100 percent. In younger adult patients with noncalcified valves, mitral valve areas from 2 to 3 cm² can be achieved. In the cardiac catheterization laboratory, the opening of the mitral valve is associated with rapid and progressive decrease in the pulmonary artery pressures, even in patients with severe pulmonary hypertension.

These impressive hemodynamic changes are achieved at the cost of some procedure-related risks, as listed in Table 10–5. Mortality ranges from 0 to 4 percent. Embolic events despite careful screening by echocardiography may occur in 2 percent of patients. Cardiac perforation may occur in 0 to 4 percent of cases and is usually related to transseptal complications or perforation of the left ventricular apex during balloon inflation. In approximately one-third of cases, there is a mild increase in the amount of mitral regurgitation. Mitral regurgitation of hemodynamic significance requiring surgical treatment occurs in only 1 to 3 percent of the cases. This results from tears in the posterior mitral leaflet, tears of the posterior calcified mitral annulus, or guidewire traction and tears on the chordae as the wires are placed out of the aorta. It should be noted that these represent early results with

Table 10–5. Immediate Major Risks of Mitral Balloon Valvuloplasty

Author	Ref	# of Pts	Procedure Death	CVA or Emboli	Perforation and Tamponade	↑MR	ASD	Comments
Lock	13	8	0	0	1	—	—	1 25 mm balloon
Palacios	20	100	1	2	2	1	20	2 pts w/AV block
Al Zaibag	21	41	—	—	—	15	—	
McKay CR	19	27	1	0	0	4	4	
Mullins	12	5	—	—	—	1	—	
McKay RG	22	18	0	0	0	5	5	Single balloon
Vahanian	23	200	0	8	2 to OR	8	16	8 technical failures
Babic	24	76	2	3	0	20	0	6 arterial complications; 4 technical failures
Chen	72	23	—	—	—	3	3	25 mm single, then 18 + 20 double
Nobuyoshi	73	64	0	0	0	14 3 to OR	—	Inoue balloon; 4 technical failures
Block (NHLBI-BVR)	74	72	3	3	4	2 to OR		

CVA = cerebrovascular accident, ↑ MR = number of patients with any increase in mitral regurgitation, to OR = number of patients taken to the operating room for mitral valve replacement, ASD = iatrogenic atrial septal defect after valvuloplasty detected by oximetry.

first-generation catheter equipment. Current experience with improved catheters demonstrates improved safety of the technique.

The beneficial immediate hemodynamic results after valvuloplasty are often associated with remarkably decreased symptoms. Especially in younger patients, relief of dyspnea and orthopnea can be immediate. These patients may be ambulatory the day after the procedure and discharged from hospital within 48 to 72 hours. The functional limitations experienced by these younger patients immediately after the procedure are often due to the chronic deconditioning that they experienced during their prevalvuloplasty symptomatic period. This condition is rapidly reversible. On early clinical follow-up, there is often a remarkably increased sense of well-being, associated with increased activity over two weeks, and increased appetite and weight gain over three months. In middle-aged and elderly patients the symptom relief is associated with improved clinical status and slowly progressive functional ability over several months.

MORPHOLOGIC STUDIES: MECHANISM OF IMPROVED MITRAL VALVE FUNCTION

Morphologic studies at surgery and autopsy have demonstrated that the hemodynamic improvement after mitral balloon valvuloplasty is due to splitting of the commissures, allowing wider opening of the anterior leaflet during diastole. In minimally calcified valves (Fig. 10–1), the fibrosed commissures are split and the valve is widely patent, just as was achieved by closed commissurotomy techniques. In about three-quarters of the younger patients treated with balloon valvuloplasty, both commissures are split. In valves with heavier calcification and thickening, one or both of the commissures may also be partially split, leading to some increase in

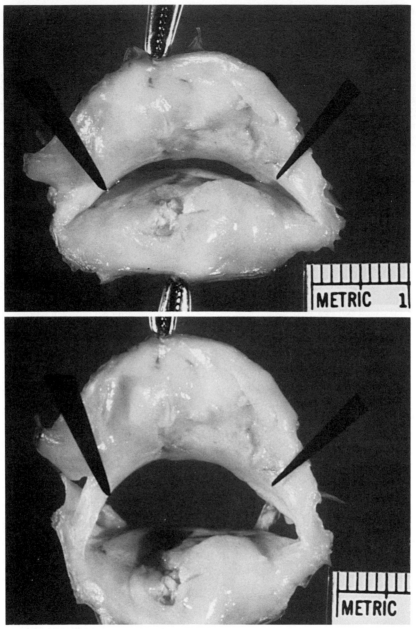

Figure 10–1. (*A*) Partially calcified mitral valve stenosis is primarily due to commissural fusion with minimal leaflet thickening, calcification, or subvalvular disease. Black arrowheads mark limits of commissural fusion. Calcific nodules are seen at the base of the anterior leaflet. (*B*) After double-balloon valvuloplasty, the commissures are split and the valve opening is greatly increased.

anterior leaflet mobility. This mechanism has been confirmed *in vivo* by quantitative two-dimensional echo Doppler studies before and after the valvuloplasty procedure (Fig. 10–2). After valvuloplasty, the transverse diameter of the mitral valve orifice is wider, the commissures are split, and the angles of opening of both the anterior and posterior commissures are increased.[76]

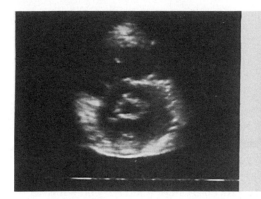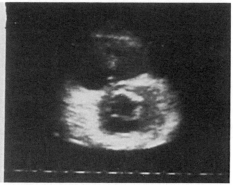

Figure 10–2. (*A*) Two-dimensional echocardiogram (parasternal short axis view) of a stenotic mitral valve before valvuloplasty. Note the small area (1.2 cm^2) and the acute angles of opening in diastole. (*B*) After valvuloplasty, the valve opens to 2.2 cm^2, the transverse diameter increases from 20 to 27 mm, and the angles of opening of the commissures have increased. The anterior commissure opens more widely than the posterior, as was often reported after closed surgical commissurotomy,[76] with permission.

IMPROVED EXERCISE CAPACITY AND EXERCISE HEMODYNAMICS

In our early experience with balloon valvuloplasty, we demonstrated that the reported symptomatic improvement was associated with improved exercise treadmill performance and exercise hemodynamics. In a consecutive series of 24 patients receiving double balloon mitral valvuloplasty, progressive improvement in exercise treadmill time was documented over the 3-month follow-up period.[19] Even those patients with modest improvements in mitral valve area demonstrated some improvement in maximum exercise tolerance. The improvement in exercise treadmill time was corroborated by supine bicycle exercise tests during cardiac catheterization before the valvuloplasty and three months after the mitral balloon valvuloplasty procedure. The mitral valve area before valvuloplasty averaged 1.0 cm^2 and increased to 2.2 cm^2 after valvuloplasty. The mitral valve gradient was 17 mmHg at rest and increased to 24 mmHg at symptom-limited exercise. Immediately after the valvuloplasty, the gradient at rest decreased to 6 mmHg and was 7 mmHg at follow-up. After 3 months, we exercised each patient during repeat cardiac catheterization to the same work level that she or he achieved before valvuloplasty. We demonstrated that despite higher cardiac outputs, the mitral gradients increased only to 14 mmHg. Continuing this exercise to a new symptom-limited end point in each patient demonstrated that the mean mitral valve gradient of 17 mmHg at peak exercise was also significantly lower than that noted before valvuloplasty. This study demonstrated that the hemodynamic improvements found at rest immediately after the procedure persisted over a three month follow-up and that the reported improved symptoms were associated with objective improvements in exercise treadmill time and improved supine exercise hemodynamics.

This study has now been confirmed by subsequent studies. Kraus[77] compared mitral balloon valvuloplasty patients with surgical patients with mitral valve replacement. This study demonstrated that six months after relief of mitral stenosis, the peak exercise heart rates and stroke volumes were greater and the pulmonary artery and pulmonary arterial wedge pressures were lower in both patient groups.

Similar results were also obtained in patients evaluated 6 months after open mitral commissurotomy.[78]

MIDTERM FOLLOW-UP STUDIES

Limited data on midterm follow-up studies are now available. As shown in Table 10–6, many patients remain symptom-free over a 6- to 24-month follow-up period. Hemodynamics at late follow-up have been difficult to document in these patients either by echo Doppler studies or by cardiac catheterization. Convincing asymptomatic patients to travel and to return to referral centers for cardiac catheterization studies is problematic. However, these data will be needed to assess the long-term effects of balloon valvuloplasty procedures adequately. The survival of patients after balloon valvuloplasty is excellent, ranging from 80 to 95 percent at 24 months. The incidence of recurrent symptoms is small—from 5 to 10 percent—and it has been distinctly unusual for these patients to require surgical commissurotomy or mitral valve replacement.

Important potential long-term problems concern (1) the incidence and clinical importance of small reductions in mitral valve areas, (2) the persistence of iatrogenic atrial septal defects, and (3) the persistence of mild mitral regurgitation documented by echo-Doppler immediately after the procedure. Therefore, it is of great importance to follow the results of the NHLBI Balloon Valvuloplasty Registry. In this study, over 700 patients will be followed for four years after mitral balloon valvuloplasty treatment using serial clinical and echocardiographic examinations. These data will be critical in determining the persistent long-term benefits of this procedure.

PATIENT SELECTION FOR MITRAL BALLOON VALVULOPLASTY

Clinical and hemodynamic criteria that can be used to select patients for mitral balloon valvuloplasty are outlined in Table 10–7. Patients should be symptomatic with physical findings and echo-Doppler findings consistent with moderate to severe mitral stenosis (mitral valve area less than or equal to 1.5 cm^2). In cases in which associated significant coronary disease[79] or valvular disease is in question, cardiac catheterization and angiography are necessary. *The younger symptomatic patient with a loud first heart sound and opening snap and a pliable valve on echocardiogram is an ideal candidate for mitral balloon valvuloplasty.* An accurate *preoperative* assessment of mitral valve morphology, of associated valve lesions, and the presence of left atrial thrombus is of critical importance. The presence of left atrial thrombus remains an absolute contraindication to balloon valvuloplasty and can be assessed by transthoracic echocardiography. Currently the usefulness of transesophageal echo, magnetic resonance image scanning, and cine computerized tomography scanning modalities are being investigated and may improve the detection of atrial thrombi.

With respect to the mitral valve morphology, several authors have evaluated the usefulness of formally *scoring* specific morphologic features of the mitral valve.[21,25] These scores assess anterior leaflet mobility, leaflet calcification, leaflet thickening, and fusion and shortening of the subvalvular chordae tendineae. Studies have demonstrated positive correlations between the high-pliability, low-calci-

Table 10–6. Midterm Follow-Up After Mitral Balloon Valvuloplasty

Author	Ref #	# of Pts	Mean F/U (Mo)	30 Day Death (%)	MVA(cm²)			Pts at F/U				Comments
					Pre	Post	F/U	↑Sx %	To OR	Repeat MBV	Death	
Lock	13	8	15	0	0.7	1.3	1.3	1	0	0	0	Restenosis in 1 pt at 6 wk cath.
Palacios	20	100	13	2	0.9	1.8	*	0	9(9)	—	7	F/U cath in 39 pts; * = MVA decreased with echo score >8
Al Zaibag	21	41	12	0	0.8	1.6	1.7	0	0	0	0	
McKay	19	27	3	0	0.9	2.2	2.0	0	0	0	1	Treadmill time ↑
Vahanian	23	100	9	0	1.0	1.9	1.8	6(6)	9(9)	—	0	
Babic	24	76	30	0	0.8	2.1	2.2	2(3)	5(7)	2	0	18 pts recath. at 6–18 mo.
Levine	75	105	14	1	1.0	1.9	1.5	4(4)	3(3)	2	8	7 technical failures; 20 pts f/u cath.
Bonan (NHLBI-BVR)	26	47	6	4	—	—	—	3(6)	—		1	Pooled data

fication scores and superior hemodynamic results. These echocardiographic criteria parallel the older clinical and intraoperative criteria used by surgeons to assess patients. Data in Table 10–5 show that mitral balloon valvuloplasties have been performed successfully in many patients. These patients are mostly younger and middle-aged; in other words, patients who achieve the best hemodynamic results

Table 10–7. Criteria for Recommending Mitral Balloon Valvuloplasty or Surgical Commissurotomy to Adult Patients with Rheumatic Mitral Stenosis

Candidates for Balloon Valvuloplasty or Surgery
Patient symptomatic—NYHA FC II-IV
Documented severe mitral stenosis—Physical exam, echo-Doppler
  (possibly cardiac catheterization). (MV Area < 1.5 cm²)

Indications for Mitral Balloon Valvuloplasty
No left atrial thrombus on echocardiography
No severe MR (0 to 2+ by angiography is acceptable)
No significant aortic or tricuspid valve disease
No significant coronary artery disease
First intervention—younger patients
Repeat intervention after previous surgical commissurotomy
Late intervention—elderly patients with high operative risks
Adequate oral anticoagulation prior to valvuloplasty procedure

Indications for Open Mitral Commissurotomy (with Optional Mitral Valve Replacement)
Presence of left atrial thrombus
Presence of severe mitral regurgitation (3+ or 4+)
Presence of heavily calcified valve commissures
Presence of significant multivalve disease
Presence of significant coronary artery disease
Repeat intervention—after failed balloon valvuloplasty

are also the same patients who are good surgical candidates. It is surprising therefore that some authors who perform balloon valvuloplasty on these younger patients still advocate restricting the use of mitral balloon valvuloplasty treatment to patients who are *high risk surgical candidates.*

SUMMARY

This review of the surgical and valvuloplasty literature demonstrates that mitral valve morphology rather than the type of intervention determines the therapeutic results after surgical commissurotomy or balloon valvuloplasty treatment of mitral stenosis. The mechanism of dilatation and hemodynamic results of transventricular mitral commissurotomy and of mitral balloon valvuloplasty are similar. Both techniques should be considered palliative. Because the balloon catheter technique can achieve hemodynamic results similar to surgery and may delay the trauma and expense of surgery, it can be offered to patients as a primary treatment for relief of symptomatic mitral stenosis.

REFERENCES

1. Brunton, L: Preliminary note on the possibility of treating mitral stenosis by surgical methods. Lancet 1:352, 1902.
2. Cutler, EC and Levine, SA: Cardiotomy and valvulotomy for mitral stenosis: Experimental observations and clinical notes concerning an operated case with recovery. Boston Med Surg J 188:1023, 1923.
3. Souttar, HS: The surgical treatment of mitral stenosis. Br Med J 1:603, 1925.
4. Bailey, CP: The surgical treatment of mitral stenosis (mitral commissurotomy). Dis Chest 15:377, 1949.
5. Harken, DE, Ellis, LB, Ware, PF, et al: The surgical treatment of mitral stenosis. I. Valvuloplasty. N Engl J Med 239:801, 1948.
6. Baker, C, Brock, RC, and Campbell, M: Valvotomy for mitral stenosis: Report of six successful cases. Br Med J 4665:1283, 1950.
7. Lillehei, CW, Gott, VL, DeWall, RA, et al: Surgical correction of pure mitral insufficiency by annuloplasty under direct vision. Lancet 77:446, 1957.
8. Nichols, HT, Blanco, G, Morse, DG, et al: Open mitral commissurotomy: Experience with 200 consecutive patients. JAMA 182:268, 1962.
9. Starr, A and Edwards, ML: Mitral replacement: Clinical experience with a ball-valve prosthesis. Ann Surg 154:726, 1961.
10. Mullin, EM, Glancy, DL, Higgs, LM, et al: Current results of operation for mitral stenosis: Clinical and hemodynamic assessment in 124 consecutive patients treated with closed commissurotomy, open commissurotomy, or valve replacement. Circulation 41:298, 1972.
11. Inoue, K, Owaki, T, Nakamura, T, et al: Clinical application of transvenous mitral commissurotomy by a new balloon catheter. J Thorac Cardiovasc Surg 87:394, 1984.
12. Mullins, CE, Nihill, MR, Vick, GW, et al: Double balloon technique for dilation of valvular or vessel stenosis in congenital and acquired heart disease. J Am Coll Cardiol 10:107, 1987.
13. Lock, JE, Khalilullah, M, Shrivastava, S, et al: Percutaneous catheter commissurotomy in rheumatic mitral stenosis. N Engl J Med 313:1515, 1985.
14. Al Zaibag, MA, Kasab, SA, Ribeiro, PA, et al: Percutaneous double-balloon mitral valvotomy for rheumatic mitral-valve stenosis. Lancet 1:757, 1986.
15. McKay, CR, Kawanishi, DT, and Rahimtoola, SH: Catheter balloon valvuloplasty of the mitral valve in adults using a double-balloon technique. JAMA 257:1753, 1987.
16. McKay, RG, Lock, JE, Keane, JF, et al: Percutaneous mitral valvuloplasty in an adult patient with calcific mitral stenosis. J Am Coll Cardiol 7:1410, 1986.
17. Palacios, I, Lock, JE, Keane, JF, et al: Percutaneous transvenous balloon valvuloplasty in a patient with severe calcific mitral stenosis. J Am Coll Cardiol 7:1416, 1986.

18. Roberts, W: Goodbye to thoracotomy for cardiac valvuloplasty. Am J Cardiol 59:198, 1987.
19. McKay, CR, Kawanishi, DT, Kotlewski, A, et al: Improvement in exercise capacity and exercise hemodynamics three months after double-balloon, catheter balloon valvuloplasty treatment of patients with symptomatic mitral disease. Circulation 77:1013, 1988.
20. Palacios, IF, Block, PC, Wilkins, GT, et al: Follow-up of patients undergoing percutaneous mitral balloon valvotomy: Analysis of factors determining restenosis. Circulation 79:573, 1989.
21. Al Zaibag, MA, Ribeiro, PA, Kasab, SA, et al: One-year follow-up after percutaneous double balloon mitral valvotomy. Am J Cardiol 63:126, 1989.
22. McKay, RG, Lock, JE, Safian, RD, et al: Balloon dilation of mitral stenosis in adult patients: Postmortem and percutaneous mitral valvuloplasty studies. J Am Coll Cardiol 9:723, 1987.
23. Vahanian, A, Michel, PL, Cormier, B, et al: Results of percutaneous mitral commissurotomy in 200 patients. Am J Cardiol 63:847, 1989.
24. Babic, U, Pejcic, P, Djurisic, Z, et al: Percutaneous transarterial balloon mitral valvuloplasty: 30 months' experience. Herz Kardiovask Erkrankungen 13:91, 1988.
25. Kisslo, J: Doppler echo evaluation of mitral stenosis pre and post balloon valvuloplasty. J Am Coll Cardiol 13:114A, 1989.
26. Bonan, R: Six month follow-up of mitral balloon valvuloplasty. J Am Coll Cardiol 13:17A, 1989.
27. Johnson, SL: The History of Cardiac Surgery, 1896–1955. Johns Hopkins Press, Baltimore, 1970, p 88.
28. Bland, EF and Jones, TD: Rheumatic fever and rheumatic heart disease: A twenty year report on 1000 patients followed since childhood. Circulation 4:836, 1951.
29. Wilson, MG and Lim, WN: Natural history of rheumatic heart disease in the third, fourth, and fifth decades of life. I. Prognosis with special reference to survivorship. Circulation 16:700, 1957.
30. Rowe, JC, Bland, EF, Sprague, HB, et al: The course of mitral stenosis without surgery: Ten and twenty year perspective. Ann Intern Med 52:741, 1960.
31. Grant, RT: After histories for 10 years of a thousand men suffering from heart disease. Heart 16:275, 1933.
32. Olesen, KH: The natural history of 271 patients with mitral stenosis under medical treatment. Br Heart J 24:349, 1962.
33. Bannister, RG: The risks of deferring valvotomy in patients with moderate mitral stenosis. Lancet 1:329, 1960.
34. Ward, C and Hancock, BW: Extreme pulmonary hypertension caused by mitral heart disease: Natural history and results of surgery. Br Heart J 37:74, 1975.
35. Rusted, IE, Scheifley, CH, and Edwards, JE: Studies of the mitral valve. II. Certain anatomic features of the mitral valve and associated structures in mitral stenosis. Circulation 14:398, 1956.
36. Wood, P: An appreciation of mitral stenosis. Br Med J I:1051, 1954.
37. Wade, OL, Bishop, JM, and Donald, KW: The effect of mitral valvotomy on cardiorespiratory function. Clin Sci 13:511, 1954.
38. Lyons, WD, Tompkins, RG, Kirklin, JW, et al: Early and late hemodynamic effects of mitral commissurotomy. J Lab Clin Med 53:499, 1959.
39. Ellis, LB, Singh, JB, Morales, DD, et al: Fifteen- to twenty-year study of one thousand patients undergoing closed mitral valvuloplasty. Circulation 48:357, 1973.
40. Glenn, WWL, Calabrese, C, Goodyear, AVN, et al: Mitral valvulotomy. II. Operative results after closed valvulotomy: A report of 500 cases. Am J Surg 117:493, 1969.
41. Ellis, LB, Benson, H, and Harken, DE: The effect of age and other factors on the early and late results following closed mitral valvuloplasty. Am Heart J 75:743, 1968.
42. Ellis, LB and Harken, DE: Closed valvuloplasty for mitral stenosis: A twelve-year follow-up study of 1571 patients. N Engl J Med 270:643, 1964.
43. Ellis, LB, Harken, DE, and Black, H: A clinical study of 1000 consecutive cases of mitral stenosis two to nine years after mitral valvuloplasty. Circulation 19:803, 1959.
44. Black, H and Harken, DE: Mitral valvuloplasty in patients past fifty. N Engl J Med 259:361, 1958.
45. Fraser, K, Kerr, IF, and McGuinness, JB: Mitral stenosis: Unexpected improvement after inadequate valvotomy. Br Med J 2:421, 1964.
46. Logan, A and Turner, R: Surgical treatment of mitral stenosis with particular reference to the transventricular approach with a mechanical dilator. Lancet 2:874, 1959.
47. John, S, Bashi, VV, Jairaj, PS, et al: Closed mitral valvotomy: Early results and long-term follow-up of 3724 consecutive patients. Circulation 68:891, 1983.
48. Manteuffel-Szoege, L, Nowicki, J, Wasniewska, M, et al: Mitral commissurotomy: Results in 1700 cases. J Cardiovasc Surg 11:350, 1970.

49. Commerford, PJ, Hastie, T, and Beck, W: Closed mitral valvotomy: Actuarial analysis of results in 654 patients over 12 years and analysis of preoperative predictors of long-term survival. Ann Thorac Surg 33:473, 1982.
50. Hoeksema, TD, Wallace, RB, and Kirklin, JW: Closed mitral commissurotomy: Recent results in 291 cases. Am J Cardiol 17:825, 1966.
51. Otto, TJ: Surgical treatment of mitral stenosis. Thorax 19:541, 1964.
52. Turina, M, Messmer, BJ, and Senning, A: Closed mitral commissurotomy: Operative results and late follow-up in 137 patients. Surgery 72:812, 1972.
53. Lowther, CP and Turner, RWD: Deterioration after mitral valvotomy. Br Med J 1:1027, 1962.
54. Fraser, K, Turner, MA, and Sugden, BA: Closed mitral valvotomy. Br Med J 2:352, 1976.
55. Austen, WG and Wooler, GH: Surgical treatment of mitral stenosis by the transventricular approach with a mechanical dilator. N Engl J Med 263:661, 1960.
56. Salerno, TA, Neilson, IR, Charrette, EJP, et al: A 25-year experience with the closed method of treatment in 139 patients with mitral stenosis. Ann Thorac Surg 31:300, 1981.
57. Grantham, RB, Daggett, WM, Cosimi, AB, et al: Transventricular mitral valvulotomy: Analysis of factors influencing operative and late results. Circulation 49, 50(Suppl II):200, 1974.
58. Kulbertus, HE and Kirk, AR: Mitral valvotomy in elderly patients. Br Med J 1:274, 1968.
59. Skagen, K, Hansen, JF, and Olesen, KH: Closed mitral valvulotomy after the age of fifty. Scand J Thorac Cardiovasc Surg 12:85, 1978.
60. Lillehei, CW, Gott, VL, DeWall, RA, et al: The surgical treatment of stenotic or regurgitant lesions of the mitral and aortic valves by direct vision utilizing a pump-oxygenator. J Thorac Surg 35:154, 1958.
61. Kay, EB, Nogueira, C, Martins de Oliveira, J, et al: Surgical treatment of mitral insufficiency: Direct vision correction with use of mechanical pump oxygenator and extracorporeal perfusion. Am J Cardiol 32:281, 1958.
62. Nichols, HT, Blanco, G, Morse, DP, et al: Open mitral commissurotomy: Experience with 200 cases. JAMA 182:148, 1962.
63. Kay, PH, Belcher, P, Dawkins, K, et al: Open mitral valvotomy: Fourteen years' experience. Br Heart J 50:4, 1983.
64. Laschinger, JC, Cunningham, JN, Baumann, FG, et al: Early open radical commissurotomy: Surgical treatment of choice for mitral stenosis. Ann Thorac Surg 34:287, 1982.
65. Housman, LB, Bonchek, L, Labert, L, et al: Prognosis of patients after open mitral commissurotomy: Actuarial analysis of late results in 100 patients. J Thorac Cardiovasc Surg 73:742, 1977.
66. Smith, WM, Neutze, JM, Barratt-Boyes, BG, et al: Open mitral valvotomy: Effect of preoperative factors on result. J Thorac Cardiovasc Surg 82:738, 1981.
67. Vega, JL, Fleitas, M, Martinez, R, et al: Open mitral commissurotomy. Ann Thorac Surg 31:266, 1981.
68. Nakano, S, Kawashima, Y, Hirose, H, et al: Long-term results of open mitral commissurotomy for mitral stenosis with severe subvalvular changes: A ten-year evaluation. Ann Thorac Surg 37:159, 1984.
69. Cohn, LH, Alfred, EN, Cohn, LA, et al: Long-term results of open mitral valve reconstruction for mitral stenosis. Am J Cardiol 55:731, 1985.
70. Finnegan, JO, Gray, DC, MacVaugh, H, III, et al: The open approach to mitral commissurotomy. J Thorac Cardiovasc Surg 67:75, 1974.
71. Munoz, S, Gallardo, J, Diaz-Gorrin, J, et al: Influence of surgery on the natural history of rheumatic mitral and aortic valve disease. Am J Cardiol 35:234, 1975.
72. Chen, C, Wang, Y, Qing, D, et al: Percutaneous mitral balloon dilatation by a new sequential single- and double-balloon technique. Am Heart J 116:1161, 1988.
73. Nobuyoshi, M, Hamasaki, N, Nosaka, H, et al: Percutaneous transvenous mitral commissurotomy: Early clinical outcome. J Am Coll Cardiol 11:14A, 1988.
74. Block, PC: Early results of mitral balloon valvuloplasty (MBV) for mitral stenosis: Report from the NHLBI registry. Circulation 78:II489, 1988.
75. Levine, MJ, Erny, RE, Leonard, BM, et al: Long-term follow-up in 105 patients undergoing percutaneous balloon mitral valvuloplasty. J Am Coll Cardiol 13:18A, 1989.
76. Reid, CL, McKay, CR, Chandraratna, PAN, et al: Mechanisms of increase in mitral valve area and influence of anatomical features in double-balloon, catheter balloon valvuloplasty in adults with rheumatic mitral stenosis: A Doppler and two-dimensional echocardiographic study. Circulation 79:628, 1987.

77. Kraus, F, Dacian, S, Rudolph, C, et al: Early and long-term results after mitral valvuloplasty as compared with valve replacement. J Am Coll Cardiol 13:18A, 1989.
78. Kraus, F, Dacian, D, Rudolph, C, et al: Early and long-term results after mitral valvuloplasty as compared with open commissurotomy. J Am Coll Cardiol 13:55A, 1989.
79. Chun, PKC, Gertz, E, Davis, JE, et al: Coronary atherosclerosis in mitral stenosis. Chest 81:36, 1982.

Commentary

By Melvin D. Cheitlin, M.D.

Until recently, the field of interventional cardiovascular procedures was dominated by balloon angioplasty, first of peripheral vessels and later, as developed by Gruentzig, of obstructed coronary arteries. Over time, procedures were developed not only to open but also to close vessels with coils, chemicals, and detachable balloons. Within the last decade the technique of balloon valvuloplasty has been introduced, first for use in children with pulmonary valvular stenosis, then in children and adults for aortic stenosis, and most recently in patients with mitral stenosis. In adults balloon valvuloplasty for calcific aortic stenosis has proved to be palliative at best and is associated with a high mortality on follow-up in elderly patients and a high recurrence rate of severe symptomatic aortic stenosis. Furthermore, the severely obstructed valve is opened by only about 0.5 cm^2, so that in most series the valve area is changed only from extremely to severely obstructed, frequently remaining after valvuloplasty with a valve area we consider an indication for surgery.

The problem with calcific aortic stenosis as opposed to congenital aortic stenosis or even rheumatic aortic stenosis is that the mechanism for obstruction is fibrosis and calcification of the valve rather than fusion of the commissures. In calcific aortic stenosis the mechanism of opening the valve is that of cracking the calcific plates of the leaflets, the benefit of which apparently is rather rapidly reversed with time. With mitral stenosis the mechanism of obstruction is commissural fusion. The excellent long-term results of operative mitral commissurotomy are related to separating the commissures, and the best candidates are usually young patients with flexible valves and no or minimal mitral regurgitation. Dr. McKay points out in this chapter that in the reported series of patients who had balloon valvuloplasty for mitral stenosis the predictors of good results are exactly the same as those that predict good results with operative commissurotomy. Although patients who have severe mitral stenosis and are not surgical candidates because of severe calcification or subvalvular obstruction are often mentioned as candidates for balloon valvuloplasty, these patients also are not likely to have good results from balloon valvuloplasty.

Balloon valvuloplasty therefore must be compared with mitral commissurotomy in mortality, morbidity, and late results. From the studies already reported, I believe that mortality and early morbidity probably will be similar to those of closed commissurotomy. The problems resulting from residual mitral regurgitation probably will be similar to those occurring after operative mitral commissurotomy. What the natural history of the small atrial defects encountered in some of these

196

patients will be is unknown, but because the shunt is usually small, this probably will not be a serious problem. The questions remaining are what the long-term follow-up results will be in terms of symptom-relief, recurrence of stenosis, embolism, and mortality. Closed mitral commissurotomy long-term results have been excellent—on 10- to 15-year follow-up, an 85 percent survival in class III and IV patients, a low embolic rate, and a repeat commissurotomy rate of 0.4 percent in a remarkable series of patients reported by John and associates.[1] In 1000 patients followed for 15 years, Ellis and colleagues[2] found a 2.7 percent late embolic rate and a 25 to 40 percent total survival of class III and IV patients at 15 years. With balloon valvuloplasty, with the exception of the series studied by Babic and colleagues[3] in which the mean follow-up was 30 months, the follow-up time has been less than two years, with incomplete hemodynamic restudy in these initial series. Nevertheless, apparently the stenotic mitral valve is opened to double the stenotic area by balloon valvuloplasty, which is better than that seen after aortic valvuloplasty, and in the range expected of mitral valve replacement—about 2 cm^2. Like balloon valvuloplasty, the increased valve area with mitral commissurotomy also results from physically separating the fused commissures. Whether the long-term results will be equal to closed mitral commissurotomy remains to be seen; however, because in the United States closed commissurotomy now is rarely done, balloon valvuloplasty will have to be compared with open mitral commissurotomy, which produces a better mitral opening than closed commissurotomy and in which the long-term results have been excellent. At the University of California at San Francisco, in 108 consecutive open valvuloplasties followed for 1 to 15 years and a mean of 6.5 years, a life-table analysis has shown the cumulative survival at 15 years to be 89 percent, the cumulative reoperation-free rate to be 75 percent, and cumulative embolism-free rate to be 89 percent. Cohn and colleagues[4] reported that the actuarial probability of survival after open commissurotomy was 95 percent at 10 years, that thromboemboli occurred in 9 of 120 patients, and that the annual reoperation rate was 1.7 percent. How well balloon valvuloplasty will compete with open commissurotomy in these results remains to be seen; at present we can say only that balloon valvuloplasty is a way of postponing mitral commissurotomy, not replacing it.

Another problem is that of operator competence. Compared with other countries, especially Third World countries, the United States has a limited number of patients with mitral stenosis. It is unlikely, therefore, for any one of our operators to have sufficient experience with cases of mitral stenosis to be proficient in this procedure, as opposed to cases of aortic stenosis, which are much more common. Hence, consideration should be given to regionalizing the procedure for mitral valvuloplasty so that it can be done in only a few centers and proficiency can be maintained.

REFERENCES

1. John, S, Bashi, VV, Jairaj, PS, et al: Closed mitral valvotomy: Early results and long-term follow-up of 3724 consecutive patients. Circulation 68:891, 1983.
2. Ellis, B, Singh, JB, Morales, DD, et al: Fifteen-to-twenty-year study of one thousand patients undergoing closed mitral valvuloplasty. Circulation 48:357, 1973.
3. Babic, U, Pejcic, P, Djurisic, Z, et al: Percutaneous transarterial balloon mitral valvuloplasty: thirty months' experience. Herz Kardiovask Erkrankungen 13:91, 1988.
4. Cohn, LH, Alfred, EN, Cohn, LA, et al: Long-term results of open mitral valve reconstruction for mitral stenosis. Am J Cardiol 55:731, 1985.

CHAPTER 11

Is Valve Replacement Indicated in Asymptomatic Patients with Aortic Stenosis or Aortic Regurgitation?

Annmarie Errichetti, M.D.
Joshua M. Greenberg, M.D.
William M. Gaasch, M.D.

Aortic valve disease in adults generally progresses slowly and insidiously, with a very low mortality during a long asymptomatic phase. When symptoms eventually develop, however, the outlook changes dramatically, and mortality exceeds 50 percent within a few years. Thus, the development of symptoms identifies a distinct and important point in the natural history of the disease. Therapeutic decisions, therefore, require an understanding of this natural history, as well as of the left ventricular response to chronic pressure overload (aortic stenosis) or volume overload (aortic regurgitation) and the surgical mortality and complications associated with prosthetic heart valves. As will be discussed, valve replacement is almost always recommended in symptomatic patients. However, the asymptomatic or minimally symptomatic patient occasionally may present a difficult management problem. In this chapter, emphasis will be on asymptomatic patients.

AORTIC STENOSIS

Isolated aortic stenosis in the adult is due usually to a congenital deformity and/or degenerative calcific changes. Over many years, the valve becomes increasingly deformed and calcified. Whereas the rate of progression appears to be gradual in some patients, others–especially those with degenerative calcific disease—may show important changes in the valve area within a few years.[1,2] As a result of these changes in the aortic valve leaflets, left ventricular outflow resistance gradually increases, as does left ventricular systolic pressure. Systolic pressure overload leads to a compensatory increase in myocardial mass, and function is preserved, so that there is little or no clinical disability during this benign, asymptomatic phase.[3-5] Eventually, left ventricular failure ensues and symptoms develop. At that time—

or occasionally earlier—the severity of the aortic valve stenosis can be evaluated with hemodynamic and/or echocardiographic techniques.

The widely recognized definition of *hemodynamically significant* aortic stenosis is a calculated effective aortic valve area of 0.7 cm^2 or less.[6] This critical value derived from cardiac output and pressure gradient measurements requires invasive cardiac catheterization procedures. Although the accuracy of this area calculation may be limited under some circumstances, it remains a standard for the assessment of the severity of aortic stenosis.

In recent years, echocardiographic techniques have been shown to provide an accurate assessment of the severity of aortic stenosis. Although M-mode and two-dimensional (2-D) echocardiography permit qualitative assessment of structural changes involving the aortic root and aortic valve leaflets, both fail to provide quantitative hemodynamic information. By contrast, continuous-wave Doppler echocardiography allows an accurate noninvasive assessment of pressure gradients across stenotic valves.[7-11] From measurement of the maximal flow velocity across the aortic valve, the peak instantaneous pressure gradient can be estimated via the modified Bernoulli equation, expressed as $p = 4 \times V^2$, in which p is the pressure drop or gradient across a stenotic orifice and V is the peak transvalvular velocity.

Numerous studies have confirmed a good correlation between continuous-wave Doppler and catheterization-derived pressure gradients.[8-13] It should be emphasized that the Doppler gradient (derived from peak velocity) represents a maximum instantaneous pressure difference, whereas the *peak-to-peak* gradient (derived from cardiac catheterization) reflects the difference between peak left ventricular and aortic pressures, which are nonsimultaneous events.[10] As a result, the Doppler-derived pressure gradient is generally higher than the peak-to-peak gradient; with severe obstruction, these differences are minimal. By averaging multiple measurements along the Doppler spectral waveform, mean pressure gradients also can be calculated.

Aortic valve area can be estimated from 2-D and Doppler echocardiography using the continuity equation. The continuity equation is based on the principle that, in a continuous flow circuit at a constant rate of flow, the product of flow area and velocity will remain constant on both sides of an obstruction: $A_1V_1 = A_2V_2$. Therefore, if the velocity and flow are known, the area of the stenotic orifice can be derived as flow divided by the velocity of the stenotic jet. The continuity equation is rearranged to yield the aortic valve area: in which A_1 is the cross-sectional area of the left ventricular outflow tract, V_1 is the velocity of blood flow in the left ventricular outflow tract, V_2 is the velocity of blood flow distal to the obstruction, and A_2 is the cross-sectional area of the aortic valve. Several investigators have demonstrated an excellent correlation between the aortic valve area estimated by this technique and that determined at catheterization by application of the Gorlin equation.[14-16]

Echocardiography also provides information on the left ventricular size and function, the degree of hypertrophy, and associated lesions such as mitral regurgitation. Thus, echocardiography has had a major impact on our ability to assess the severity of aortic stenosis and particularly to follow its progression without the need for serial cardiac catheterization. Having assessed the severity of the aortic stenosis and the status of the left ventricle, the next stop in the decision analysis depends on the presence or absence of symptoms.

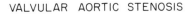

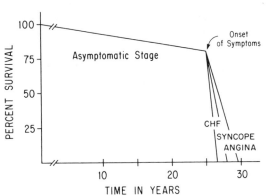

Figure 11–1. Survival in patients with aortic stenosis. During a prolonged asymptomatic stage the annual mortality is very low; after the onset of symptoms the prognosis is substantially worsened.

SYMPTOMATIC PATIENTS

After the onset of symptoms, patients with aortic stenosis exhibit a predictably poor prognosis (Fig. 11–1). Congestive heart failure carries the worst prognosis, whereas syncope, angina, and exertional dyspnea are somewhat less ominous. Aortic valve replacement is almost always followed by symptomatic improvement and a substantial improvement in survival rate, even in patients with impaired left ventricular function. In patients with modest depression of ventricular function (i.e., ejection fractions of 40 to 50 percent), the results of valve replacement are similar to those in patients with normal function. Patients with severely depressed ventricular function (i.e., ejection fractions of 20 to 30 percent) may not experience complete symptomatic improvement, but some improvement can be expected, and these patients also should undergo valve replacement.[17–19] Thus, all symptomatic patients with isolated aortic stenosis should undergo aortic valve replacement; the only exception might be the elderly patient with severe end-stage left ventricular dysfunction, due usually to associated coronary artery disease. Under some circumstances, balloon aortic valvuloplasty might be considered an alternative (albeit palliative) procedure.[20]

ASYMPTOMATIC PATIENTS

Inasmuch as the natural history of asymptomatic aortic stenosis is generally benign, why should aortic valve replacement be considered? Two reasons are commonly mentioned. First, it has been suggested that irreversible myocardial depression may develop during the compensated asymptomatic phase and that this might preclude an optimal surgical result. Although irreversible plastic changes in the myocardium do occur in the large dilated hearts found in patients with chronic aortic regurgitation, such irreversibility has not proved to be a significant problem in patients with aortic stenosis. Second, aortic valve replacement might be considered in an asymptomatic patient to reduce the risk of sudden death. If valve replacement is considered for this reason, the risk of sudden death must be weighed against the surgical mortality and the known complications of prosthetic heart valves.

Sudden Death

In an attempt to estimate the frequency of sudden death in asymptomatic patients with aortic stenosis, it is useful to examine the overall profile of patients with aortic stenosis who die suddenly. Whereas sudden death is known to occur in hemodynamically significant aortic stenosis, it has been extremely difficult to document sudden death in a patient without prior symptoms.[3–5,21] Among all patients dying of aortic stenosis, death is sudden in less than 20 percent, and approximately three fourths of these patients exhibit preexisting angina, congestive heart failure, or syncope. Thus, it appears that sudden death may occur in 3 to 5 percent of patients with aortic stenosis without preexisting symptoms.[5] This is not an annual mortality but, rather, the overall prevalence of sudden death in the population studied. The frequency of sudden death on an annual basis must therefore be substantially lower. In addition, it should be recognized that most of the data on this subject were compiled from literature that did not exclude the coexistence of other lesions. If associated valvular or coronary disease is excluded, the frequency of sudden death in asymptomatic patients with aortic stenosis must be extremely low. This conclusion is consistent with the observations of Chizner and associates,[3] who followed eight patients with moderate to severe aortic stenosis for an average of 70 months; there were no deaths. Kelly and associates[21] have recently reported data that further support our conclusions regarding the benign nature of asymptomatic aortic stenosis. They identified 51 asymptomatic and 39 symptomatic patients with significant transvalvular pressure gradients (50 to 130 mmHg by Doppler echocardiography) and followed them conservatively for an average of 17 months (range 1 to 45 months). During this period, 41 percent of the asymptomatic group developed symptoms; dyspnea was considerably more frequent than angina or syncope. Two patients (4 percent) of the initially asymptomatic group developed symptoms and died. Sudden death did not occur in any asymptomatic patient.

Surgical Risk

Perioperative mortality varies in different series.[17,22–24] If it is not well under 5 percent,[3] the surgical risk clearly exceeds the risk of sudden death in an asymptomatic patient who does not undergo operation. Perioperative complications and morbidity should also be considered in any decision to proceed with aortic valve replacement, but a discussion of these factors is beyond the scope of this chapter.

Complications of Prosthetic Valves

The serious complications of prosthetic heart valves are also an important consideration in designing optimal therapy for a patient with aortic stenosis. Valve-related thromboembolism and thrombotic occlusion of the valve occur at the rate of 1 to 2 percent per year. The incidence of serious hemorrhagic complications secondary to the required anticoagulation is approximately the same. The risk of prosthetic valve dysfunction or serious paravalvular regurgitation is at least 1 percent per year, and these problems generally require reoperation. Infectious endocarditis occurs at the rate of approximately 1 percent per year; the overall mortality of this complication approaches 50 percent. Thus, the frequency of serious complications of prosthetic valves is approximately 5 percent per year, and the mortality due to prosthetic valve–related complications is in the range of 1 to 2 percent per year.[25]

It appears, therefore, that the risks of aortic valve replacement in the asymptomatic patient outweigh the single potential benefit (which is the prevention of sudden death). If, for example, the surgical mortality is 2 to 3 percent and the risk of fatal prosthetic-valve–related complications is 1 percent per year, the surgical risk clearly exceeds the possibility of sudden death (1 to 2 percent per year) in the unoperated patient. It can be argued, therefore, that there is no indication for aortic valve replacement in the asymptomatic patient with pure aortic stenosis.

High-Risk Patients

Our discussion has not yet considered the patient who, after a long asymptomatic phase, manifests new symptoms that rapidly progress to pulmonary edema, hypotension, and cardiogenic shock; this ominous clinical presentation carries a very high mortality.[3] Occasionally, patients exhibit such rapid progression that they die within hours or days of the onset of symptoms. This generally occurs in patients with associated coronary disease or depressed left ventricular function. Thus, the decision to proceed with aortic valve replacement depends in part on special efforts to identify patients who might be at exceptionally high risk.

The presence of associated coronary artery disease, abnormal ventricular function, and, especially, pulmonary hypertension are markers of the patient at high risk.[26] A markedly abnormal response to exercise is another marker, as is the presence of degenerative calcific disease because of its tendency to progress. These potential risk factors have not been statistically validated, but the presence of one or more of these factors could be considered a reason to proceed with valve replacement in the asymptomatic patient with aortic stenosis. Lacking valid information on such risk factors, it would seem prudent to follow such patients and to postpone surgery until symptoms develop. The patient's understanding of the risks and benefits is also important. Commonly the risks are nearly equal to the potential benefits.[27]

AORTIC REGURGITATION

Compensated aortic regurgitation is characterized by left ventricular chamber dilatation, an appropriate increase in myocardial mass, and normal myocardial contractility. As a consequence, left ventricular systolic wall stress (afterload) and the systolic ejection fraction are normal or near normal and the patient remains asymptomatic.[28] With progression (i.e., increased regurgitant volume and/or progressive chamber dilatation), fiber shortening tends to decline. Eventually there is gross left ventricular enlargement with inadequate hypertrophy, high wall stress, and depressed shortening (decompensated aortic regurgitation); elevated left ventricular diastolic pressures and systolic dysfunction result in dyspnea and fatigue. Aortic valve replacement is generally recommended in symptomatic patients, but the optimal approach to the asymptomatic patient has not been defined to everyone's satisfaction. As will be discussed, left ventricular function is closely related to survival, and, thus, a careful assessment of ventricular function is of signal importance in patients with chronic aortic regurgitation (Fig. 11–2).

As with aortic stenosis, cardiac catheterization and angiography have been the standards for evaluation of aortic insufficiency. Unfortunately, the invasive approach is not ideally suited for serial evaluations. Echocardiography is useful in this regard. The principal echocardiographic findings on M-mode examination

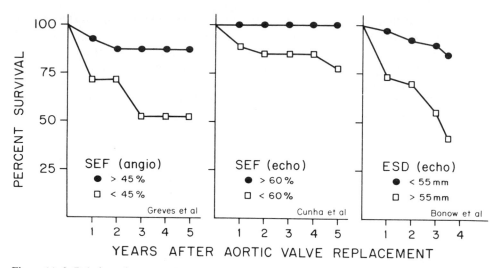

Figure 11–2. Relation of preoperative ventricular function to postoperative survival. Data of Greves, et al[43] *(left)* and those of Bonow, et al[51] *(right)* show remarkable agreement; both groups incorporated limits clearly in abnormal range. Cunha, et al[50] *(center)* selected a limit that was well within normal range. These and other published data *(see text)* indicate that preoperative ventricular function is an important determinant of postoperative survival. SEF indicates systolic ejection fraction; ESD, echocardiographically measured dimension at end-systole; angio = angiography; echo = echocardiography.

include diastolic fluttering of the anterior mitral leaflet, fluttering of the interventricular septum (or rarely the chordae tendineae), and a typical left ventricular volume overload pattern. However, these signs are neither sensitive nor specific as to the hemodynamic significance of the regurgitant leak.[29] Perhaps the most useful M-mode sign of aortic insufficiency is the premature closure of the mitral valve, indicating a marked increase in left ventricular diastolic pressure and generally a sign of severe aortic insufficiency.[30] Structural abnormalities of the aortic valve leaflets and aortic annulus as well as dilatation of the aortic root can be identified by 2-D echocardiography. However, changes in the echocardiographic appearance of the aortic valve leaflets generally are not specific nor do they provide quantitative information.

Recently there has been increasing interest in employing Doppler techniques to provide a semiquantitative assessment of the severity of aortic insufficiency. Pulsed Doppler has been shown to be useful in describing the regurgitant jet.[31,32] This method uses a flow-mapping technique that describes the extent of the regurgitant jet from the aortic valve plane into the left ventricle. The accuracy of this technique is imperfect because of the absence of standard landmarks, which is particularly a problem in dilated ventricles; the eccentric patterns of some jets; and interference from mitral valve flow. Color flow mapping also has been used to assess the severity of aortic insufficiency.[33,34] The technique allows an evaluation of the aortic regurgitation in multiple planes, even in the presence of mitral valve disease or eccentric jets. Some investigators have reported that the width of the aortic regurgitant jet at the valve orifice relative to the size of the left ventricular outflow tract is a better predictor of severity than is the area of the regurgitant jet or the depth to which it extends in the left ventricle.[33]

Pulsed Doppler also has been used to assess the regurgitant volume and regurgitant fraction.[35,36] One method calculates a regurgitant fraction by comparison of antegrade systolic flow to retrograde diastolic flow at the level of the aortic arch,[35] whereas the other calculates regurgitant volume as the difference between aortic stroke volume at the level of the aortic valve and stroke volume from a remote site, such as the pulmonary artery.[36] The use of continuous-wave Doppler in the assessment of the severity of aortic regurgitation also has been reported.[37-39] The slope of the velocity decline of the spectral envelope of the regurgitant leak has been found to correlate with the angiographic severity of aortic regurgitation; more severe regurgitation results in a more rapid rate of decline as the pressure difference between the aorta and left ventricle equilibrates. These methods, however, have had limited clinical application.

Although absolute quantitation of the severity of the aortic regurgitant lesion is not possible with echocardiography, the secondary effects of chronic aortic insufficiency can be determined. Serial measurements of left ventricular chamber size and systolic function are known to be useful in following patients with chronic aortic insufficiency. Review of data from essentially all published studies indicates that the frequency of persistent left ventricular dilatation after aortic valve replacement is highest in patients with preoperative left ventricular dysfunction.[40] This is usually translated into a suboptimal prognosis.

SYMPTOMATIC PATIENTS

Symptoms in patients with pure aortic regurgitation are almost always the consequence of elevated pulmonary venous pressure. In some patients, the initial symptom is effort dyspnea; in others, it is acute pulmonary edema. Angina pectoris in the absence of coronary artery disease is relatively uncommon, and syncope in the absence of arrhythmia occurs rarely.[41] Aortic valve replacement uniformly results in symptomatic improvement, due primarily to a reduction in left ventricular diastolic pressure. Although excellent surgical results are encountered in patients with preserved ventricular function, markedly abnormal ventricular function does not preclude substantial symptomatic improvement.

Although the notion of improved survival in surgically treated patients has been questioned,[42] most long-term follow-up data[22 24,43,44] indicate that aortic valve replacement enables longer survival than medical therapy. It does appear, however, that survival differences (medical versus surgical treatment) are minimal in the patient with only mildly depressed ventricular function. In patients with clearly depressed ventricular function, the difference between medical and surgical therapy is more apparent.

In conclusion, aortic valve replacement should be performed in essentially all symptomatic patients with aortic regurgitation. Despite impressive symptoms and marked left ventricular dysfunction, almost all patients exhibit symptomatic improvement after valve replacement surgery (even though left ventricular enlargement and dysfunction persist).[40] Thus it is almost never *too late* to proceed with valve replacement surgery.[45] Our goal, however, should be earlier identification of the patient who might benefit from surgery; this requires a careful assessment of the natural history of asymptomatic patients.

ASYMPTOMATIC PATIENTS

It is widely held that asymptomatic patients with chronic aortic regurgitation have a good prognosis;[41,46] consequently, there appears to be little reason to proceed with aortic valve replacement. However, if asymptomatic patients are divided into populations with normal and abnormal ventricular function, two distinct groups emerge, each with a different prognosis. In this section, these two subgroups will be discussed in an attempt to identify which patients might benefit from aortic valve replacement, despite the absence of significant symptoms.

Normal Left Ventricular Function

Asymptomatic patients with normal left ventricular systolic performance have an excellent prognosis despite considerable chamber enlargement. Symptoms develop in these patients at the rate of only a few percent per year,[46] and surgery easily can be postponed until the patient complains of symptoms. When corrective surgery is eventually performed, the duration of symptoms will have been relatively short and the postoperative results should be excellent.[47]

Abnormal Left Ventricular Function

There is a large body of evidence to support the hypothesis that prognosis is related to ventricular function. Thus it would seem important to identify asymptomatic patients with left ventricular dysfunction. Before proceeding with this discussion, however, we should consider how frequently patients with abnormal ventricular function remain asymptomatic. Data from echocardiographic studies indicate that as many as 25 percent of all patients with a large left ventricular end-systolic diameter remain asymptomatic (New York Heart Association functional class I).[48,49] More than half of the patients with depressed systolic shortening (echocardiographic fractional shortening less than 30 percent) are in New York Heart Association functional class I or II.[50] This is also true in patients with an angiographic ejection fraction of less than 50 percent.[43] Thus, many patients with abnormal ventricular function remain asymptomatic; many more have only minimal symptoms.

Many cardiologists recommend aortic valve replacement when there is reliable evidence of left ventricular dysfunction, even if important symptoms are absent. The rationale of this approach is as follows: Asymptomatic patients with ventricular dysfunction usually develop symptoms within a few years; as many as two thirds experience symptoms and require surgery within three years.[51] Therefore, it may seem reasonable to postpone surgery in these patients until symptoms develop. It can be argued, however, that the optimal time for aortic valve replacement is *before* the development of this ominous combination of symptoms and left ventricular dysfunction. Postponing surgery only increases the likelihood of a suboptimal postoperative result. For this reason, many cardiologists believe that, if operative mortality and the complications of prosthetic valves can be minimized, aortic valve replacement should be performed in patients with definite and reliable evidence of left ventricular dysfunction, even in the absence of symptoms.

If important clinical decisions are to be made on the basis of measured parameters of left ventricular function, it is of signal importance to develop a precise definition of compensated and decompensated chronic aortic regurgitation.[52] Cardiac catheterization and angiography, radionuclide techniques, and echocardiography have all been used to define the functional state of the left ventricle in chronic aortic regurgitation. Several parameters have been used to identify the high-risk patient. These include a large end-diastolic volume,[43,50,53−55,58,59] a large end-systolic volume,[48,50,53,55,56] an elevated end-diastolic pressure,[56,57] a subnormal ejection fraction,[43,50,53,55,59] increased indices of systolic wall stress,[48,56,60,61] a low ratio of regurgitant volume to end-diastolic volume,[62] and reduced exercise capacity.[63]

Follow-up of Asymptomatic Patients

A substantial number of asymptomatic patients who are not yet candidates for aortic valve replacement are best followed with serial noninvasive tests; these are generally patients with left ventricular enlargement and compensated or borderline ventricular function. After the initial or baseline studies, patients with preserved systolic function (i.e., end-systolic dimension less than 2.5 cm/m^2, normal ejection fraction, and so on) should be evaluated approximately every twelve months. Those in a borderline category should be studied every six months, at least until there is evidence that the left ventricular size and function are stable; afterward, less frequent studies might be possible. Those patients with ventricular dysfunction (i.e., end-systolic dimension greater than 2.6 cm/m^2, reduced ejection fraction, and so on) should undergo repeat studies, and if the diagnosis of left ventricular dysfunction is confirmed, cardiac catheterization and angiography should be performed in preparation for surgery. Our practice is to rely heavily on echocardiographic techniques and to use radionuclide ventriculography less frequently, usually on a confirmatory basis. Decisions regarding surgery should not be made on the basis of a single test or measurement; indeed, a combination of all echocardiographic, radionuclide, and other clinical data should be used.[64]

In a recent commentary, Bonow and Epstein[65] noted that "survival and functional results in patients with preoperative LV dysfunction are related to the severity of preoperative symptoms, exercise tolerance, and both the severity and duration of impaired left ventricular dysfunction."[65] They then indicated their preference for early operation when left ventricular dysfunction is clearly demonstrated, even in the absence of symptoms. Lacking data from a prospective study of aortic valve replacement and medical treatment in asymptomatic patients, we likewise recommend valve replacement in such patients.

SUMMARY

With rare exceptions, aortic valve replacement should be performed in all symptomatic patients with hemodynamically significant aortic stenosis; however, the asymptomatic patient requires a difficult risk-benefit analysis. In most asymptomatic patients the risks of aortic valve replacement outweigh the risks of conservative therapy and careful follow-up.

Symptomatic patients with chronic aortic regurgitation should undergo aortic valve replacement. Asymptomatic patients with normal left ventricular function are not surgical candidates, but aortic valve replacement should be performed in most patients with reliable evidence for left ventricle dysfunction, even if symptoms are not yet present.

REFERENCES

1. Cheitlin, MD, Gertz, EW Brundage, BH, et al: Rate of progression of severity of valvular aortic stenosis in the adult. Am Heart J 98:689, 1979.
2. Wagner, S and Selzer, A: Patterns of progression of aortic stenosis: A longitudinal hemodynamic study. Circulation 65:709, 1982.

3. Chizner, MA, Pearle, DL, and de Leon, AC, Jr: The natural history of aortic stenosis in adults. Am Heart J 99:419, 1980.
4. Frank, S, Johnson, A, and Ross, J, Jr: Natural history of valvular aortic stenosis. Br Heart J 35:41, 1973.
5. Ross, J, Jr and Braunwald, E: Aortic stenosis. Circulation 35:61, 1968.
6. Carabello, BA and Grossman, W: Calculation of stenotic valve orifice area. In Grossman, W (ed): Cardiac Catheterization and Angiography, ed 3. Lea & Febiger, Philadelphia, 1986.
7. Hatle, L, Angelson, BA, and Tromsdal, A: Non-invasive assessment of aortic stenosis by Doppler ultrasound. Br Heart J 43:284, 1980.
8. Stamm, RB and Martin, RP: Quantification of pressure gradients across stenotic valves by Doppler ultrasound. J Am Coll Cardiol 2:707, 1983.
9. Berger, M, Berdoff, RL, Gallerstein, TE, et al: Evaluation of aortic stenosis by continuous wave Doppler ultrasound. J Am Coll Cardiol 3:150, 1984.
10. Currie, PJ, Seward, JB, Reeder, GS, et al: Continuous-wave Doppler echocardiographic assessment of severity of calcific aortic stenosis: A simultaneous Doppler-catheter correlative study in 100 adult patients. Circulation 71:1162, 1985.
11. Smith, MD, Dawson, PL, Elion, JL, et al: Correlation of continuous wave Doppler velocities with cardiac catheterization gradients: An experimental model of aortic stenosis. J Am Coll Cardiol 6:1306, 1985.
12. Williams, GA, Labovitz, AJ, Nelson, JG, et al: Value of multiple echocardiographic views in the evaluation of aortic stenosis in adults by continuous wave Doppler. Am J Cardiol 55:445, 1985.
13. Yeager, M, Yock, PG, and Popp, RL: Comparison of Doppler-derived pressure gradient to that determined at cardiac catheterization in adults with aortic valve stenosis: Implications for management. Am J Cardiol 57:644, 1986.
14. Skjaerpe, T, Hegrenaes, L, and Hatle, L: Noninvasive estimation of valve area in patients with aortic stenosis by Doppler ultrasound and two-dimensional echocardiography. Circulation 72:810, 1985.
15. Zoghbi, WA, Farmer, KL, Soto, JG, et al: Accurate noninvasive quantification of stenotic aortic valve area by Doppler echocardiography. Circulation 73:452, 1986.
16. Oh, JK, Taliercio, CP, Holmes, DR, Jr, et al: Prediction of the severity of aortic stenosis by Doppler aortic valve area determination: Prospective Doppler-catheterization correlation in 100 patients. J Am Coll Cardiol 11:1223, 1988.
17. Murphy, ES, Lawson, RM, Starr, A, et al: Severe aortic stenosis in patients 60 years of age and older: Left ventricular function and 10-year survival after valve replacement. Circulation 64 (Suppl 2): 184, 1981.
18. Schwarz, F, Flameng, W, Langebartels, F, et al: Impaired left ventricular function in chronic aortic valve disease: Survival and function after replacement by Bjork-Shiley prosthesis. Circulation 60:48, 1979.
19. Smith, N, McAnulty, JH, and Rahimtoola, SH: Severe aortic stenosis with impaired left ventricular function and clinical heart failure: Results of valve replacement. Circulation 58:255, 1978.
20. Safian, RD, Berman, AD, Diver, DJ, et al: Balloon aortic valvuloplasty in 170 consecutive patients. N Engl J Med 319:125, 1989.
21. Kelly, TA, Rothbart, RM, Cooper, CM, et al: Comparison of outcome of asymptomatic to symptomatic patients older than 20 years of age with valvular aortic stenosis. Am J Cardiol 61:123, 1988.
22. Barnhorst, DA, Oxman, HA, Connolly, DC, et al: Long term follow-up of isolated replacement of the aortic or mitral valve with the Starr-Edwards prosthesis. Am J Cardiol 35:228, 1975.
23. Copeland, JG, Griepp, RB, Stinson, EB, et al: Long-term follow-up after isolated aortic valve replacement. J Thorac Cardiovasc Surg 74:875, 1977.
24. Macmanus, Q, Grunkemeier, GL, Lambert, LE, et al: Year of operation as a risk factor in the late results of valve replacement. J Thorac Cardiovasc Surg 80:843, 1980.
25. Kloster, FE and Murphy, ES: Late results and complications of prosthetic aortic valves. In Gaasch, WH and Levine, HJ (eds): Chronic Aortic Regurgitation. Klewer Academic Publishers, Boston/Dordrecht/London, 1988.
26. McHenry, MM, Rice, J, Matlof, HJ, et al: Pulmonary hypertension and sudden death in aortic stenosis. Br Heart J 41:463, 1979.
27. Kassirer, JP and Pauker, SG: The toss-up. N Engl J Med 305:1467, 1981.
28. Ross, J, Jr: Left ventricular function and the timing of surgical treatment in valvular heart disease. Ann Intern Med 94:498, 1981.
29. Skorton, DJ, Child, JS, and Perloff, JK: Accuracy of the echocardiographic diagnosis of aortic regurgitation. Am J Med 69:377, 1980.

30. Botvinick, EH, Schiller, NB, Wickramasekaran, R, et al: Echocardiographic demonstration of early mitral valve closure in severe aortic insufficiency. Circulation 51:836, 1975.
31. Ciobanu, M, Abbasi, A, Allen, M, et al: Pulsed Doppler echocardiography in the diagnosis and estimation of aortic insufficiency. Am J Cardiol 49:339, 1982.
32. Grayburn, PA, Smith, MD, Handshoe, R, et al: Detection of aortic insufficiency by standard echocardiography, pulsed Doppler echocardiography, and auscultation: A comparison of accuracies. Ann Intern Med 104:599, 1986.
33. Perry, GJ, Helmche, F, Nanda, NL, et al: Evaluation of aortic insufficiency by Doppler color flow mapping. J Am Coll Cardiol 9:952, 1987.
34. Smith, MD, Greyburn, PA, Spain, MG, et al: Observer variability in the quantitation of Doppler color flow jet areas for mitral and aortic regurgitation. J Am Coll Cardiol 11:579, 1988.
35. Touche, T, Prasquier, R, Nittenberg, A, et al: Assessment and follow-up of patients with aortic regurgitation by an updated Doppler echocardiographic measurement of the regurgitant fraction in the aortic arch. Circulation 72:819, 1985.
36. Kitabatake, A, Ito, H, Inoue, M, et al: A new approach to noninvasive evaluation of aortic regurgitant fraction by two-dimensional Doppler echocardiography. Circulation 72:523, 1985.
37. Labovitz, AJ, Ferrara, RP, Kern, MJ, et al: Quantitative evaluation of aortic insufficiency by continuous wave Doppler echocardiography. J Am Coll Cardiol 8:1341, 1986.
38. Masuyama, T, Kodama, K, Kitabatake, A, et al: Noninvasive evaluation of aortic regurgitation by continuous wave Doppler echocardiography. Circulation 73:460, 1986.
39. Grayburn, PA, Handshoe, R, Smith, MD, et al: Quantitative assessment of the hemodynamic consequences of aortic regurgitation by means of continuous wave Doppler recordings. J Am Coll Cardiol 10:135, 1987.
40. Gaasch, WH and Levine, HJ (eds): Chronic Aortic Regurgitation. Kluwer Academic Publishers, Boston/Dordrecht/London, 1988.
41. Goldschlager, N, Pfeifer, J, Cohn, K, et al: The natural history of aortic regurgitation: A clinical and hemodynamic study. Am J Med 54:577, 1973.
42. Schwarz, F, Baumann, P, Manthey, J, et al: The effect of aortic valve replacement on survival. Circulation 66:1105, 1982.
43. Greves, J, Rahimtoola, SH, McAnulty, JH, et al: Preoperative criteria predictive of late survival following valve replacement for severe aortic regurgitation. Am Heart J 101:300, 1981.
44. Rapaport, E: Natural history of aortic and mitral valve disease. Am J Cardiol 35:221, 1975.
45. Fioretti, P, Roelandt, J, Bos, RJ, et al: Echocardiography in chronic aortic insufficiency: Is replacement too late when left ventricular end systolic dimension reaches 55 mm? Circulation 67:216, 1983.
46. Bonow, RO, Rosing, DR, McIntosh, CL, et al: The natural history of asymptomatic patients with aortic regurgitation and normal left ventricular function. Circulation 68:509, 1983.
47. Bonow, RO, Rosing, DR, Maron, BJ, et al: Reversal of left ventricular dysfunction after aortic valve replacement for chronic aortic regurgitation: Influence of duration of preoperative left ventricular dysfunction. Circulation 70:570, 1984.
48. Gaasch, WH, Carroll, JD, Levine, HJ, et al: Chronic aortic regurgitation: Prognostic value of left ventricular end-systolic dimension and end-diastolic radius/thickness ratio. J Am Coll Cardiol 1:775, 1983.
49. Henry, WL, Bonow, RO, Rosing, DR, et al: Observations on the optimum time for operative intervention for aortic regurgitation: II. Serial echocardiographic evaluation of asymptomatic patients. Circulation 61:484, 1980.
50. Cunha, CLP, Giuliani, ER, Fuster, V, et al: Preoperative M-mode echocardiography as a predictor of surgical results in chronic aortic insufficiency. J Thorac Cardiovasc Surg 79:256, 1980.
51. Bonow, RO, Rosing, DR, Kent, KM, et al: Timing of operation for chronic aortic regurgitation. Am J Cardiol 50:325, 1982.
52. Gaasch, WH, Levine, HJ, and Zile, MR: Chronic aortic and mitral regurgitation: Mechanical consequences of the lesion and the results of surgery. In Gaasch, WH and Levine, HJ (eds): The Ventricle. Martinus Nijhoff, Boston, 1985.
53. Borow, KM, Green, LH, Mann, T, et al: End-systolic volume as a predictor of postoperative left ventricular performance in volume overload from valvular regurgitation. Am J Med 68:655, 1980.
54. Clark, RD, Korcuska, KL, and Cohn, K: Serial echocardiographic evaluation of left ventricular function in valvular disease, including reproducibility guidelines for serial studies. Circulation 62:564, 1980.

55. Henry, WL, Bonow, RO, Borer, JS, et al: Observations on the optimum time for operative intervention for aortic regurgitation: I. Evaluation of the results of aortic valve replacement in symptomatic patients. Circulation 61:471, 1980.

56. Kumpuris, AG, Quinones, MA, Waggoner, AD, et al: Importance of preoperative hypertrophy, wall stress and end-systolic dimension as echocardiographic predictors of normalization of left ventricular dilation after valve replacement in chronic aortic insufficiency. Am J Cardiol 49:1091, 1982.

57. Hirshfeld, JW, Jr, Epstein, SE, Roberts, AJ, et al: Indices predicting long-term survival after valve replacement in patients with aortic regurgitation and patients with aortic stenosis. Circulation 50:1190, 1974.

58. Mirsky, I, Henschke, C, Hess, OM, et al: Prediction of postoperative performance in aortic valve disease. Am J Cardiol 48:295, 1981.

59. Cohn, PF, Gorlin, R, Cohn, LH, et al: Left ventricular ejection fraction as a prognostic guide in surgical treatment of coronary and valvular heart disease. Am J Cardiol 34:136, 1974.

60. Goldman, ME, Packer, M, Horowitz, SF, et al: Relation between exercise-induced changes in ejection fraction and systolic loading conditions at rest in aortic regurgitation. J Am Coll Cardiol 3:924, 1984.

61. Lewis, SM, Riba, AL, Berger, HJ, et al: Radionuclide angiographic exercise left ventricular performance in chronic aortic regurgitation: Relationship to resting echocardiographic ventricular dimensions and systolic wall stress index. Am Heart J 103:498, 1983.

62. Levine, HJ, and Gaasch, WH: Ratio of regurgitant volume to end-diastolic volume: A major determinant of ventricular response to surgical correction of chronic volume overload. Am J Cardiol 52:406, 1983.

63. Bonow, RO, Borer, JS, Rosing, DR, et al: Preoperative exercise capacity in symptomatic patients with aortic regurgitation as a predictor of postoperative left ventricular function and long-term prognosis. Circulation 62:1280, 1980.

64. Hoshino, PK and Gaasch, WH: When to intervene in chronic aortic regurgitation. Arch Intern Med 146:349, 1986.

65. Bonow, RO and Epstein, SE: Is preoperative left ventricular function predictive of survival and functional results after aortic valve replacement for chronic aortic regurgitation? J Am Coll Cardiol 10:713, 1987.

Commentary

By Melvin D. Cheitlin, M.D.

A general rule that serves us well is that in asymptomatic patients with valve disease or, for that matter, almost any heart disease, surgery should be recommended only if there is overwhelming evidence that the patient will benefit. In most cases the most obvious benefit of surgery is relief of symptoms and an increase in exercise capacity, which can lead to a marked change in the patient's life. In the asymptomatic patient, it is true that it is impossible to make the patient feel better by surgery. Because in the adult, aortic valve surgery for either aortic stenosis or aortic regurgitation involves valve replacement, we must balance the dangers of valve replacement—including both preoperative and late mortality and morbidity—against those of the medically managed patient.

Because symptoms develop late in the course of aortic valve disease, the onset of symptoms is usually ominous, and it is generally agreed that surgical intervention is indicated. In the case of aortic stenosis, surgery probably prolongs life better than continued medical management. In the asymptomatic patient with aortic stenosis the fear is that sudden death can be the first manifestation. As Errichetti and colleagues indicate in this chapter, it is probable that with significant aortic stenosis in the truly asymptomatic patient, the incidence of sudden death as the *first manifestation* is probably of the same magnitude, or perhaps less likely, than death at or within a short period after surgery. Although there is no randomized study in patients with severe aortic stenosis who are asymptomatic that compares survival with medical management to that of surgical intervention, many cardiologists, for the reasons stated, refuse to recommend surgery for an asymptomatic patient with aortic stenosis.[1,2] Others, however, believe that in the asymptomatic patient with aortic stenosis, quantifying the degree of aortic stenosis is probably useful. Patients with very severe aortic stenosis—that is, valve area less than 0.75 cm^2—have the greatest left ventricular afterload burden and therefore are most likely to develop subendocardial ischemia and probably more likely to be among the patients who die suddenly. Without data to support either decision, knowledgeable cardiologists reasonably could choose either course of action.

With chronic aortic regurgitation, the problem is more difficult. The regurgitant volume increases end-diastolic wall tension, which is the stimulus for the development of left ventricular eccentric hypertrophy, that is, increasing left ventricular muscle mass around a larger left ventricular cavity. As long as hypertrophy keeps up with the increasing left ventricular volume, wall stress will remain normal and heart failure will not occur; that is, systolic function will be well preserved. It

212

is abundantly clear from many studies that if left ventricular function is good, prognosis is good.[3] Therefore, if ventricular function is normal, only the development of symptoms would be an indication for surgery.

In the truly asymptomatic patient with chronic aortic regurgitation, left ventricular function is usually normal. However, in some asymptomatic patients, left ventricular function can be depressed. Because aortic regurgitation presents both a preload and an afterload burden to the left ventricle, it might be expected that when left ventricular systolic dysfunction begins, it might be related to the increased afterload and therefore could be expected to normalize after this afterload is removed by surgery. Bonow and colleagues[4] have shown that even in symptomatic patients with aortic regurgitation, survival after aortic valve replacement can be good, with return of the ventricular function and size toward normal if preoperative exercise capacity is maintained.

What, then, is the rationale for recommending surgery in chronic aortic regurgitation in the asymptomatic patient? In analyzing predictors of poor outcome in patients with aortic valve replacement for chronic aortic regurgitation, increased left ventricular size is important. As the heart size increases, there is increasing difficulty in maintaining myocardial preservation during surgery, and the possibility of intraoperative myocardial damage increases.

Determining whether a patient is asymptomatic or not is sometimes difficult. After all, symptoms are subjective, requiring the patient to sense that there is something wrong and to verbalize that complaint to a physician. The physician must listen to the patient and associate the symptoms with the aortic regurgitation. Because it is very unusual to encounter poor left ventricular function in a patient doing normal or more than normal activity, it is probable that when decreasing left ventricular function on serial measurements is observed, then surgery is probably indicated even in the asymptomatic patient.

Finally, the question of whether surgery in patients with aortic regurgitation really prolongs life is a reasonable one. In symptomatic patients, because surgery decreases or eliminates symptoms, it is unjustifiable to randomize symptomatic patients to medical or surgical management. In asymptomatic patients, such a randomized study would have to be a very large one with a long follow-up time in order to show benefit of surgery over medical management. I am impressed with the study by Schwarz and colleagues,[5] who reported a large number of patients with aortic valve disease, both aortic stenosis and regurgitation, all of whom were judged to be surgical candidates. Most were operated upon, but for various nonrandomized reasons some were not operated. On the follow-up, there was a striking benefit of surgery over medical management in the patients with aortic stenosis, whereas there was an identical survival for at least three years with medical and surgical management in the patients with aortic regurgitation. Inasmuch as this is the case with symptomatic patients, it is probably also the case with asymptomatic patients.

REFERENCES

1. Chizner, MA, Pearle, DL, and de Leon, AC, Jr: The natural history of aortic stenosis in adults. Am Heart J 99:419, 1980.
2. Kelly, TA, Rothbart, RM, Cooper, CM, et al: Comparison of outcome of asymptomatic to symptomatic patients older than 20 years of age with valvular aortic stenosis. Am J Cardiol 61:123, 1988.

3. Greves, J, Rahimtoola, SH, McAnulty, JH, et al: Preoperative criteria predictive of late survival following valve replacement for severe aortic regurgitation. Am Heart J 101:300, 1981.
4. Bonow, RO, Borer, JS, Rosing, D, et al: Preoperative exercise capacity in symptomatic patients with aortic regurgitation as a predictor of postoperative left ventricular function and long-term prognosis. Circulation 62:1280, 1980.
5. Schwarz, F, Baumann, P, Manthey, J, et al: The effect of aortic valve replacement on survival. Circulation 66:1105, 1982.

CHAPTER 12

Does the Patient with Infective Endocarditis and a Large Vegetation on the Mitral or Aortic Valve Need Surgery?

Howard S. Lewis, M.D.
Barry H. Greenberg, M.D.

The management of infective endocarditis (IE) is influenced by many factors, including the clinical status of the patient, the microbiology of the infecting organism, and, often, descriptive data from noninvasive and invasive tests that help characterize the site and extent of the infection. Integration of these factors enables clinicians caring for patients with IE to define severity and to determine the necessity for and timing of surgery.

Prior to the development of echocardiography, decisions regarding medical and surgical therapy in patients with IE were based on clinical assessment and microbiologic findings. In some instances, cardiac catheterization played an important role in management.[1] Criteria that were found to be predictive of an adverse outcome included evidence of hemodynamic compromise, persistent bacteremia, infection with a highly pathogenic organism, recurrent embolization, and infection of either a native aortic or a prosthetic valve.[2-6]

The development of echocardiography, however, has permitted a much better appreciation of the characteristics of infection of the heart valves. This noninvasive technology enables physicians to study the site, morphology, and extent of intracardiac vegetations; to determine valvular competence; and to assess ventricular function. Echocardiography also allows assessment of size of vegetations. Overall, this technology has added considerably to our ability to define the optimal timing for surgery. In addition, it has greatly enhanced the understanding of the natural history of vegetations in IE. However, the improved ability to visualize vegetations has given rise to an important controversy—whether patients with echocardiographic evidence of a vegetation, especially a large vegetation, should undergo surgery early in their clinical course. Using M-mode techniques, some investigators have reported that patients with a diagnosis compatible with IE and evidence of a vegetation had a worse prognosis than did patients without an identifiable vegetation; based on these observations it has been suggested that such *high risk* patients should be treated surgically.[7-10] Subsequent studies using two-dimensional techniques demonstrated that the presence of vegetations were predictive of an adverse outcome.[11-13] Although there are conflicting reports in the literature, some authors have concluded that the presence of large, as opposed to small, vegetations identifies patients who are at increased risk for complications such as heart failure and death.[11,14-17]

The issue here is whether or not it is advisable to recommend surgery in patients with IE who have large vegetations on left-sided heart valves. Another way of stating this is, Should the presence of a large vegetation on either the aortic or mitral valve be a separate and distinct criterion for recommending surgery early, or should the more traditional criteria be applied before offering surgery as an adjunct to medical therapy? In order to fully discuss this issue, *large* vegetation will be defined, the methods of diagnosing IE will be reviewed, and the available information regarding incidence of large vegetations will be summarized. We will identify the clinical characteristics of patients who have vegetations and address aspects of both medical and surgical therapies that are relevant to these issues. The complications, consequences, and management issues in prosthetic valve and right-sided IE are different from those concerning infections of the left side of the heart. These have been reviewed elsewhere and will not be addressed in the present chapter.[18-23]

DEFINITION

The clinical diagnosis of IE is based on traditional criteria, which generally include at least two positive blood cultures with the same organism and a new or changing heart murmur. Many clinicians also include the appearance of classical peripheral stigmata or laboratory results compatible with IE (e.g., elevated sedimentation rate, active urinary sediment) as part of their diagnostic criteria.[24] Series of patients with IE reported in the literature do not apply these criteria uniformly, and this has made comparison of studies difficult in some instances.

Culture-negative IE also has been described, most commonly in patients who have taken antibiotics or when an unusual organism is involved.[25] Unfortunately, there are not adequate data to analyze the predictive value of the size of vegetations in regard to outcome in this clinical setting.

The definition of *large* vegetation IE has not been applied uniformly. Firstly, an accurate appreciation of the size of a lesion requires two-dimensional echocardiography. Although some groups use planimetry of the largest two-dimensional area of the vegetation, lesions are usually measured at their longest diameter. Vegetations are considered as large (larger than 10 mm), medium (5 to 10 mm), or small (smaller than 5 mm). Because of the limited numbers of patients who have been described in the available literature, we have catergorized lesions less than 10 mm at their longest diameter as small and those which are greater than or equal to 10 mm as large. Our discussion applies to infections of the aortic and mitral valves, and not to intramyocardial or aortic root abscesses.

In addition to size, vegetations also can be described with regard to mobility, extent, and texture. A recent retrospective series from the Massachusetts General

Hospital assessed these characteristics in a series of patients with IE.[26] They also graded these variables on a scale of 1 to 4 and created an echocardiographic score in order to predict clinical events. They found that these variables contributed significantly to the prediction of risk for major complications, such as heart failure, embolism, death, or the need for surgery. Although additional echocardiographic characteristics such as the aforementioned ones may prove to be important independent variables in predicting outcome, this issue requires further study, and the prognostic value of such variables will have to be determined before routinely incorporating them in the description of vegetations.

DIAGNOSIS

The clinical diagnosis of IE is based on the aforementioned criteria. Echocardiography has expanded that definition to include a more detailed morphologic description of the infection. The initial descriptions of IE by M-mode echocardiography included the presence of a shaggy, *echogenic* mass that was attached to the valve leaflet.[7] The sensitivity of M-mode for the detection of vegetations varies from 30 to 60 percent, depending on the particular laboratory and patient population.[7-10] In a prospective analysis that included a large group of patients, Come and coworkers[9] reported that M-mode echocardiography had a sensitivity of only 37 percent and a specificity of 96 percent. The diagnostic accuracy for a positive test was 76 percent, and the diagnostic accuracy for a negative test was 80 percent. In addition to its limited ability to detect vegetations, M-mode does not allow quantitation of lesion size or an appreciation of morphology. The sensitivity of two-dimensional echocardiography is estimated to be higher, ranging from 40 to 85 percent.[11-15,27] However, the reported studies include patients with both right- and left-sided infections. The actual sensitivity is subject to debate because most studies have been based on the clinical diagnosis of IE as opposed to anatomic (or pathologic) findings.[29] The more difficult cases to diagnose will usually be ones with vegetations in the 1- to 2-mm range because this approaches the limits of resolution of the system. As the size of the lesion increases, the sensitivity of the test is likely to improve substantially. The specificity of the test, which is an indicator of how often a positive test correctly defines the presence of vegetations, is quite good. In certain laboratories specificity can approach 100 percent, even when smaller lesions are present.[12] In addition, two-dimensional echocardiography allows a more precise definition of the lesion than does M-mode and has been shown to correlate with pathologic findings at surgery or autopsy.[28]

Other diagnostic tests available to help characterize IE include transesophageal, Doppler, and color-flow Doppler echocardiography. Transesophageal echocardiography offers a unique window to assess the morphology of lesions and may improve the sensitivity and diagnostic accuracy of noninvasive testing.[30] This would be of particular value when the technical quality of a transthoracic study is inadequate. Doppler echocardiography permits definition of the direction and velocity of blood flow and thus allows characterization of complications of intracardiac infections, such as valvular insufficiency, cusp perforation, or functional valvular stenosis[31-33] (Fig. 12–1).

The role of cardiac catheterization is controversial. This invasive test may play an important role when clinical and echocardiographic findings are discordant or when there is uncertainty regarding the hemodynamic status of the patient.[1,34]

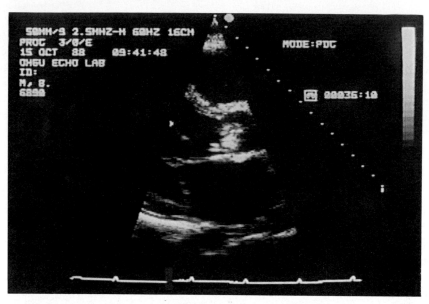

Figure 12–1. Echocardiography in a 27-year-old male with aortic valve infective endocarditis. Blood cultures and pathologic specimens grew strep viridans. At surgery, he was found to have multiple large valvular vegetations with extensive erosions of the cusps. The infection extended to the sinuses and sub-aortic curtain. 2-D echocardiography shows large vegetations on the valve. The longest dimension of the largest lesion is 1.2 mm.

Although two-dimensional echocardiography provides superior morphologic descriptions of lesions, catheterization may contribute to the delineation of an abscess or annular infection, and it can clarify hemodynamics. It is also useful in defining the coronary anatomy in preparation for surgery.[1,35]

INCIDENCE

The incidence of large lesions in left-sided IE varies, depending on patient selection and referral patterns (Table 12–1). In a series from the University of Michigan Hospital, 50 patients who fit strict clinical and bacteriologic criteria for IE were described.[15] Evidence of valvular vegetations was detected by two-dimensional echocardiography in 21 patients (42 percent), and in 18 patients (38 percent) these lesions involved left-sided valves. Overall, 11 patients (22 percent) had vegetations that were considered to be large (greater than or equal to 10 mm). In a series from Los Angeles County Hospital, Long Beach Veterans Administration Hospital, and University of California in Irvine Hospital, Wong and associates[16] identified 31 patients with clinical IE who had two-dimensional echocardiograms. As noted in Table 12–1, this group reports a higher incidence of IE with vegetations, especially those involving the left side, although it is unclear whether this is a consecutive series of patients. One of the most widely cited studies is from Duke University Medical Center, where Stewart and colleagues[11] prospectively identified 87 patients with clinical IE. Forty-seven (54 percent) of the patients had echocardiographic evidence of vegetations, and 41 (47 percent) patients had involvement of at least the mitral or aortic valve. Sixty-three lesions were identified, and only 10 (16 percent) were large. However, it is unclear from their data whether the relatively low inci-

Table 12–1. Incidence of Infective Endocarditis in Selected Populations

Patient Population	% with IE and Veg	% with IE and Left-Sided Veg	% with IE and Large Left-sided Veg
University of Michigan[15] (n = 50)	42	36	22
University of Southern California[16] (n = 21)	87	58	35
Duke University[11] (n = 87)	54	47	16*

*The number of these that involved the tricuspid valve is unclear. IE = infective endocarditis; veg = vegetation.

dence of large lesions was due to inclusions of patients with right-sided or nonvalvular sites of endocarditis. A preliminary report from Strom and coworkers[17] reported 45 consecutive cases of left-sided IE in 43 patients. Nineteen (42 percent) of these episodes involved large vegetations.

After pooling these somewhat disparate patient populations, one can conclude that echocardiographic evidence of either mitral or aortic vegetations will be present in about 35 to 45 percent of patients with a clinical diagnosis of IE. Of patients with left-sided lesions demonstrable by echocardiogram, roughly one third to one half will have a vegetation classified as large.

EPIDEMIOLOGY

It is not clear by echocardiography which patients with IE develop large, small, or even no vegetations. One variable to examine would be the microbiology of the infection in order to determine whether certain organisms are more likely to result in large lesions. Another variable to consider is whether patients with large vegetations are likely to have preexisting structural abnormalities of the valves.

The microbiology of patients with IE has been extensively studied and is the subject of numerous reviews.[24,36] The studies describing the microbiology of patients with large, left-sided lesions report a spectrum of organisms that are similar to those causing IE in patients without large vegetations. In a series of 10 patients with large lesions, Stewart and associates[11] reported that all 10 had infection with a gram-positive coccus. In the report by Wong and colleagues,[16] 10 of 11 patients with large, left-sided lesions were infected with a gram-positive coccus. In another series describing 45 consecutive episodes of left-sided IE in 43 patients,[17] a streptococcus species was associated with 58 percent of the large vegetations and accounted for 69 percent of the smaller lesions (nonsignificant difference). Staphylococci were also equally represented in the two groups. Without distinguishing between large and small lesions, other investigators have reported that in patients with echocardiographic evidence of vegetations, streptococci and staphylococci account for 70 to 85 percent of cases.[13–15]

It is noteworthy that in virtually all series there is only a small incidence of infections with gram-negative and fungal organisms. This could be attributed to various reasons, for example, (1) these patients may have presented earlier in their illness and a large lesion had not yet developed, (2) such patients may have been referred to surgery early in their course before a large lesion developed, (3) they may have died earlier, sometimes before an echocardiogram could be obtained. There are reports of fungal IE being characterized by large vegetations; however, there are no controlled data to suggest that fungal IE is more likely to result in large, as opposed to small, lesions. In any given series of patients with IE, cases of fungal disease or gram-negative infection comprise a relatively small proportion. Therefore, it is not possible to state whether patients with a clinical diagnosis of IE and a non-gram-positive organism are more likely to have large as opposed to small vegetations. With the increasing use of immunosuppressive agents, parenteral nutrition, and the intravenous use of illicit drugs, there likely will be more cases of IE with exotic organisms, which will allow further study of this issue.

In attempting to identify clinical variables that place patients with IE at higher risk for large vegetations, one can also examine whether the presence of preexisting valvular abnormalities is important. Unfortunately, most of the studies that describe extensive series of patients with large left-sided lesions have not rigorously reported the relationship between the specific patient characteristics and the subsequent clinical course. A few of the studies indicate that roughly one quarter to one half of the patients with IE have a *predisposing* factor, such as a history of intravenous drug use, rheumatic heart disease, or mitral valve prolapse.[15,16] However, it is not clear that the presence of such factors predisposes a patient to a large versus a small vegetation.

Pathologic studies by Roberts and Buchbinder[37,38] state that vegetations in left-sided IE occur on previously anatomically normal valves in 53 percent of cases. Their classical studies, however, did not report the size of the lesions, and unfortunately these studies were conducted at a time when two-dimensional echocardiography was not available to supplement the clinical diagnosis.

Thus, it is difficult to discern which patients are more likely to develop larger lesions. The microbiology in patients with large lesions seems to be similar to that in patients with small lesions. Also, one cannot conclude that patients with preexisting valvular abnormalities or a history of intravenous drug use are more likely to develop larger vegetations during the course of IE. It is also possible that the size of the lesion in left-sided IE may be more a function of the duration of the illness or the host's immune response to infection than a characteristic of the organism involved or the presence and extent of preexisting valve pathology. There is no available evidence, however, to support or to refute this concept.

CLINICAL MANIFESTATIONS

The presentation of IE can be protean, but it is classically characterized by fever, heart murmur, and occasionally peripheral stigmata of infection, such as splenomegaly or splinter hemorrhages. The initial clinical manifestations of individuals with IE and large vegetations appear to be similar to those of patients with smaller lesions.

In comparing the natural history of patients with IE and large versus small valvular vegetations, most authors have reported the incidence of major complications, defined as heart failure, embolism, need for surgery, or death. Absolute conclusions are difficult to reach based on the available literature because there is no single series that is sufficiently large or representative. Pooling of the data may not be valid because indications for one of the major interventions in the disease process—namely, valve surgery—are not necessarily applied uniformly. For instance, if the presence of a large vegetation led some clinicians to alter their recommendations for the timing of surgery, this approach might skew the data reported in that series.

Despite this limitation, it is possible to determine whether or not the presence of a vegetation, especially a large one, identifies patients at increased risk for the occurrence of a major complication. A series of 42 patients from the University of Michigan demonstrated that the presence of a vegetation was associated with a higher incidence of major complications (100 percent versus 67 percent in the absence of a vegetation).[15] Although the presence of a large vegetation was associated with a higher likelihood of progression to congestive heart failure and death, it did not appear to be associated with an increased incidence of embolic events. Although the numbers are small, the death rate was higher in patients with evidence of vegetations on the aortic valve. Another series of 45 patients with left-sided IE described 19 individuals with large lesions.[17] In this latter group, urgent surgery was necessary in 58 percent of patients, and a medical cure was achieved in only 16 percent of cases. Of the 26 patients with small lesions, 88 percent were cured medically—how many of these patients had nonfatal complications, however, is not clear. This issue has also been addressed by Wong and associates,[16] who described the course of 21 patients who had left-sided IE and two-dimensional echocardiograms. The clinical description suggests that these patients were more critically ill than those reported in other series. The incidence of major complications, although high in both groups, was similar in patients with large and small lesions—73 percent versus 80 percent, respectively. The authors state that the four patients in their series with large aortic valve lesions may have been at the highest risk: All developed heart failure; two underwent valve replacement (but one died); one had a stroke and died; and the fourth was referred to surgery but refused valve replacement. In a prospective study from Duke University that included 47 patients with echocardiographic evidence of vegetations, 30 percent had embolic events, 32 percent developed congestive heart failure, and 25 percent required surgery.[11] The mortality was 11 percent. Although the data were not completely presented, the authors concluded that neither size nor morphology, nor location of the lesions predicted the occurrence of clinically important complications. However, there were only 10 cases with large vegetations, and it is not clear whether they involved left- or right-sided valves.

A preliminary report from Sanfilippo and colleagues[26] analyzed the clinical course of 53 patients with left-sided IE in relation to lesion size, mobility, extent, and texture. Using logistic regression analysis, they reported that mobility and extent (i.e., beyond the valve leaflet into the adjacent structures) were the only statistically significant variables that predicted the likelihood of major complications. By tabulating an *echo* score that included all of the characteristics, the clinical outcome could be predicted in 78 percent of cases.

Thus, the majority of reports tend to favor the notion that patients with IE and echocardiographic evidence of a vegetation—particularly of a large vegetation—are at increased risk for the occurrence of heart failure, death, and a need for surgery. The recent preliminary report by Sanfilippo and colleagues[26] is provocative in that it suggests that there may be other features of a vegetation, specifically morphology and extent, that may be more predictive of an adverse outcome than size alone. Although patients with vegetations are at higher risk for systemic embolization than those without, size of the lesion does not seem to predict which individuals are more or less prone to this complication. There may be other features of vegetations—for example, whether they are multiple, pedunculated, or extend onto the extravalvular structures[39]—that will better predict the risk of embolization. However, these criteria neither have been rigorously defined nor have been applied to series of patients with IE that have been reported in the literature.

TREATMENT

The cornerstone of medical therapy for IE is the administration of antimicrobial agents. This subject has been extensively reviewed elsewhere and will not be addressed here.[24,36] Briefly, though, appropriate therapy should be based on identification of the culprit organism, sensitivity to various drugs, and the clinical setting. Several factors, including infection with fungal organisms or the presence of an intramyocardial abscess, are known to decrease the likelihood that medical therapy alone will be sufficient to cure the infection. When present, these factors should be indicators that early surgical treatment may be needed. In contrast, there are no data to suggest that the principles and practice of medical treatment of IE are influenced by the size of a vegetation alone.

The natural history of vegetations treated medically has been studied by serial echocardiography. In a prospective report from Duke University Medical Center,[11] patients were followed with serial two-dimensional echocardiograms during the treatment period and then during a convalescent period that spanned at least one month (most patients had studies at least six months later). As shown in Table 12–2, a small number of lesions either increased or decreased in size, but over two thirds remained unchanged. Of interest was the finding that vegetations tended to persist well into the convalescent period. It is unclear from this report whether the relative size of the lesion helped predict whether or not it would involute after appropriate medical therapy. Other authors report that approximately two thirds of vegetations will not change in size after bacteriologic cure has been achieved.[40] However, distal embolization is one means by which a vegetation can change size dramatically;[41] and we have noted this unfortunate sequence of events in some of our patients.

During the 1960s advances in cardiovascular surgery allowed for damaged heart valves in patients with IE to be replaced. Subsequently, there have been numerous reports of successful valve replacement in patients with both active and healed infection.[6,42–45] There have not been—and probably never will be—controlled, randomized, prospective trials comparing surgical therapy with medical

Table 12–2. Changes in the Size of Vegetations during Therapy and Convalescence (3- to 6-month Follow-up)[11]

	New	Increase	Decrease	Stable	Gone
Treatment (43 patients, 63 lesions)	5	6	4	45	3
Convalescence (29 patients, 47 lesions)	0	7	4	34	2

therapy for patients with IE. However, there have been noncontrolled series that demonstrate lower mortality among those treated surgically.[6,46] In a report from the University of Alabama at Birmingham, patients with IE who had emergent or urgent valve replacement had a 14 percent in-hospital mortality compared with a 44 percent mortality in patients treated medically.[6] The percentages were similar when subgroups with mitral and aortic valves were analyzed. The difference in death rates between surgical and medical groups was greatest in patients with advanced heart failure (Table 12–3). Interestingly, in patients who survived hospitalization, long-term survival was comparable in the two groups. Another smaller series of patients reported by Croft and associates[46] demonstrated similar findings. In all patients who survive, the likelihood of relapse or reoperation is significantly less in those treated surgically (as low as 15 percent in 5-year follow-up).[6] There is no evidence that the presence or the size of vegetations on echocardiography will affect either the likelihood of successful valve replacement or posthospitalization survival in either surgical or nonsurgical groups.

The available studies demonstrate that surgery can be performed at relatively low risk in many patients with active IE. As already noted, those with advanced heart failure at the time of surgery are at the greatest risk for perioperative complications and mortality. Consequently, the ability to identify patients with IE who are at high risk for heart failure is of importance. Such patients can be carefully watched, and at the first sign of hemodynamic deterioration, valve replacement can be recommended. It is hoped that this approach would decrease the need for emergency surgery in critically ill patients and would increase likelihood of a successful outcome. For instance, in a large series from the University of Alabama, in-hospital mortality rose from 5 percent when surgery was elective to 33 percent when the procedure was emergent.[6]

One additional issue is whether there is a role for prophylactic surgery to prevent an embolic event. A meta-analysis of the published reports that used echocardiography to characterize vegetations suggests that roughly one third of patients with left-sided vegetations will suffer a clinically significant systemic embolic episode.[13] There are no data to suggest that infection of either the aortic or the mitral valve is more likely to result in this complication. In addition, the published series report that there is no significant increase in rates of embolization in patients with large lesions. Last, there are no firm data to support the concept that a patient who has had one embolic event is at increased risk of another.

Table 12–3. Relationship of Mortality to Preoperative Status[6]

	Medical Therapy		Surgical Therapy	
	Hospital Deaths		**Hospital Deaths**	
	n	*# (%)*	*n*	*# (%)*
Heart failure				
Absent/mild	22	3 (14)	49	3 (6)
Moderate	30	19 (63)	20	4 (20)
Severe	2	2 (100)	12	4 (33)
Total	54	24	81	11

SUMMARY AND RECOMMENDATIONS

Two-dimensional echocardiography is the most accurate method of determining the presence and the size of vegetations. Patients with a clinical diagnosis of IE will have about a 20 to 35 percent likelihood of having a large vegetation on either the aortic or mitral valve when this methodology is used. It does not appear that the presence of preexisting structural valvular disease or specific microorganisms predispose patients to this complication.

There is convincing and consistent evidence from several institutions that echocardiographic visualization of vegetations places patients at higher risk for major complications such as heart failure, embolism, death, or the need for surgery.[7-13] Although the literature is conflicting as to whether a large, as opposed to small, left-sided lesion places additional risk on patients for the occurrence of any of these complications, this is probably the case. There are supporting data from two of the larger, consecutive series, which show that the presence of large vegetations identify patients at increased risk for heart failure, death, and the need for surgery.[15,17] However, there is no evidence to support the hypothesis that patients with large lesions have an increased incidence of systemic embolic events.[15]

We approach the management of a patient with IE in a stepwise fashion. While the diagnosis is being secured with the appropriate clinical and laboratory examinations, adequate visualization and characterization of the valves involved, as well as a determination of the presence and size of vegetations, should be obtained with two-dimensional echocardiography. This information, with the addition of data from hemodynamic and angiographic studies in selected cases in which uncertainties exist, can then be assessed to determine whether there are indications for urgent surgery. Although the presence of a large lesion places the patient at increased risk, information to support the concept that such patients should undergo urgent surgery based on this finding alone is lacking. We believe that in the absence of other risk factors (such as heart failure, persistent bacteremia, intramyocardial abscess, recurrent large artery emboli, or fungal infection), the presence of a large vegetation alone is not an indication for surgery. However, the presence of a large lesion alerts us to the fact that the individual should be followed with extreme vigilance and with a lower threshold for using noninvasive and invasive tests to determine valvular integrity, ventricular function, and overall hemodynamic status. If there is hemodynamic deterioration or if other traditional criterial apply, then surgery is recommended. Although patients with IE can progress with frightening rapidity from a stable condition to an unstable one, we believe that careful observation along with judicious use of diagnostic tests allows the clinician to determine when changes are occurring in the patient's hemodynamic status.

Because the value of two-dimensional echocardiography in following the natural history of the vegetations is limited, we do not perform serial studies on a routine basis but, rather, repeat the test when clinical parameters suggest that the course has changed or that the response to therapy is different from what has been anticipated. Whether additional features of a vegetation, such as mobility or morphology, are predictive of embolization is an area in need of further investigation. If additional studies determine that there are certain types of lesions that have an unacceptably high rate of embolism, then preventive surgery in those instances would be recommended.

REFERENCES

1. Hosenpud, JD and Greenberg, BH: The preoperative evaluation in patients with endocarditis: Is cardiac catheterization necessary? Chest 84:690, 1983.
2. Kaye, D: Changes in the spectrum, diagnosis, and management of bacterial and fungal endocarditis. Med Clin North Am 57:941, 1973.
3. Pelletier, LL and Petersdorf, RG: Infective endocarditis: A review of 125 cases from the University of Washington Hospitals, 1963–72. Medicine 56:287, 1977.
4. Garvey, GJ and Neu, HC: Infective endocarditis—an evolving disease. Medicine 57:105, 1978.
5. Stinson, EB: Surgical treatment of infective endocarditis. Prog Cardiovasc Dis 22:145, 1979.
6. Richardson, JV, Karp, RB, Kirklin, JW, et al: Treatment of infective endocarditis: A 10-year comparative analysis. Circulation 58:589, 1978.
7. Wann, LS, Dillon, JC, Weyman, AE, et al: Echocardiography in bacterial endocarditis. N Engl J Med 295:135, 1976.
8. Davis, RS, Strom, JA, Frishman, W, et al: The demonstration of vegetations by echocardiography in bacterial endocarditis: An indication for early surgical intervention. Am J Med 69:57, 1980.
9. Come, PC, Isaacs, RE, and Riley, MF: Diagnostic accuracy of M-mode echocardiography in active infective endocarditis and prognostic implications of ultrasound-detectable vegetations. Am Heart J 103:839, 1982.
10. Markiewicz, W, Moscovitz, M, Edoute, Y, et al: Prognostic implication of detecting vegetations by M-mode echocardiography. Cardiol 70:194, 1983.
11. Stewart, JA, Silimperi, D, Harris, P, et al: Echocardiographic documentation of vegetative lesions in infective endocarditis: Clinical implications. Circulation 61:374, 1980.
12. Martin, RP, Meltzer, RS, Chia, BL, et al: Clinical utility of two dimensional echocardiography in infective endocarditis. Am J Cardiol 46:379, 1980.
13. O'Brien, JT, and Geiser, EA: Infective endocarditis and echocardiography. Am Heart J 108:386, 1984.
14. Lutas, EM, Roberts, RB, Devereux, RB, et al: Relation between the presence of echocardiographic vegetations and the complication rate in infective endocarditis. Am Heart J 112:107, 1986.
15. Buda, AJ, Zotz, RJ, Lemire, MS, et al: Prognostic significance of vegetations detected by two-dimensional echocardiography in infective endocarditis. Am Heart J 112:1291, 1986.
16. Wong, D, Chandraratna, PAN, Wishnow, RM, et al: Clinical implications of large vegetations in infectious endocarditis. Arch Intern Med 143:1874, 1983.
17. Strom, JA, Frishman, WH, Klein, N, et al: Effective of vegetation size on the outcome patients with infective endocarditis (abstr). Circulation 66:II103, 1982.
18. Wilson, WR, Danielson, GK, Giulani, ER, et al: Prosthetic valve endocarditis. Mayo Clin Proc 57:155, 1982.
19. Arnett, EN and Roberts, WC: Prosthetic valve endocarditis. Clinicopathological analysis of 22 necropsy patients with active infective endocarditis involving natural left-sided cardiac valves. Am J Cardiol 38:281, 1976.
20. Masur, H and Johnson, WD: Prosthetic valve endocarditis. J Thorac Cardiovasc Surg 80:31, 1980.
21. Calderwood, SB, Swinski, LA, Waternaux, CM, et al: Risk factors for the development of prosthetic valve endocarditis. Circulation 72:31, 1985.
22. Manolis, AS and Melita, H: Echocardiographic and clinical correlates in drug addicts with infective endocarditis: Implications of vegetation size. Arch Intern Med 148:2461, 1988.
23. Robbins, MJ, Frater, RWM, Soeiro, R, et al: Outcome of right-sided infective endocarditis. Am J Med 80:165, 1986.
24. Weinstein, L: Infective endocarditis. In Braunwald, E (ed):Heart Disease: A Textbook of Cardiovascular Medicine. WB Saunders, Philadelphia, 1988, pp 1093–1134.
25. Rubenson, DS, Tucker, CR, Stinson, EB, et al: The use of echocardiography in diagnosing culture-negative endocarditis. Circulation 64:641, 1981.
26. Sanfilippo, AJ, Picard, MH, Davidoff, R, et al: Prediction of risk for complications in patients with left-sided infectious endocarditis (abstr). J Am Coll Cardiol 13:72A, 1989.
27. Mintz, GS, Kotler, MN, Segal, BL, et al: Comparison of two-dimensional and M-mode echocardiography in the evaluation of patients with endocarditis. Am J Cardiol 43:738, 1979.
28. Gilbert, BW, Haney, RS, Crawford, F, et al: Two-dimensional echocardiographic assessment of vegetative endocarditis. Circulation 55:346, 1977.
29. Plehn, JF: The evolving role of echocardiography in management of bacterial endocarditis (editorial). Chest 94:904, 1988.

30. Gussenhoven, EJ, Taams, MA, Roelandt, JRTC, et al: Transesophageal two-dimensional echocardiography: Its role in solving clinical problems. J Am Coll Cardiol 8:975, 1986.
31. Chow, LC, Dittrich, HC, Dembitsky, WP, et al: Accurate localization of ruptured sinus of Valsalva aneurysm by real-time two-dimensional Doppler flow imaging. Chest 94:462, 1988.
32. Copeland, JG, Salomon, NW, Stinson, EB, et al: Acute mitral valvular obstruction from infective endocarditis: Echocardiographic diagnosis and report of the second successfully treated case. J Thorac Cardiovasc Surg 78:128, 1979.
33. Roberts, WC, Ewy, GA, Glancy, DL, et al: Valvular stenosis produced by active infective endocarditis. Circulation 36:449, 1967.
34. Cheitlin, MD and Mills, J: Infective endocarditis: Is cardiac catheterization usually needed before cardiac surgery (editorial)? Chest 86:4, 1984.
35. Mills, J, Abbott, J, Utley, JR, et al: Role of cardiac catheterization in infective endocarditis. Chest 72:576, 1977.
36. Larsen, G and Greenberg, B: Infective endocarditis. In Rakel, RE (ed): Conn's Current Therapy 1988. WB Saunders, Philadelphia, 1988, pp 218–225.
37. Roberts, WC and Buchbinder, NA: Healed left-sided infective endocarditis: A clinicopathologic study of 59 patients. Am J Cardiol 40:876, 1977.
38. Buchbinder, NA and Roberts, WC: Left-sided valvular active infective endocarditis: A study of forty-five necropsy patients. Am J Med 53:20, 1972.
39. Greenberg, BH, Hoffman, P, Schiller, NB, et al: Sudden death in infective endocarditis. Chest 71:794, 1977.
40. Roudaut, R, Billes, MA, Ginestes, J, et al: Echocardiographic vegetations in bacterial endocarditis. Arch Mal Coeur 75:1061, 1982.
41. Sharma, S, Desai, A, Kumar, A, et al: Two dimensional echocardiographic documentation of disappearance of mobile vegetations following fatal embolization. Ind Heart J 35:247, 1983.
42. Jung, JY, Saab, SB, and Almond, CH: The case for early surgical treatment of left-sided primary infective endocarditis: A collective review. J Thorac Cardiovasc Surg 70:509, 1975.
43. Lewis, BS, Agathangelou, NE, Colsen, PR, et al: Cardiac operation during active infective endocarditis: Results of aortic, mitral, and double valve replacement in 94 patients. J Thorac Cardiovasc Surg 84:579, 1982.
44. Bortolotti, U, Milano, A, Livi, U, et al: Aortic valve replacement in active infective endocarditis. Thorac Cardiovasc Surg 29:303, 1981.
45. Wilson, WR, Danielson, GK, Giuliani, ER, et al: Valve replacement in patients with active infective endocarditis. Circulation 58:585, 1978.
46. Croft, CH, Woodward, W, Elliott, A, et al: Analysis of surgical versus medical therapy in active complicated native valve infective endocarditis. Am J Cardiol 51:1650, 1983.

Commentary

By Melvin D. Cheitlin, M.D.

Since 1973 when Dillon and colleagues[1] described the detection of valvular vegetations in patients with infective endocarditis, attempts have been made to relate complications to the presence, size, location, mobility, and texture of these vegetations. Numerous studies summarized in papers by O'Brien and Geiser[2] and Buda and colleagues[3] have shown an increase in the incidence of complications in patients with echocardiographically detected vegetations compared with those without. In a meta-analysis summarizing 159 patients reported in the literature with vegetations and 165 without, in those with vegetations versus those without there was an increase of death (23 percent versus 12 percent), of congestive heart failure (66 percent versus 25 percent), of embolism (42 percent versus 17 percent), and of surgery (63 percent versus 16 percent).[3] Combining series of patients in the literature is difficult because most cases are nonconsecutive and because uniformity is lacking with regard to diagnosis, inclusion versus exclusion of tricuspid valve involvement, definitions of congestive heart failure and embolism and criteria defining indications for surgery. Despite these problems, there is general agreement that the presence of vegetations is a predictor of complications. Inasmuch as anywhere from 40 to 80 percent of patients diagnosed as having infective endocarditis may have vegetations definable by echocardiography, the presence of vegetations alone cannot be an indication for surgery.

In most series, by far the most frequent indication for surgery is the presence of congestive heart failure. More infrequently the presence of resistant organisms (including most fungi), recurrent emboli to large vessels, and evidence of extravalvular infection serve as the primary indications for surgery.

Inasmuch as the mere presence of a vegetation cannot help decide who needs surgery, the question arises as to whether the size of the vegetation by echocardiography can allow subgrouping into high-risk and low-risk patients. One problem with deciding this question is the difficulty in separating the presence of the underlying valve disease, which can cause vegetationlike thickening of the valve leaflet, from vegetations that are frequently described as mobile, attached to the leaflet, not uniformly thickening the leaflet, and so on. These definitions limit our ability to detect vegetations as separate from valvular abnormality, as may be encountered in rheumatic heart disease, ruptured chordae tendineae, mitral valve prolapse, or aortic valve dysplasia. A second problem with determining the *size* of the vegetation is that its *size* depends upon the variable gain or number of echo signals, and because there is no agreed-upon standardization, comparing the *size* of the echo density from one study to another is quite difficult.

227

In this chapter, Lewis and Greenberg address the question of whether the apparent *size* of the vegetation should in itself be a determinant of surgery. There is no study in the literature that specifically addresses this question prospectively. In the echocardiographic studies reported, large vegetations are usually defined as greater than or equal to 10 mm in largest diameter; medium-sized, 5 to 10 mm; and small, less than 5 mm. Using these arbitrary definitions, which are not uniform from study to study, attempts have been made to relate the size of the lesions to complications. In their 18 patients with left-sided vegetations, Buda and colleagues[3] found 11 greater than or equal to 1 cm^2 and 7 less than 1 cm^2, and the larger vegetations had a higher incidence of death (36 percent versus 14 percent), congestive heart failure (64 percent versus 14 percent), and surgery (55 percent versus 43 percent) but a smaller of incidence of embolization (55 percent versus 57 percent). In an earlier study, Stewart and colleagues[4] did not find a relation between vegetation size and clinical outcome.

In a preliminary report, Sanfilippo and colleagues[5] retrospectively evaluated morphologic features such as vegetative size, mobility, extravalvular extent, and texture of vegetations and related them to the clinical outcome as indicated by peripheral or central embolization, congestive heart failure, necessity for valve surgery, and death. In 53 patients with left-sided native endocarditis, they found that vegetative extravalvular extent (p = 0.002) and mobility (p = 0.01) were significant predictors of complications, but size (p = 0.15) and texture (p = 0.41) were not. An echo score based on extravalvular extent and mobility predicted complications with even greater power (p = 0.0007) and correctly predicted outcome in 78 percent of cases. The conclusion that Lewis and Greenberg reach is that neither the size of the vegetation nor its presence is an indication in itself for surgery; however, the presence of a vegetation is an indication that the patient is more likely to become a candidate for surgical intervention for the more classic indication of congestive heart failure and therefore should be watched very closely. In the future, other characteristics of the lesion may provide an earlier indication for surgery, thus avoiding the problem of the higher operative mortality in the patient who has developed severe congestive heart failure.

REFERENCES

1. Dillon, JC, Feigenbaum, H, Konecke, LL, et al: Echocardiographic manifestations of valvular vegetations. Am Heart J 86:698, 1973.
2. O'Brien, JT and Geiser, EA: Infective endocarditis and echocardiography. Am Heart J 108:386, 1984.
3. Buda, AJ, Zotz, RJ, LeMire, MS, et al: Prognostic significance of vegetations detected by two-dimensional echocardiography in infective endocarditis. Am Heart J 112:1291, 1986.
4. Stewart, JA, Silimperi, D, Horris, P, et al: Echocardiographic documentation of vegetative lesions in infective endocarditis: Clinical implications. Circulation 61:374, 1980.
5. Sanfilippo, AJ, Picard, MH, Davidoff, R, et al: Prediction of risk for complications in patients with left-sided infectious endocarditis (abstr). J Am Coll Cardiol 13:72A, 1989.

PART 3

Other Cardiovascular Challenges

CHAPTER 13

Should Patients with Atrial Fibrillation Be Anticoagulated Prior to and Chronically Following Cardioversion?

Bernardo Stein, M.D.
Jonathan L. Halperin, M.D.
Valentin Fuster, M.D.

Atrial fibrillation (AF) is a relatively common arrhythmia with a prevalence of 21.5 per 1000 men and 17.1 per 1000 women, according to the Framingham Heart Study.[1] In this epidemiologic study, the incidence of AF was found to increase markedly with age, and most affected individuals had some form of underlying cardiac disease, including rheumatic heart disease (RHD), coronary artery disease, hypertensive cardiovascular disease, or heart failure.[1]

Atrial fibrillation is one of the most common underlying cardiac disorders predisposing to systemic arterial embolism.[2] Emboli involve the cerebral circulation in up to 70 percent of cases but may also affect the coronary circulation, the spleen, the kidneys, the splanchnic bed, and the limbs. Because acute stroke is the most common and devastating manifestation of embolism in AF, it is important to analyze briefly the etiologic factors related to stroke. Approximately 85 percent of strokes are ischemic in origin, and only 15 percent are due to hemorrhage (Fig. 13–1).[3,4] Of all ischemic strokes, 80 percent are atherothrombotic in nature and can be attributed to advanced cerebrovascular disease. Fifteen percent of ischemic strokes are due to cardiogenic embolism, and only 5 percent are due to other unusual causes such as vasculitis, systemic hypotension, and hypercoagulable states.[3]

Of all cardiogenic emboli encountered in this country, 45 percent are associated with nonvalvular AF; the rest occur in patients with acute myocardial infarction (15 percent), chronic left ventricular dysfunction (10 percent), rheumatic heart disease (10 percent), prosthetic heart valves (10 percent), and other causes. In underdeveloped countries, rheumatic heart disease may be the predominant cause of systemic embolism. Most cardiogenic emboli affect the middle cerebral artery circulation and commonly present as an abrupt onset of a maximal neurologic deficit in an awake, active individual.

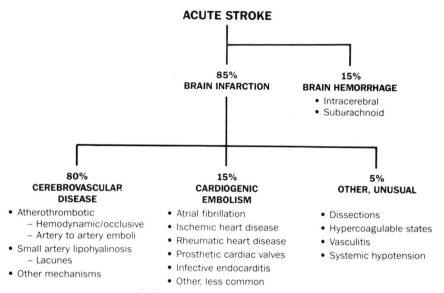

Figure 13–1. Diagram shows different causes of acute stroke; only 15 percent of cases are due to embolism from a cardiac source. (From Sherman, et al,[3] with permission).

Whereas the significant morbidity and mortality attributed to arterial embolism in patients with AF are not in doubt, treatment and preventive strategies are still controversial and empiric.[5] Although the focus of this chapter is mainly on the indications for anticoagulation prior to cardioversion in AF, it is essential to begin this discussion by analyzing the currently available data on the risk of embolism in AF associated with different cardiac disorders. We will discuss (1) pathophysiology of embolism in AF and following cardioversion, (2) incidence of embolism, (3) risk stratification of patients with AF, (4) embolic risk in cardioversion, and (5) recommendations for anticoagulant therapy.

PATHOPHYSIOLOGY OF EMBOLISM IN ATRIAL FIBRILLATION

In patients with AF, systemic emboli probably originate from thrombi formed in the left atrial cavity or the left atrial appendage.[6] Given that fibrillating atria are devoid of significant mechanical activity, the presence of a zone of circulatory stasis is probably the most important mechanism for the formation of thrombi. This may explain also why other forms of supraventricular tachyarrhythmias, such as atrial tachycardia or atrial flutter, in which some degree of mechanical activity is preserved, are not as commonly associated with thromboembolic phenomena as AF. Furthermore, thrombi are commonly present in enlarged atrial appendages, where blood stasis is usually present.

The presence of a hypercoagulable state may predispose to thromboembolism in AF.[7] However, rather than a systemic hypercoagulable state, the presence of an intracavitary clot may itself be a highly thrombogenic stimulus, as has been demonstrated experimentally.[8] This is possibly due to the fact that thrombin, bound to fibrin, is commonly present within thrombi;[9] therefore, when embolism occurs, the thrombin in the remaining intracavitary thrombus is exposed to the circulating blood, which predisposes it to further platelet aggregation and thrombosis.[8]

In addition, the dynamic forces of the circulation are responsible for the migration of thrombotic material into the circulation. Thus, although blood stasis or a procoagulant state predispose to thrombosis, isolation from the circulation, such as occurs in the atrial appendage, may protect against embolic migration.

With respect to embolism in patients with AF undergoing cardioversion, several issues need to be addressed. First, after the onset of AF, it probably takes several days for thrombi to form in the left atrium, and therefore, anticoagulation has not been routinely recommended in AF less than 2 days duration.[10] Furthermore, it is not clear how long it takes for thrombi to form in fibrillating atria, which probably depends on multiple factors, including the type of underlying heart disease, atrial size, ventricular function, coagulability, and so on.[11] Second, once thrombi are formed it may take approximately 2 weeks of anticoagulant therapy to allow the thrombus to undergo fibrotic organization and to become more adherent to the atrial wall, while simultaneously preventing the formation of new thrombi. Although these theories are attractive, there are no scientific data available to fully support them.[11]

Third, what is the mechanism of embolism following cardioversion? Conceivably, regaining atrial mechanical activity facilitates the propulsion of an intracavitary thrombus into the atrial outlet, resulting in embolism. If this is true, why does paroxysmal AF carry a lower embolic risk compared with sustained AF? By definition, patients with paroxysmal AF have spontaneous recurrent conversions to sinus rhythm, yet their embolic risk is less than one half of patients with sustained AF.[12] On the other hand, embolism is a well-documented complication of chemical or electrical cardioversion. One possible explanation for this paradox is that patients with paroxysmal AF have associated organic heart disease that is usually less severe than that of patients with the sustained form of the arrythmia. Therefore, the embolic potential may be influenced more by the degree of underlying cardiac pathology than by the presence of sustained or intermittent AF. Changes in blood flow patterns or in blood viscosity or coagulability also may exert some influence.[5] Clear answers to the aforementioned pathogenetic issues require further research.

RELATION OF ETIOLOGY TO EMBOLIC RISK IN ATRIAL FIBRILLATION

VALVULAR HEART DISEASE

Most of the patients with AF in association with rheumatic valvular heart disease have mitral valve involvement. Without anticoagulation, these patients have an incidence of embolism that approximates 4 to 6 percent per year. The embolic risk appears higher in mitral stenosis than in pure mitral regurgitation, and the presence of AF increases the embolic risk by three to seven times over that of sinus rhythm.[13,14] The majority of these embolic events affect the brain[4] and are associated with severe neurologic functional deficits and a 25 percent mortality. Furthermore, these events are not preceded by warning signs (such as transient ischemic attacks), which makes preventive therapy the more important. Cerebral emboli tend to recur in 30 to 75 percent of patients, at an approximate rate of 10 percent per year, with the highest risk of recurrence being in the first year following the initial embolic event.[4]

Dunn and coworkers[10] analyzed the results of several studies of anticoagulants in AF associated with rheumatic mitral valve disease; most were small, nonrandomized, and retrospective. Nonetheless, these studies showed a 4 to 72 percent (mean of 24 percent) reduction in systemic and pulmonary embolism in anticoagulated patients as compared with controls.[10] Although no large, randomized trials of anticoagulation in rheumatic mitral valve disease have been done, the available data warrant the use of chronic anticoagulation in these patients.[4,10]

A different form of valvular disease, which also has been associated with an increased risk of stroke (particularly in young adults), is mitral valve prolapse.[4] Embolism from valvular thrombi is probably the mechanism of stroke, although other factors such as atrial thrombi associated with AF, septic emboli from endocarditis, and thrombosis due to platelet hyperaggregability have been implicated.[4] In a follow-up study of 237 patients with mitral valve prolapse, Nishimura and associates[15] found 10 embolic events at a mean of 6.2 years of follow-up. Two of these patients had other risk factors for stroke; of the remaining patients, six were in AF and two in sinus rhythm. A more recent retrospective study[16] confirmed the risk of stroke in patients with mitral valve prolapse. Even though over one third of the patients in this study had associated atrial arrhythmias, it is unclear whether the presence of arrhythmias constituted an additional risk for stroke. The formation of platelet-fibrin thrombi on the abnormal valve is probably the most important factor in the genesis of embolism. The presence of associated AF, mitral regurgitation, or left ventricular dysfunction contributes additional risk. No randomized trial of antithrombotic therapy in patients with mitral valve prolapse has been conducted; given the low incidence of embolism, prophylactic anticoagulation in the absence of other risk factors is not recommended.

Thromboembolism associated with aortic valve disease (rheumatic or congenital) is much less frequent than with mitral valve disease and usually occurs in patients with AF, endocarditis, or associated mitral valve disease.[17] Most emboli in aortic stenosis are calcareous, small, and clinically silent.[18] Because there is no available medical therapy for the prevention of embolism in this setting, patients with significant aortic stenosis and recurrent emboli probably should undergo valve replacement.[17]

NONVALVULAR HEART DISEASE

The most common causes of AF include cardiac disorders other than rheumatic heart disease (RHD). Furthermore, nonvalvular AF is currently the most common cardiac disease associated with cerebral emoblism.[4,19] The Framingham data[19] revealed that the risk of stroke in nonvalvular AF was 41.5 per 1000 patient-years, or five to six times more frequent than in age-matched controls without AF. Given their high prevalence, coronary disease and hypertension are the most common underlying disorders associated with AF. Other diseases include cardiomyopathy, thyrotoxicosis, and congenital heart disorders. In addition, patients without an identifiable cardiac disease are considered to have *lone,* or idiopathic, AF.

Coronary Artery Disease

The actual incidence of AF is low in patients with uncomplicated coronary disease but increases significantly in the presence of heart failure.[1] Ischemic heart disease accounts for almost 50 percent of AF cases in some series.[20,21] Clinical[22] and autopsy[23] studies have found ischemic heart disease in association with AF to be a common predisposing factor for stroke and systemic embolism.

There have been no prospective randomized trials of anticoagulation in AF associated with coronary artery disease. Based on the beneficial effects of anticoagulation in RHD, some investigators have advocated the use of chronic anticoagulation for these patients. While awaiting the completion of randomized studies, it seems prudent to recommend chronic anticoagulation to patients with AF at high embolic risk, namely, those with congestive heart failure or history of embolism within the previous 2 years.[4]

Cardiomyopathy

Autopsy studies have shown a high incidence of mural thrombi in patients with dilated cardiomyopathy.[24] Clinical studies also have demonstrated an increased incidence of systemic and pulmonary embolism in patients with dilated cardiomyopathy.[25] The source of embolism in these patients is usually a ventricular mural thrombus, but the presence of atrial arrhythmias constituted an additional risk factor for embolism.[25] With respect to preventive antithrombotic therapy, a nonrandomized study showed that patients on anticoagulant therapy had no embolic events during a follow-up of 101 patient-years, whereas embolism occurred in 18 percent of nonanticoagulated patients, for an event rate of 3.5 per 100 patient-years.[25] Based on this trial, chronic anticoagulation is recommended to patients with dilated cardiomyopathy and clinical heart failure, whether or not AF is present.

Atrial fibrillation is usually a late complication of hypertrophic cardiomyopathy and is commonly associated with heart failure and a definite increase in embolic risk.[26,27] Nevertheless, no studies have evaluated the role of anticoagulation in the prevention of embolism in these patients, and thus, the decision to use antithrombotic therapy should be individualized.

Hypertension

Hypertension alone was not a strong precursor of AF in the Framingham Study,[1] whereas the presence of left ventricular hypertrophy was associated with a 2.4 to 3-fold increase in the risk of AF. On the other hand, given its high prevalence in the general population, hypertensive heart disease was found in 23 percent of subjects with AF in one study.[20] Although patients with hypertension and AF are more prone to develop systemic emboli, there are no data regarding the use of anticoagulants in this group.[10] Moreover, hypertensive patients have an increased risk for cerebral hemorrhage, which may be enhanced by the use of anticoagulants.

Thyrotoxicosis

Paroxysmal or chronic AF may occur in 10 to 28 percent of patients with thyrotoxicosis.[28-30] In these patients, the incidence of systemic thromboembolism is high, ranging from 8 to 39 percent, with an average of 14 percent.[10] Embolism can occur in individuals with persistent AF after hyperthroidism has been controlled, as well as shortly after reversal to sinus rhythm.[29] In one study,[31] the presence of heart failure was an additional risk of embolism.

A recent retrospective study challenged the widespread opinion that thyrotoxic patients with AF have an increased embolic risk, when compared with patients with hyperthyroidism in sinus rhythm.[32] In this study, 13 percent of patients with AF had a cerebrovascular event, whereas this complication occurred in only 3 percent of those in normal sinus rhythm. However, by logistic regression analysis, only age was found to be an independent predictor of cerebral ischemic events. On the other hand, when only strokes were considered (i.e., transient ischemic attacks excluded), AF patients were at increased risk, compared with those in sinus rhythm (p = 0.03).[32]

Although no prospective randomized trials of anticoagulation in thyrotoxic AF have been done, given the risk of systemic embolism, anticoagulation is recommended as soon as the combination of AF and hyperthyroidism is recognized. This therapy should be continued until the patient becomes euthyroid and reversion to sinus rhythm has been achieved.[28-31]

LONE ATRIAL FIBRILLATION

Lone or idiopathic AF occurs in 2.7 to 11.4 percent of cases of AF,[33,34] depending on the criteria used to exclude patients with possible underlying heart disease. In the Mayo Clinic study,[33] 97 patients under the age of 60 with lone AF were followed for a mean of 14.8 years. There were eight embolic events (four strokes and four myocardial infarctions in patients without significant coronary disease) for an overall embolic rate of 0.55 per 100 patient-years. Based on their low incidence of embolic events and their excellent survival, the investigators did not recommend the use of anticoagulants in these patients.

In contrast, in the Framingham Heart Study,[34] patients with lone AF had a significant increase in the age-adjusted incidence of stroke (28 percent versus 7 percent in controls). The difference in the results of these two studies can be explained partially by the fact that the Mayo Clinic study involved a larger number of lone AF cases, was limited to younger patients (under the age of 60), and excluded those with systemic hypertension.

Based on the available data, patients with lone AF under the age of 60 have a very low embolic risk, and, therefore, chronic anticoagulation is not indicated. Older patients and those with hypertension are at higher risk of stroke, and, thus, decisions to anticoagulate should be individualized.

STRATIFICATION OF EMBOLIC RISK

Identification of subgroups of patients with AF depending on their risk of embolism would definitely influence their management and would allow us to implement a more rational preventive strategy. Some patients clearly belong to the *high-risk* and the *low-risk* categories; however, a high proportion of them have an intermediate yet uncertain risk of embolism, and it is in this group in whom decisions regarding antithrombotic therapy are most difficult. For the purpose of our discussion, we will classify patients into four different risk categories for thromboembolism: high, medium-high, medium-low, and low (Table 13-1). However, it should be emphasized that the division into risk groups is not rigid, and the risk of the patient may change with time.

HIGH RISK

These patients have an embolic risk of 6 percent or higher per year. This group predominantly includes patients with a history of embolism (within the previous two years) and those with old mechanical heart valve prostheses.

Table 13–1. Stratification of Thromboembolic Risk in Atrial Fibrillation

	Thromboembolic Risk (per Year)			
	High (>6%)	Medium-High (4–6%)	Medium-Low (2–4%)	Low (<2%)
Underlying heart disease	Prior embolism Old mechanical prostheses	Mitral stenosis Thyrotoxicosis Heart failure Modern mechanical prostheses	Mitral regurgitation Aortic valve disease Coronary disease Hypertensive disease Bioprostheses	Lone AF (age < 60) Isolated mitral valve prolapse
Long-term A/C therapy	A/C (INR = 3.0–4.5)*	A/C (INR = 2.0–3.0)†	A/C (INR = 2.0–3.0)‡	No therapy

*In high-risk patients with old mechanical prostheses, dipyridamole may be added to warfarin.

†In patients with mechanical prostheses, INR range should be 3.0–4.5.

‡The decision for anticoagulation in this group should be individualized.

AF = Atrial fibrillation; A/C = Anticoagulant; INR = International Normalized Ratio of pro-thrombin suppression.

The presence of a previous embolic event clearly predisposes the patient for recurrent embolism, at a rate that can be as high as 15 to 20 percent in the first year alone.[3,35,36] Furthermore, there is evidence that suggests that the high recurrence rate of stroke persists beyond the first year of the initial event.[35] This group of patients with prior embolic stroke constitutes a particularly difficult population for management, given their advanced age, residual neurologic deficits, and relatively high risk of major bleeding complications in the range of 3 to 5 percent per year.[3] The proper time to initiate anticoagulation following cardiogenic brain embolism is controversial. It appears that small- to moderate-sized embolic strokes can be safely anticoagulated if computed tomography shows no evidence of hemorrhage 24 to 48 hours after the event. However, in case of large embolic stroke, anticoagulation should probably be postponed for 5 to 7 days, owing to the risk for delayed hemorrhagic transformation.[4]

Patients with mechanical prosthetic heart valves are at increased risk of thrombosis and embolism, particularly those with prostheses implanted before the mid-1970s.[37] Although older studies did not show that AF was an independent risk factor for thromboembolism, more recent studies have found that atrial arrhythmias contribute to additional embolic risk in patients with mechanical as well as bioprosthetic valves.[37]

Patients in this group should receive chronic anticoagulants, aimed at an International Normalized Ratio (INR) of prothrombin suppression of 3.0 to 4.5 (equivalent prothrombin time of 1.5 to 2.0 × control using conventional North American rabbit-brain thromboplastin reagent). In addition, patients with mechanical prostheses at high risk of embolism (e.g., those with old devices or previous emboli) may benefit from the addition of a platelet inhibitor (e.g., dipyridamole) to the anticoagulant regimen.[37]

MEDIUM-HIGH RISK

Patients in this group have a risk of embolism between 4 and 6 per 100 patient-years. This category includes patients with rheumatic mitral stenosis, thyrotoxicosis, dilated cardiomyopathy, and those with modern mechanical valve implantation. Among patients with RHD, those with mitral stenosis have the highest embolic risk. About 20 percent of patients with mitral stenosis experience a clinically significant embolic event.[4] In addition, the presence of AF increases the risk of embolism by three- to seven-fold over sinus rhythm. These patients, as well as those with recent mechanical prostheses, should receive long-term warfarin therapy. The dose should be adjusted to an INR of 3.0 to 4.5 (PT ratio = 1.5 to 2.0 $\times$ control) for patients with mechanical valves, and to an INR of 2.0 to 3.0 (PT ratio = 1.3 to 1.5) for those with mitral stenosis.

Although less well defined in terms of embolic risk, the subgroup of patients with nonvalvular AF at a higher risk includes those with uncontrolled hyperthroidism or decompensated heart failure. Strong consideration of anticoagulation should be given to these patients, aimed at an INR of 2.0 to 3.0 (PT ratio = 1.3 to 1.5). In patients with dilated cardiomyopathy, warfarin should probably be continued indefinitely. However, in cases of thyrotoxicosis, this therapy may be stopped once hyperthyroidism is under control and the atria have regained adequate mechanical activity.[38]

MEDIUM-LOW RISK

This is a heterogeneous group, which contains the largest number of patients. Within this category are patients with an embolic risk of 2 to 4 per 100 patient-years. The underlying organic heart disease associated with AF in these patients includes mitral regurgitation, aortic valve disease, coronary artery disease, hypertension, congenital heart disease, and mitral valve replacement with a bioprosthesis.

The indications for antithrombotic therapy have not been clearly established, because risk subgroups within this category have been difficult to define. There is some evidence that suggests that there is a clustering of stroke events in the inital months following the onset of AF.[4,12,36] In addition, chronic AF appears to carry a higher embolic risk when compared with paroxysmal AF.[12,39,40] In a retrospective study,[12] the annual incidence of embolism was 2.5 times higher in patients with sustained versus paroxysmal AF. In another, smaller, study of patients with clinical emboli, three fourths had sustained AF, and only one fourth had the paroxysmal form of the arrhythmia.[39] Stratification of patients with nonvalvular AF into different embolic risk groups based on echocardiographic criteria has not been well settled. Although one study[41] showed that left atrial size was a predictor for embolism, other studies[39,42,43] have not been able to confirm this finding. However, it should be noted that most patients with sustained AF have enlarged left atria.

As discussed later, recent evidence suggests that long-term anticoagulation effectively reduces the incidence of embolism in patients with nonvalvular AF.[70] However, subgroups of patients that stand to gain most from chronic anticoagulation have not yet been well-defined.

Low Risk

The embolic risk of these patients is less than two events per 100 patient-years. This group primarily includes patients under the age of 60 with either lone[33] or paroxysmal AF. Included in this group also are patients with mitral valve prolapse in the absence of other risk factors for embolism, such as endocarditis or significant mitral regurgitation. In these patients, the risk of bleeding from long-term anticoagulation probably outweighs benefits in terms of prevention of embolism, and therefore this therapy is not recommended.

Although the classification of AF patients into different risk categories has not been completely established, stratification of these patients would clearly influence preventive efforts. Knowledge of the risk of bleeding with chronic anticoagulation therapy is essential. According to several studies,[4,44,45] the risk of major noncerebral bleeding is 2 to 3 per 100 patients per year of exposure. The risk of brain hemorrhage approximates 1 percent per year (an eightfold increase over controls).[4] Therefore, before the decision to institute chronic anticoagulation is made, an analysis of the risks and the benefits of such therapy as it pertains to the individual patient should be made.

RISK OF EMBOLISM IN RELATION TO CARDIOVERSION

Since Lown and associates[46] introduced the method of electrical cardioversion for the termination of atrial and ventricular arrhythmias, systemic embolism has emerged as one of the complications of the procedure. There are numerous reports in the literature that have addressed this issue, but the data on prophylactic anticoagulation prior to cardioversion are imprecise. It appears that the risk of embolism is similar with pharmacologic and electric means of cardioversion. In the following section, we will review the available data on embolism following cardioversion for AF. These studies are summarized in Table 13–2.

Sokolow and Ball[47] studied 177 patients, most of whom had AF and only a few atrial flutter. Rheumatic disease was the underlying pathology in 53 percent. All patients were treated with quinidine, and only those with prior embolism received anticoagulation prior to cardioversion. Only two embolic events were found; one occurred among 30 patients with prior embolism. Interestingly, three patients successfully converted to sinus rhythm had embolic events at the time of relapse to AF.

In his review article of 1960, Goldman[48] described six cases of embolism in 400 patients successfully reverted to sinus rhythm with quinidine, for an incidence of embolism of 1.5 percent. None of his patients was anticoagulated. The author proposed that it takes 14 days for an atrial thrombus to undergo fibroblastic infiltration and to become adherent to the endocardium, thus preventing its dislodgement following resumption of sinus rhythm. Although there is no proof for this theory, Goldman suggested consideration be given to anticoagulation for 2 weeks prior to cardioversion with quinidine.

Lown and colleagues[49] were the first to report the results of electrical cardioversion in patients with AF; they studied 50 patients in whom 65 electrical cardioversion attempts were made. Ninty-four percent of this group had RHD. Only nonsurgical patients with mitral stenosis were anticoagulated 3 to 4 weeks prior to conversion, although the exact number of anticoagulated patients was not stated. One episode of splenic embolism was found after conversion in a patient with

Table 13–2. Embolic Risk During Cardioversion for Atrial Fibrillation

Trial (Year)	No. of Patients	(%) with RHD	Method of Conversion	A/C Therapy	Incidence of Embolism* n	%	Comments
Sokolow (1956)[47]	177	53	Quinidine	In few pts	2	(1.3)	A/C given to pts with prior embolism
Goldman (1960)[48]	400	?	Quinidine	No	6	(1.5)	
Lown (1963)[49]	50	94	Electrical	In some pts	1	(1.7)	A/C given to pts with mitral stenosis
Killip (1963)[50]	62	Most	Electrical	In 45%	0		
Freeman (1963)[51]	100	11	Quinidine	Yes	0		
Rokseth (1963)[52]	274	52	Quinidine	Yes	2	(1.6)	Additional pulmonary embolus occurred
Morris (1964)[53]	70	66	Electrical	In 6%	3	(3.4)	Embolic events in pts not on A/C
Oram (1964)[55]	100	65	Electrical	In some pts	2	(1.9)	A/C used in pts at highest embolic risk
Hurst (1964)[20]	121	27	Electrical	No	2	(1.3)	
Morris (1966)[54]	108	62	Electrical	In some pts	4	(2.5)	Embolic events in pts with RHD on no A/C
Korsgren (1965)[56]	138	58	Electrical	Yes	0		No emboli even in pts with prior embolism
Halmos (1966)[57]	175	80	Electrical	No	1	(0.4)	
Selzer (1966)[58]	189	?	Electrical	No	4	(2.1)	
Lown (1967)[59]	350	70	Electrical	In 29%	3	(0.9)	Embolic events in pts not on A/C
Resnekov (1967)[60]	204	50	Electrical	In some pts	2	(0.6)	Additional embolus in pt post-infarction
Hall (1968)[61]	142	68	Electrical	In 39%	1	(0.8)	Embolic event in pt not on A/C
Radford (1968)[62]	156	56	Electrical	In 17%	0		Only pts with prior emboli received A/C
Aberg (1968)[63]	207	58	Electrical	In most pts	2	(0.7)	Embolus in pt with low A/C dosage
Bjerkelund (1969)[66]	437	58	Electrical	Yes	2	(1.1)	A/C reduced embolic incidence by 86% (p =0.012)
				No	11	(5.6)	
McCarthy (1969)[64]	149	44	Electrical	In some pts	2	(1.6)	Embolic events in pts not on A/C
Henry (1976)[26]	37	65	Electrical	In some pts	3	(5.6)	Emboli in pts with HCM, despite A/C
Roy (1986)[45]	152	?	Electrical	In 72%	2	(1.3)	Emboli in atrial flutter pts not on A/C

*Calculated per successful cardioversion attempts. HCM = hypertrophic cardiomyopathy, RHD = rheumatic heart disease, A/C = anticoagulants, pts = patients.

mitral stenosis and AF of 4 months duration who was not anticoagulated. The authors recommended the use of anticoagulants for 3 weeks prior to and 1 week after cardioversion in all patients with RHD.

Killip[50] described 84 electric cardioversion attempts in 62 patients, most of whom had RHD. The study included some patients with atrial flutter. Forty-five percent of patients were prophylactically anticoagulated, and 55 percent were not.

No embolic events were encountered in either of the two groups. Freeman and Wexler[51] studied 100 patients treated with oral anticoagulants for at least 18 days prior to cardioversion with quinidine, and no thromboembolic events were encountered.

Rokseth and Storstein[52] used chemical cardioversion with quinidine in 274 patients with AF, half of whom had RHD. All patients were anticoagulated prior to cardioversion. They found two instances of cerebral emboli, one occurring immediately after conversion to sinus rhythm, and the other 5 days later. Therefore, anticoagulation did not prevent embolism in 1.6 percent of cases, although the duration of therapy prior to conversion was not stated.

In 1964, Morris and coworkers[53] analyzed the results of 94 electric cardioversion attempts in 70 patients (90 percent with AF and 10 percent with atrial flutter). Only four of their patients were on chronic anticoagulation therapy. The authors observed three cerebral embolic events: one occurred at the time of conversion, one 3 days after conversion, and another 10 days after conversion. Two of the three embolic events occurred in patients with prior embolism, but none was on anticoagulants. Interestingly, 18 patients with prior embolism had no recurrence of embolism after cardioversion. In 1966, a report from the same laboratory[54] depicted the results of 167 cardioversion attempts in 108 patients with AF, 62 percent of whom had RHD. Prophylactic anticoagulation was instituted only in patients with a recent embolism (less than eight weeks old) and was given for eight weeks prior to conversion and for several weeks thereafter. There were four embolic events, which occurred immediately and 3, 7, and 10 days following cardioversion. All of these patients had RHD, and none was on anticoagulants, although two patients had prior embolism. The authors concluded that if anticoagulants were to be used prophylactically, they should be used in all patients with RHD, whether or not embolism had previously occurred, and they should be continued for at least two weeks after the procedure to prevent late embolic events. In patients with recent embolism, they recommended eight weeks of anticoagulation prior to cardioversion, although no rationale for this specific length of therapy was given.

Oram and Davies[55] reported the results of electric cardioversion in 100 patients with AF, 65 of whom had RHD. Prophylactic anticoagulation was used in patients with mitral stenosis, cardiomegaly, embolic history, or recent onset AF. There were two embolic events 2 days after cardioversion, although it is not clear whether these patients were anticoagulated or not. Hurst and associates[20] reported two peripheral emboli (3 and 8 days after the procedure) in 158 attempts at electric cardioversion in 121 patients, none of whom was on anticoagulants.

Korsgren and colleagues[56] studied 138 patients with atrial arrhythmias (83 percent with AF), all of whom were on anticoagulants for three weeks prior to electric cardioversion. No embolic events occurred despite prior embolism in some patients. On the other hand, Halmos[57] did not use anticoagulants in 175 patients with AF who underwent cardioversion. Only one episode of cerebral embolism was found, a surprisingly low incidence of 0.7 percent. Selzer and colleagues[58] reported the results of 240 cardioversion attempts in 189 patients not on anticoagulants, most of whom had AF. There were four embolic events after conversion, two cerebral and two pulmonary. The authors did not recommend prophylactic anticoagulation because of the low incidence of embolism and the lack of evidence that anticoagulants were protective, except in patients with prior embolism.

In his review article of 1967, Lown[59] analyzed the outcome of 456 cardioversion attempts in 350 patients with AF, 70 percent of whom had RHD. Only 100 out of the 350 patients were on anticoagulants. The total incidence of embolism was 1.2 percent, and all embolic events occurred in nonanticoagulated patients. No mention of the specific indications for anticoagulation or the length of therapy was made. Nevertheless, Lown recommended prophylactic anticoagulation in patients with prior embolism and women with mitral valve disease and new onset AF, which should be started three weeks prior to reversion and continued for 1 week thereafter.[59]

Resnekov and McDonald[60] studied 180 patients with AF and 24 with atrial flutter, half of whom had RHD. An unspecified number of patients were on chronic anticoagulants prior to cardioversion. Only two embolic events could clearly be related to the procedure. The first case was interesting in that it occurred in a patient with lone AF who was on anticoagulants, even though such a patient has the lowest embolic potential. The second case occurred in a patient with atrial tachycardia in association with a recent myocardial infarction; in this case, the embolus may have originated in the left ventricle, as opposed to the atrium. The authors recommended the use of prophylactic coumarin derivatives in patients with an increased thromboembolic risk, including those with a recent infarction, chronic ischemic heart disease, mitral valve disease, cardiomyopathy, and prior embolism.

In the study by Hall and Wood,[61] 142 patients with AF or flutter underwent cardioversion. Fifty-five patients were put on anticoagulants prophylactically for 3 weeks, including those with prior emboli, left atrial thrombus found at surgery, or recent onset of AF. Only one patient not on anticoagulants had cerebral embolism 18 hours after conversion.

Radford and Evans[62] found no incidence of embolism in 120 patients with AF electrically reverted to sinus rhythm. Only 17 percent of their patients were chronically on anticoagulants because of previous embolism. Aberg and Cullhed[63] found two embolic events, 2 and 18 days after cardioversion, in 207 patients with AF or flutter. Most of their patients received anticoagulation for an unspecified length of time. Interestingly, one of the embolic events occurred in a patient with mitral and aortic valve disease who had a subtherapeutic level of anticoagulation.

McCarthy and associates[64] studied 149 patients with AF and flutter, 44 percent of whom had RHD. Patients with prior emboli and most of those with mitral valve disease were receiving anticoagulants. Two systemic emboli occurred following cardioversion in patients not receiving anticoagulants who did not have mitral valve disease. The proportion of patients on anticoagulants and the duration of therapy was not specified. Henry and coworkers[26] described 54 cardioversion attempts in 37 patients with AF and mitral valve disease (24 patients) or asymmetric septal hypertrophy (13 patients). No patients with mitral valve disease had an embolic event, whereas 3 of 13 patients with asymmetric septal hypertrophy did, despite the fact that two were receiving anticoagulants. Therefore, patients with hypertrophic cardiomyopathy and AF constitute a high-risk group for embolism.

In a more recent report, Roy and coworkers[45] described 152 attempts of cardioversion in patients with AF or flutter, of whom 72 percent received prophylactic anticoagulation. There were only two embolic events in two patients with paroxysmal AF not receiving anticoagulants who, interestingly enough, had atrial flutter at the time of cardioversion. The authors recommended prophylactic anticoagulation prior to cardioversion in patients with AF and in those with atrial flutter in whom AF had previously been documented.

One of the most important studies that addressed the risk of embolism following cardioversion is the one by Bjerkelund and Orning[65,66] from Norway. These authors prospectively studied 437 patients (58 percent with RHD), referred for electrical treatment of atrial arrhythmias. Patients already on anticoagulants were maintained on them, whereas those not on anticoagulants did not receive anticoagulant prophylaxis. Despite the fact that patients on anticoagulants had a higher embolic risk due to cardiomegaly, heart failure, and higher incidence of RHD and of prior embolism, there were only two embolic events in this group, a low incidence of 0.8 percent. In contrast, 11 patients not on anticoagulants suffered an embolic event, an incidence of 5.3 percent (p = 0.016). When only successfully cardioverted patients were considered, the embolic rate was 1.1 percent versus 6.8 percent, respectively (p = 0.012). Moreover, none of the patients with prior emboli receiving anticoagulation had a recurrence, whereas 3 out of 11 patients not receiving anticoagulation had a prior embolic event. Half of the embolic events occurred in patients with nonrheumatic heart disease. Although this was a nonrandomized study, its significance is strengthened by the fact that the patients on anticoagulants were at higher risk, which introduced a bias against this therapy. Inasmuch as this is an important study, we agree with the criticisms of Mancini and Goldberger[11] that the effects of short-term prophylactic anticoagulation cannot be assessed from this study, because patients were receiving chronic anticoagulant therapy. In addition, not all studied patients had AF; some had atrial tachycardia and flutter, although no subgroup analysis was made.

RECOMMENDATIONS FOR ANTICOAGULATION PRIOR TO AND AFTER CARDIOVERSION

PROPHYLACTIC ANTICOAGULATION FOR CARDIOVERSION

The risk of embolism following cardioversion in patients with AF ranges from as low as 0 to as high as 7 percent, and depends on whether or not underlying heart disease is present, and on the duration of AF. There is not a single randomized study of prophylactic anticoagulation prior to cardioversion; therefore, the decision must be based on assessment of the embolic risk of the individual patient. As discussed previously, two groups of patients can be clearly defined: the high-risk and the low-risk. For patients at high risk of embolism (those with prior embolism, mechanical valve prosthesis, or mitral stenosis), long-term anticoagulant therapy should be instituted, regardless of the need for cardioversion. In contrast, for patients at low risk (those without underlying heart disease under the age of 60), the incidence of embolism is extremely low, and anticoagulation does not seem necessary.

Between these two extremes are the majority of patients with AF. For this intermediate risk group we currently recommend anticoagulation for several weeks before and up to four weeks after conversion to sinus rhythm.[67] This recommendation is mainly based on two arguments: (1) There is clinical evidence from nonrandomized trials, which suggests that anticoagulants reduce the risk of embolism after cardioversion. [45,59,66] (2) The risk of bleeding associated with short-term anticoagulation is low, and is probably outweighed by the risk of embolism postcardioversion. The rationale to continue anticoagulation for several weeks postconversion is based on the studies by Ikram,[68] Rowlands,[69] Manning[38] and their coworkers who have shown that the mechanical activation of the atria may be delayed for several weeks after the resumption of electrical atrial activity.

The consensus of the American College of Chest Physicians[10] provided the following guidelines with respect to prophylactic anticoagulation prior to cardioversion: (1) In cases of AF of more than three days duration, warfarin therapy aimed at an INR of 2.0–3.0 (PT ratio = 1.3–1.5 × control) should be given for three weeks prior to elective cardioversion. (2) This therapy should be continued for two to four weeks following reversion to sinus rhythm. (3) No anticoagulation is necessary for AF of shorter duration (<2 days) or for cardioversion of patients with atrial flutter or supraventricular tachycardia. However, patients with atrial flutter, in whom intermittent episodes of AF have been present, should be regarded as having an embolic risk similar to patients with AF, and should be considered for prophylactic anticoagulation.[45] (4) In cases of emergency cardioversion in patients with ischemia or hemodynamic compromise, anticoagulation with heparin started on the day of cardioversion is advisable for patients with AF of several days duration, those at high risk of arrhythmia recurrence, and those with additional risk factors such as mitral valve disease. Chronic oral anticoagulation should be considered, depending on the patient's embolic risk as discussed later.

A novel approach to the intermediate-risk patient not receiving chronic anticoagulant therapy could conceivably be based on the findings of transesophageal echocardiography. This technique is clearly superior to transthoracic echocardiography for the detection of thrombi within the left atrial cavity or appendage. If a thrombus is found on echocardiography, anticoagulant therapy could then be given for several weeks prior to cardioversion. If, on the other hand, no thrombus is found, cardioversion could be performed immediately, without the need for anticoagulants. This approach requires clinical testing; if it is shown to be safe, it could potentially eliminate the unnecessary delay, cost, and small risk involved in anticoagulation.

LONG-TERM ANTICOAGULATION

A more difficult problem is the development of guidelines for long-term anticoagulation in patients with AF associated with different forms of heart disease (see Table 13–1). Our approach to this problem is based on stratifying patients with AF according to risk of embolism, whether or not cardioversion is to be performed. High-risk patients have an incidence of embolism over six percent per year and should be on chronic anticoagulant therapy. This group includes patients with previous embolism and those with older mechanical prostheses. At the lower end of the spectrum of embolic risk are patients under the age of 60 with AF but no evidence of organic heart disease (lone fibrillators). Their risk of embolism is well under two percent per year, and no anticoagulation is necessary.

Between these two poles exists a large group of patients with an intermediate but incompletely defined risk of embolism. Because the rationale for chronic anticoagulant therapy is based on the stratification of embolic risk, we have attempted to classify this heterogeneous group further into two risk categories: medium-high and medium-low, although the boundaries between subgroups cannot be rigid and may change with time. The medium-high-risk patients—those with mitral stenosis, uncompensated hyperthyroidism, congestive heart failure, or recent mechanical prostheses—have substantial embolic risk of 4 to 6 percent per year. In these patients, the benefits of anticoagulation outweigh its risks, and, thus, long-term warfarin therapy is indicated.

The medium-low-risk subgroup includes patients with valvular disease other than mitral stenosis, those with bioprostheses, and those with other forms of organic heart disease (coronary, hypertensive, congenital). Their embolic risk ranges from 2 to 4 percent per year, and the decision to use anticoagulants on a chronic basis should be made only after careful analysis of the benefit-to-risk ratio of the individual patient. If elective cardioversion is planned and the patient is not on chronic anticoagulant therapy, we recommend warfarin for 3 weeks prior to the procedure and for 4 weeks following conversion, in order to prevent embolism at the time of restoration of atrial mechanical activity. At this point, the clinician must decide whether or not chronic anticoagulation is warranted. There has been only one large, prospective, randomized trial of chronic anticoagulation in patients with nonvalvular AF.[70] In this study, patients whose mean age was 74 years were randomized to warfarin, aspirin, or placebo and followed for 2 years. The total incidence of stroke and transient ischemic attacks was reduced by 75 percent with warfarin (INR = 2.8 to 4.2), although the rate of severe and fatal strokes was similar in both groups. No advantage of aspirin over placebo in prevention of embolism was found. This study suggests that long-term anticoagulation may be beneficial for prevention of embolic stroke in patients with chronic, nonvalvular AF. Another study that addresses this problem is the Stroke Prevention in Atrial Fibrillation (SPAF) trial. This ongoing, large, multicenter, prospective study is comparing warfarin, aspirin, and placebo in patients with nonvalvulopathic AF. When available, the results of this trial may help us determine which subgroups of patients with AF are most likely to benefit from chronic anticoagulant therapy. The role of aspirin in this group of patients remains to be determined.

In conclusion, the ability to stratify patients into different subgroups depending on their risk of embolism, and a thorough knowledge of the risks of short-term and long-term anticoagulation, will allow the treating physician to make a more rational decision regarding the antithrombotic management of patients with atrial fibrillation.

REFERENCES

1. Kannel, WB, Abbott, RD, Savage, DD, et al: Epidemiologic features of chronic atrial fibrillation: The Framingham Study. N Engl J Med 306:1018, 1982.
2. Wolf, PA, Abbott, RD, and Kannel, WB: Atrial fibrillation: A major contributor to stroke in the elderly: The Framingham Study. Arch Intern Med 147:1561, 1987.
3. Sherman, DG, Dyken, ML, Fisher, M, et al: Cerebral embolism. Chest 89 (Suppl S):82S, 1986.
4. Sherman, DG, Dyken, ML, Fisher, M, et al: Antithrombotic therapy for cerebrovascular disorders. Chest 95(Suppl):140S, 1989.
5. Halperin, JL and Hart, RG: Atrial fibrillation and stroke: New ideas, persisting dilemmas. Stroke 19:937, 1988.
6. Shrestha, NK, Moreno, FL, Narciso, FV, et al: Two-dimensional echocardiographic diagnosis of left-atrial thrombus in rheumatic heart disease: A clinicopathologic study. Circulation 67:341, 1983.
7. Gustafsson, C, Blomback, M, Britton, M, et al: Haemostatic function and the increased risk of stroke in nonvalvular atrial fibrillation (abstr). Stroke 18:299, 1987.
8. Fuster, V, Badimon, L, Cohen, M, et al: Insights into the pathogenesis of acute ischemic syndromes. Circulation 22:1213, 1988.
9. Francis, CW, Markham, RE, Jr, Barlow, GH, et al: Thrombin activity of fibrin thrombi and soluble plasmic derivatives. J Lab Clin Med 102:220, 1983.
10. Dunn, M, Alexander, J, de Silva, R, et al: Antithrombotic therapy in atrial fibrillation. Chest 95(Suppl):118S, 1989.

11. Mancini, GBJ and Goldberger, AL: Cardioversion of atrial fibrillation: Consideration of embolization, anticoagulation, prophylactic pacemaker, and long-term success. Am Heart J 104:617, 1982.
12. Petersen, P and Godtfredsen, J: Embolic complications in paroxysmal atrial fibrillation. Stroke 17:622, 1986.
13. Coulshed, N, Epstein, EJ, McKendrick, CS, et al: Systemic embolism in mitral valve disease. Br Heart J 32:26, 1970.
14. Szekely, P: Systemic embolism and anticoagulant prophylaxis in rheumatic heart disease. Br Med J 1:1209, 1964.
15. Nishimura, RA, McGoon, MD, Shub, C, et al: Echocardiographically documented mitral-valve prolapse: Long-term follow-up of 237 patients. N Engl J Med 313:1305, 1985.
16. Marks, AR, Choong, CY, Sanfilippo, AJ, et al: Identification of high-risk and low-risk subgroups of patients with mitral-valve prolapse. N Engl J Med 320:1031, 1989.
17. Chesebro, JH, Adams, PC, and Fuster, V: Antithrombotic therapy in patients with valvular heart disease and prosthetic heart valves. J Am Coll Cardiol 8 (Suppl B):41B, 1986.
18. Brockmeier, LB, Adolph, RJ, Gustin, BW, et al: Calcium emboli to the retinal artery in calcific aortic stenosis. Am Heart J 101:32, 1981.
19. Wolf, PA, Dawber, TR, Thomas HE, et al: Epidemiologic assessment of chronic atrial fibrillation and risk of stroke: The Framingham Study. Neurology (Minneap) 28:973, 1978.
20. Hurst, JW, Paulk, EA, Proctor, HD, et al: Management of patients with atrial fibrillation. Am J Med 37:728, 1964.
21. Aberg, H: Atrial fibrillation. Acta Med Scand 184:425, 1968.
22. Abbott, WM, Maloney, RD, McCabe, CC, et al: Arterial embolism: A 44 year perspective. Am J Surg 1243:460, 1982.
23. Hinton, RC, Kistler, P, Fallon, JT, et al: Influence of etiology of atrial fibrillation on incidence on systemic embolism. Am J Cardiol 40:509, 1977.
24. Roberts, WC, Siegel, RJ, and McManus, BM: Idiopathic dilated cardiomyopathy: Analysis of 152 necropsy patients. Am J Cardiol 60:1340, 1987.
25. Fuster, V, Gersh, BJ, Giuliani, ER, et al: The natural history of idiopathic dilated cardiomyopathy. Am J Cardiol 47:525, 1981.
26. Henry, WL, Morganroth, J, Pearlman, AS, et al: Relation between echocardiographically determined left atrial size and atrial fibrillation. Circulation 53:273, 1976.
27. Glancy, DL, O'Brien, KP, Gold, HK, et al: Atrial fibrillation in patients with idiopathic hypertrophic subaortic stenosis. Br Heart J 32:652, 1970.
28. Yuen, RWM, Gutteridge, DH, Thompson, PL, et al: Embolism in thyrotoxic atrial fibrillation. Med J Aust 1:630, 1979.
29. Staffurth, JS, Gibberd, MC, and Tang Fui, SN: Arterial embolism in thyrotoxicosis with atrial fibrillation. Br Med J 2:688, 1977.
30. Bar-Sela, S, Ehrenfeld, M, and Eliakim, M: Arterial embolism in thyrotoxicosis with atrial fibrillation. Arch Intern Med 141:1191, 1981.
31. Hurley, DM, Hunter, AN, Hewett, MJ, et al: Atrial fibrillation and arterial embolism in hyperthyroidism. Aust NZ J Med 11:391, 1981.
32. Petersen, P and Hansen, JM: Stroke in thyrotoxicosis with atrial fibrillation. Stroke 19:15, 1988.
33. Kopecky, SL, Gersh, BJ, McGoon, MD, et al: The natural history of lone atrial fibrillation: A population-based study over three decades. N Engl J Med 317:669, 1987.
34. Brand, FN, Abbott, RD, Kannel, WB, et al: Characteristics and prognosis of lone atrial fibrillation: 30-year follow-up in the Framingham Study. JAMA 254:3449, 1985.
35. Sage, JI and Van Uitert, RL: Risk of recurrent stroke in patients with atrial fibrillation and nonvalvular heart disease. Stroke 14:537, 1983.
36. Wolf, PA, Kannel, WB, McGee, DL, et al: Duration of atrial fibrillation and imminence of stroke: The Framingham Study. Stroke 14:664, 1983.
37. Fuster, V, Badimon, L, Badimon, JJ, et al: Prevention of thromboembolism induced by prosthetic heart valves. Semin Thromb Hemost 14:50, 1988.
38. Manning, WJ, Leeman, DE, Gotch, PJ, et al: Pulsed Doppler evaluation of atrial mechanical function after electrical cardioversion of atrial fibrillation. J Am Coll Cardiol 13:617, 1989.
39. Wiener, I, Hafner, R, Nicolai, M, et al: Clinical and echocardiographic correlates of systemic embolization in nonrheumatic atrial fibrillation. Am J Cardiol 59:177, 1987.
40. Fortin, AH and Isner, JM: Should patients with paroxysmal atrial fibrillation receive prophylactic anticoagulation (abstr)? J Am Coll Cardiol 1:704, 1983.

41. Caplan, LR, D'Cruz, I, Hier, DB, et al: Atrial size, atrial fibrillation and stroke. Ann Neurol 19:158, 1986.
42. Ruocco, NA and Most, AS: Clinical and echocardiographic risk factors for systemic embolization in patients with atrial fibrillation in the absence of mitral stenosis (abstr). J Am Coll Cardiol 7:165A, 1987.
43. Tegeler, CH and Hart, RG: Atrial size, atrial fibrillation and stroke. Ann Neurol 21:315, 1987.
44. Levine, HJ, Pauker, SG, and Salzman, EW: Antithrombotic therapy in valvular heart disease. Chest 89 (Suppl 2):36S, 1986.
45. Roy, D, Marchand, E, Gagne, P, et al: Usefulness of anticoagulant therapy in the prevention of embolic complications of atrial fibrillation. Am Heart J 112:1039, 1986.
46. Lown, B, Amarasingham, RS and Neuman, J: New method for terminating cardiac arrhythmias. JAMA 182:373, 1962.
47. Sokolow, M and Ball, RE: Factors influencing conversion of chronic atrial fibrillation with special reference to serum quinidine concentration. Circulation 14:568, 1956.
48. Goldman, MJ: The management of chronic atrial fibrillation: Indications for and method of conversion to sinus rhythm. Prog Cardiovasc Dis 2:465, 1960.
49. Lown, B, Perlroth, MG, Kaidbey, S, et al: "Cardioversion" of atrial fibrillation. A report on the treatment of 65 episodes in 50 patients. N Engl J Med 269:325, 1963.
50. Killip, T: Synchronized DC precordial shock for arrhythmias: Safe new technique to establish normal rhythm may be utilized on an elective or an emergency basis. JAMA 186:107, 1963.
51. Freeman, I and Wexler, J: Anticoagulants for treatment of atrial fibrillation. JAMA 184:1007, 1963.
52. Rokseth, R and Storstein, O: Quinidine therapy of chronic auricular fibrillation: The occurrence and mechanism of syncope. Arch Intern Med 111:184, 1963.
53. Morris, JJ, Kong, Y, North, WC, et al: Experience with "cardioversion" of atrial fibrillation and flutter. Am J Cardiol 14:94, 1964.
54. Morris, JJ, Peter, RH, and McIntosh, HD: Electrical conversion of atrial fibrillation: Immediate and long-term results and selection of patients. Ann Intern Med 65:216, 1966.
55. Oram, S and Davies, JPH: Further experience of electrical conversion of atrial fibrillation to sinus rhythm: Analysis of 100 patients. Lancet 1:1204, 1964.
56. Korsgren, M, Leskinen, E, Peterhoff, V, et al: Conversion of atrial arrhythmias with DC shock: Primary results and a follow-up investigation. Acta Med Scand 431(Suppl):1, 1965.
57. Halmos, PB: Direct current conversion of atrial fibrillation. Br Heart J 28:302, 1966.
58. Selzer, A, Kelly, JJ, Johnson, RB, et al: Immediate and long-term results of electrical conversion of arrhythmias. Prog Cardiovasc Dis 9:90, 1966.
59. Lown, B: Electrical reversion of cardiac arrhythmias. Br Heart J 29:469, 1967.
60. Resnekov, L and McDonald, L: Complications in 220 patients with cardiac dysrhythmias treated by phased direct current shock, and indications for electroconversion. Br Heart J 29:926, 1967.
61. Hall, JI and Wood, DR: Factors affecting cardioversion of atrial arrhythmias with special reference to quinidine. Br Heart J 30:84, 1968.
62. Radford, MD and Evans, DW: Long-term results of DC reversion of atrial fibrillation. Br Heart J 30:91, 1968.
63. Aberg, H and Cullhed, I: Direct current countershock complications. Acta Med Scand 183:415, 1968.
64. McCarthy, C, Varghese, PJ, and Barritt, DW: Prognosis of atrial arrhythmias treated by electrical countershock therapy: A three-year follow-up. Br Heart J 31:496, 1969.
65. Bjerkelund, CJ and Orning, OM: An evaluation of DC shock treatment of atrial arrhythmias: Immediate results and complications in 437 patients, with long-term results in the first 290 of these. Acta Med Scand 184:481, 1968.
66. Bjerkelund, CJ and Orning, OM: The efficacy of anticoagulant therapy in preventing embolism related to DC electrical conversion of atrial fibrillation. Am J Cardiol 23:208, 1969.
67. DeSilva, RA, Graboys, TB, Podrid, PJ, et al: Cardioversion and defibrillation. Am Heart J 100:881, 1980.
68. Ikram, H, Nixon, PGF, and Arcan, T: Left atrial function after electrical conversion to sinus rhythm. Br Heart J 30:80, 1968.
69. Rowlands, DJ, Logan, WFWE, Howitt, E, et al: Atrial function after cardioversion. Am Heart J 74:149, 1967.
70. Petersen, P, Boysen, G, Godtfredsen, J, et al: Placebo-controlled, randomised trial of warfarin and aspirin for prevention of thromboembolic complications in chronic atrial fibrillation: The Copenhagen AFASAK Study. Lancet 1:175, 1989.

Commentary

By Melvin D. Cheitlin, M.D

One of the common problems that arise in clinical cardiology is whether a patient in atrial fibrillation who is to be cardioverted should be on anticoagulants and, if so, for how long before and after cardioversion. In the literature one finds varied opinions. Frequently the physician's own experience is the most powerful determinant of whether or not anticoagulants are used. Every physician in practice, of necessity, has established his or her own *modus operandi,* and the chapter by Stein, Halperin, and Fuster gives evidence on why confusion exists on this point. Although the literature contains many studies, the data are not the result of an organized prospective attempt to answer the question but, instead, are derived from a host of small studies, which are nonrandomized and retrospective for the most part and noncontrolled almost without exception. It is also important to realize that the incidence of embolization described in these studies varies. At times all recognized or suspected systemic emboli are included, but often only cerebral emboli are counted. Coronary, mesenteric, renal, and other systemic arterial emboli to the legs and arms can at times be very important and result in major problems for the patient.

Because there is a risk in prescribing anticoagulants for patients for long periods of time, the risk:benefit ratio of anticoagulation must be considered. Overall, studies indicate a low but definite incidence of emboli, varying from 0 to 7 percent at the time of or after chemical or electrical cardioversion. The concept of risk stratification in an attempt to isolate the group who will benefit most from chronic anticoagulation is a good one, and this is the approach taken by the authors.

This chapter is the most comprehensive review of the literature on this topic. The conclusion to stratify risk and not to recommend anticoagulation for patients in the low-risk group, but only for those in the moderate-to-high-risk groups is a compromise based on the best available data. The decision to put patients with atrial fibrillation on anticoagulants over the long term is somewhat harder, with a two to three percent per year complication rate of anticoagulation and even 0.5 percent per year chance of intracerebral hemorrhage. These are risks that the patient and the patient's family will need to understand. In the high-risk group, especially in patients with prosthetic valves, it is hoped that the decision to anticoagulate chronically can be made before the prosthetic valve is implanted. At other times, moderately high-risk patients, such as those with cardiomyopathy, may be at too high risk for anticoagulation owing to their unreliability for follow-up of their prothrombin times or because of their alcohol or drug abuse, which is an index to both unreliability and susceptibility to trauma. The decision to anti-coagulate patients in atrial fibrillation chronically always requires the physician's knowledge of the patient and the patient's support system. The best decision, giving the greatest advantage to the patient, can be made only on an individual basis by the physician who really knows the patient.

CHAPTER 14

Should All Patients with Congestive Heart Failure and Dilated Cardiomyopathy Be Treated with Vasodilators?

Barry M. Massie, M.D.

The question addressed by this chapter is a broad and, in some respects, controversial one; it deals with a wide spectrum of patients and therapeutic agents. At the same time, it has become a major clinical issue that could influence the treatment of several million individuals in the United States alone.

To address this question, I will define more precisely the relevant patient populations and briefly summarize the rationale for the use of vasodilators. I will examine the topic by sections—as a number of narrower questions, because the available data, and potentially the answers, vary among subsets of patients and categories of drugs. The specific questions are

1. Should patients with refractory or severe symptoms of congestive heart failure receive vasodilators?
2. Should patients with mild and moderate symptoms of congestive heart failure receive vasodilators?
3. Should patients with dilated cardiomyopathy of either ischemic or other origin with few or no symptoms receive vasodilators?
4. When should vasodilators be initiated in relation to other therapeutic agents, such as diuretics and digitalis glycosides?
5. Should a distinction be made between direct vasodilators, such as nitrates and hydralazine, and the angiotensin converting enzyme inhibitors in answering these questions?

BACKGROUND

Several terms require precise definition for this discussion. When discussing *congestive heart failure* (CHF), I will refer only to patients who have (1) symptoms of left ventricular failure, such as dyspnea at rest or with exertion, exercise intolerance due to shortness of breath or muscle fatigue, or fluid retention; *and* (2) documented evidence of left ventricular dilatation and systolic dysfunction. In general, such patients will have a left ventricular ejection fraction well below 40 percent. In using the term *dilated cardiomyopathy* (DCM), I will be referring again to patients with left ventricular dilatation and impaired systolic function, as defined by an ejection fraction below 45 percent, although symptomatic patients will usually have a much lower value. I will not make a distinction between patients whose DCM is due to ischemic heart disease and those with cardiomyopathy from other etiologies, such as postmyocarditis, alcoholic, or idiopathic. In discussing the severity of CHF, I will be referring to symptom status. Refractory and severe CHF cause hemodynamic decompensation or symptoms at rest or with ordinary daily activities. Moderate and mild CHF are associated with fewer symptoms and less activity limitation, so that the patient with very mild CHF may be symptomatic only with rather strenuous activity. It should be noted that there is often marked dissociation between the severity of symptoms and heart size, indices of left ventricular function such as ejection fraction, or even hemodynamic measurements,[1] but clinical trials have generally classified patients by clinical criteria and measurements of exercise tolerance.

The rationale for using drugs that alter the loading conditions of the left ventricle to treat CHF evolved from laboratory experiments that demonstrated that cardiac muscle performance, as measured by its velocity and magnitude of shortening, was determined as much by its initial length (reflecting its preload) and the load against which it shortened (afterload) as by its contractile state.[2] Hemodynamic studies in patients with CHF confirmed that cardiac output could be increased and left ventricular filling pressure could be reduced as effectively by agents that reduce left ventricular afterload and preload as by positive inotropic drugs. Initial experience with medications that directly relax vascular smooth muscle indicated that predominantly arteriolar vasodilators, such as hydralazine, markedly increase cardiac output, whereas venodilators, such as nitroglycerin preparations, primarily lower left and right ventricular filling pressures.[3] Often a combination of agents that produced both actions was employed.

However, research over the past two decades has made it clear that the pathophysiology of CHF is more complex than can be explained on the basis of myocardial mechanics or even by careful hemodynamic characterization of cardiac performance. Although depressed left ventricular contractility is usually the initial derangement in patients with cardiomyopathy and CHF, much of the subsequent clinical course reflects hemodynamic and neurohormonal changes affecting both the central circulation and the periphery.[1,4-6] Many of these changes initially serve an important compensatory function but may in the longer term exacerbate both the signs and symptoms of CHF and underlying cardiac dysfunction. Sympathetic nervous system activation may partially restore contractility but ultimately may depress myocardial inotropic responsiveness and even exacerbate cardiac dysfunction and arrhythmias. The increase in left ventricular end-diastolic volume, which is mediated in part by the sympathetic nervous system (as a result of increased outflow resistance and decreased venous capacitance) and the renin-angiotensin-aldosterone system (via salt and fluid retention and increased outflow resistance), initially may improve cardiac output but also depresses systolic performance and leads to pulmonary and systemic congestion. Peripheral vasoconstriction may maintain arterial pressure and perfusion to some organs, but it may impair flow to others.

In the more advanced stages of CHF, therapeutic interventions are designed as much to overcome these secondary changes as to treat the underlying disorder. Thus, diuretics remain the mainstay of treatment. Vasodilators overcome the secondary hemodynamic derangements—the excessive peripheral vasoconstriction in the venous and arteriolar beds. The angiotensin converting enzyme (ACE) inhibitors not only promote vasodilation but also interdict other neurohormonal changes and tend to *down regulate* the sympathetic nervous system.[7-9] The latter goal can be accomplished more directly with beta blockers, but this approach is experimental.

With this background, let us return to the specific questions at the beginning of this chapter.

QUESTION 1: SHOULD PATIENTS WITH REFRACTORY OR SEVERE SYMPTOMS OF CHF RECEIVE VASODILATORS?

In this group of patients, symptoms occur at rest or with very limited activity and often are associated with signs of low cardiac output and end-organ dysfunction. The rationale for administering vasodilators to these patients has been given already. The more severe the syndrome of CHF, the more severe the activation of neurohormonal systems and the more vulnerable cardiac performance is to excessive vasoconstriction. Numerous studies have demonstrated immediate and more sustained hemodynamic improvement in these patients with vasodilator therapy.[1,2,10,11] Often hospital discharge is facilitated.[12,13] However, the short- to intermediate-term prognosis of these patients remains poor when direct-acting vasodilators, such as hydralazine and nitrates, are employed.[14]

The best evidence for using vasodilators in this particular subgroup comes from the CONSENSUS Study, which randomly assigned 253 patients in this category to enalapril or placebo, while other therapies (which included diuretics, digoxin, and other vasodilators) were continued.[15] As can be seen from Figure 14–1, survival was significantly better in the enalapril group for the entire study population and also for the subgroup continued on other vasodilators. In addition, although all patients were in New York Heart Association (NYHA) class IV (symptomatic at rest), 72 percent of the survivors in the enalapril group, but only 47 percent of the survivors in the placebo group, were in a less advanced NYHA class at the end of the study.

These results strongly support the use of vasodilators, and ACE inhibitors in particular, in patients with advanced CHF, based upon evidence of improved cardiac performance, reduced symptoms, and, most importantly, improved survival.

QUESTION 2: SHOULD PATIENTS WITH MILD AND MODERATE SYMPTOMS OF CHF RECEIVE VASODILATORS?

This group of patients is characterized primarily by intermittent symptoms, especially with exertion. Although usually they are asymptomatic at rest and during activities of daily living, they may have very poor cardiac function by standard indices, such as ejection fraction. The rationale for vasodilator therapy is somewhat

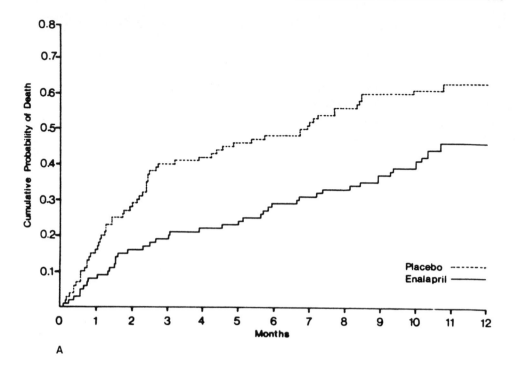

A

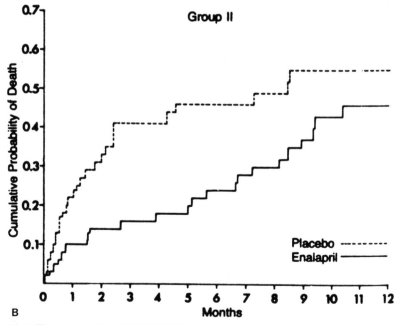

B

Figure 14–1. The results of the CONSENSUS trial, which evaluted the effect of enalapril on survival in refractory, NYHA Class IV heart failure patients are illustrated. (*A*) In the overall group of 253 patients enalapril treatment was associated with a significantly lower mortality rate. (*B*) This difference was also observed in patients who were taking other vasodilators (primarily nitrates). (From Massie, BM, et al,[13] with permission.)

less obvious in this group, because resting hemodynamics may be relatively normal and neurohormonal activation is less common. Nonetheless, hemodynamic responses during exercise are consistently abnormal, and intermittent bursts of excessive sympathetic nervous system or renin-angiotensin system activity cannot be excluded.

Again, numerous clinical trials support a beneficial effect of vasodilators, especially the ACE inhibitors, in mild to moderate CHF.[16-24] Well-controlled trials with both captopril and enalapril in NYHA classes II and III CHF have documented acute and sustained improvement in hemodynamics, measured both at rest and during exercise.[18-24] More important, exercise tolerance increases significantly, while symptoms and episodes of worsening heart failure decrease. Although most controlled trials have entailed the addition of ACE inhibitors to digoxin and diuretics, a recent multicenter trial found that captopril added to diuretic alone was superior to placebo plus diuretic.[25]

Information about the effect of vasodilator therapy on survival in mild to moderate heart failure is limited but also suggests a beneficial effect. A retrospective review of the data from the Captopril Multicenter Trial, in which captopril or placebo were added to digoxin and diuretic in NYHA class II and III patients, found significantly more deaths over a 90-day follow-up period in the placebo group (11 of 52 versus 2 of 53, $P < 0.01$) (Fig. 14-2).[26] An ongoing West German study, which also has followed patients randomized to captopril or placebo in addition to digoxin and diuretics, has shown fewer deaths and fewer patients progressing to severe heart failure in the captopril group after a mean follow-up of nearly two

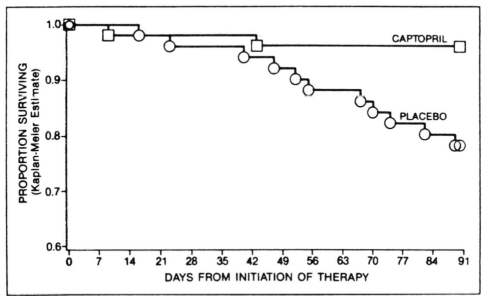

Patient survival as a function of time.

Figure 14-2. Survival curves are shown from the Captopril Multicenter Study which examined the efficacy of captopril in patients with moderate to severe CHF. Using an intent to treat analysis for the 90-day protocol, the captopril group had significantly fewer deaths than the placebo group. (From Newman, TJ, et al,[26] with permission.)

years.[27] The study population and event rate were too small to demonstrate significance for these end points individually.

The largest completed survival study in patients with mild to moderate heart failure is the Veterans Administration Cooperative Heart Failure Trial (V-HeFT).[28] This study randomized patients in NYHA class II or III on digoxin and diuretics to receive the combination of hydralazine and isosorbide dinitrate, prazosin, or placebo. Follow-up averaged 27 months, and the hydralazine-nitrate group exhibited a significantly lower mortality than the other groups. Only limited data have been presented on symptoms and exercise tolerance in this trial, but from the available data it would appear that these improved only slightly, if at all.[29]

Thus, in patients with mild and moderate CHF, ACE inhibitors improve symptoms, exercise capacity, and, probably, survival. Direct-acting vasodilators, namely hydralazine and nitrates, also appear to prolong life.

QUESTION 3: SHOULD PATIENTS WITH DILATED CARDIOMYOPATHY WITH FEW OR NO SYMPTOMS RECEIVE VASODILATORS?

This is, perhaps, the most controversial of the issues we will address here, largely because there are few applicable data. This group is, by definition, not symptom-limited, and therefore treatment cannot improve the quality of life. Nonetheless, these patients do not have a benign natural history, as is illustrated in Figure

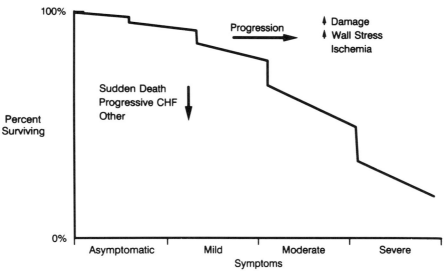

Figure 14–3. The natural history of CHF is illustrated schematically. There is a tendency for patients with CHF to progress over time from asymptomatic left ventricular dysfunction to severe CHF, as is indicated on the horizontal axis. This may occur gradually or in more abrupt episodes of deterioration. The mechanism of progression varies from patient to patient. It may be the result of ongoing damage occurring gradually (such as smoldering myocarditis or in discrete episodes (such as a new myocardial infarction). In many patients, no obvious cause for progression is apparent; in these, further deterioration may be due to left ventricular dilatation, excessive wall stress or myocardial ischemia.

The vertical axis indicates the proportion of patients surviving. Mortality rates accelerate as CHF worsens; however, sudden death may occur at any stage, and this is shown by the abrupt decreases in survival rate. Other deaths will occur from progressive CHF and a variety of related complications (for example, systemic or pulmonary emboli, renal failure, infarction).

14–3. Even at this stage, there is a very real incidence of sudden death (indicated by the abrupt declines in the schematic survival curve). In addition, many will progress to more severe CHF, either as a result of a gradual decline in left ventricular function or episodic deterioration. Mortality rates from sudden death and progressive CHF accelerate as CHF becomes more severe.[30]

The mechanism for progression of CHF is unknown. In some patients, it is progression of the underlying process, such as myocarditis or recurrent infarction. In others, the chronically elevated wall stress resulting from left ventricular dilatation may overload the already impaired myocardium, leading to further dilatation and dysfunction. Myocardial ischemia due to impaired myocardial blood flow, especially in the subendocardium, may be an additional insult even in patients without coronary artery disease.[31] Perhaps the best example of this process is the progressive left ventricular dilatation and delayed onset of CHF after an extensive myocardial infarction, which may occur even in patients with single-vessel disease and no residual jeopardized myocardium. This process of remodeling and functional deterioration is shown schematically in Figure 14–4.

Can vasodilator therapy delay or prevent this progression? Several studies in an infarct model in rats[32,33] and clinical trials in patients following myocardial infarction or with chronic volume overload suggest this possibility.[34,35] Sharpe and associates[34] studied 60 patients with recent large myocardial infarctions (EF < 45%) who were randomly assigned to therapy with captopril, furosemide, or placebo for the succeeding 12 months. Captopril prevented subsequent left ventricular dilation and improved systolic shortening (Fig. 14–5). A conceptually similar study was performed by Pfeffer and colleagues[35] who performed early and one-year left ventriculograms in patients with extensive anterior infarctions, half of whom were randomized to captopril and half to placebo. Whereas left ventricular volume rose in the latter group, it did not in captopril-treated patients. In addition, the latter

LV ENLARGEMENT POST-MI

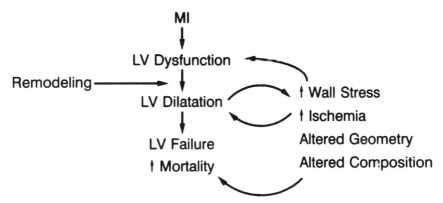

Figure 14–4. The pathophysiology of post-myocardial infarction (MI) left ventricular (LV) enlargement and dysfunction is illustrated schematically. Following MI, there is an abrupt loss of function in the affected region, which may, if large, cause a significant decline in overall LV function. Over a period of weeks to months, the geometry of the LV is altered as it remodels. In general, there is some dilatation of the chamber together with hypertrophy of the residual myocardium, with thinning and fibrosis of the infarcted segment and adjacent muscle. There may be alterations in the collagen matrix and other cellular elements as well. These changes may lead to increased wall stress and suboptimal geometry for systolic shortening. All these changes may lead to further LV enlargement and set off a progressive cycle leading to CHF and death.

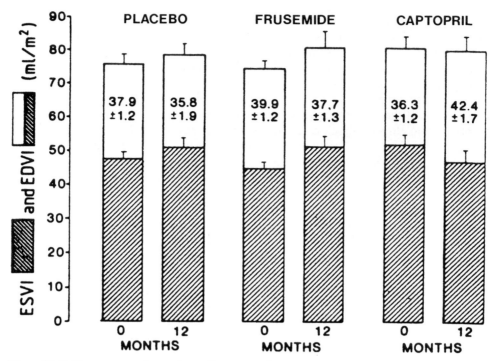

Figure 14–5. Measurements from echocardiograms performed early post-myocardial infarction and 12 months later in a group of 60 patients randomly assigned to treatment with placebo, captopril or furosemide. The bars indicate left ventricular end-diastolic volume index (EDVI), the hatched portion shows the end-systolic volume index (ESVI), and ejection fraction (EF) is enclosed. Both EDVI and ESVI rose on placebo and even on furosemide, while they fell on captopril. EF rose only on captopril. (From Sharpe, N, et al,[34] with permission.)

group maintained better hemodynamics and exercise capacity. In chronic aortic insufficiency (a very different setting), we found that oral hydralazine therapy reduced left ventricular end-diastolic and end-systolic volumes and increased ejection fraction compared with a matched placebo group during two years of follow-up.[36] The noteworthy point in each of these studies is that the patients did not have CHF and tended to be asymptomatic at entry.

Obviously, the evidence that vasodilator therapy is beneficial in mild CHF would be compelling if it could be demonstrated either to prolong life or to prevent progression to symptomatic CHF or to more severe left ventricular dysfunction. Major trials are underway in both postinfarction patients and in other forms of cardiomyopathy to determine whether this is the case. Meanwhile, prevention of progressive left ventricular enlargement, which is a potent negative prognostic indicator, is arguably a useful surrogate end point.

QUESTION 4: WHEN SHOULD VASODILATORS BE INITIATED IN RELATION TO OTHER THERAPEUTIC AGENTS, SUCH AS DIURETICS AND DIGOXIN?

This question differs from, but is closely related particularly to, the primary question of this chapter. Physicians often prefer to start one medication at a time and may be reluctant to add additional agents to patients who are doing well. Thus, the relative merits of diuretics, digoxin, and vasodilators warrant discussion.

Diuretics remain the mainstay of treatment for symptomatic patients. They produce symptomatic benefit within hours, and the successful management of patients with moderate and severe CHF, as well as mild CHF in most cases, is impossible without maintenance diuretics. However, a large study indicated that during chronic therapy, maintenance treatment with diuretic alone was not as successful as the combination of diuretic with either digoxin or an ACE inhibitor.[25] Patients who received either of these two agents in addition to diuretics showed more improvement in exercise tolerance and symptoms, had significantly fewer episodes of decompensation, and required an increase in diuretic dosage less frequently. Finally, there is little theoretic rationale and no data to justify the use of diuretics in asymptomatic patients with left ventricular dysfunction. Sharpe and colleagues'[34] postmyocardial infarction study discussed previously found that furosemide was not better than placebo in preventing further left ventricular dilation.

Digoxin is another effective agent for treating CHF. Although its value in patients in normal sinus rhythm has been debated, recent data unequivocally demonstrate a beneficial response to digoxin.[25,37–39] However, in these studies the patients with the most apparent benefit are those with the most severe left ventricular dysfunction, the largest hearts, and the most symptoms.[38–40] This latter group has clearly benefited from ACE inhibitors as well (see above); and, unless contraindicated in an individual patient, these patients should be treated with the combination of diuretics, digoxin, and ACE inhibitors. In patients with milder but still symptomatic CHF, the response to digoxin is less impressive,[38–41] and ACE inhibitors may be a better choice as adjuncts to diuretics because of their beneficial effect on survival and their potential to counter undesirable electrolyte changes from diuretics. Again, patients with residual symptoms on two agents should receive all three. There are no data available concerning the response to digoxin in asymptomatic left ventricular dysfunction. Theoretically, maintaining myocardial contractility may prevent the progression of CHF. However, balancing this potential effect is the concern that digoxin may exacerbate arrhythmias and ischemia, especially in patients with coronary artery disease. An international trial is planned to examine the effect of digoxin on survival in CHF.

Thus, although diuretics, digoxin, and vasodilators all have useful roles in the management of CHF, by synthesizing available data and our understanding of the pathophysiology of CHF, one can develop some guidelines for the use of these agents. Patients with severe CHF should receive agents from all three classes—diuretics and digoxin to manage symptoms and a vasodilator for additional clinical benefit and to prolong life. The same is probably true for most patients with moderate CHF, unless they become asymptomatic with diuretics and a second agent. Patients with mild symptom limitation should receive diuretics and a second agent. For the reasons already stated, the second agent should be an ACE inhibitor in most instances, except when digoxin is indicated for supraventricular arrhythmias or when ACE inhibitors are relatively contraindicated because of hypotension or renal dysfunction. Asymptomatic patients with dilated cardiomyopathy may benefit from ACE inhibitors, but there are no data to support the use of either diuretics or digoxin in this group.

QUESTION 5: SHOULD A DISTINCTION BE MADE
BETWEEN DIRECT VASODILATORS AND ACE INHIBITORS?

This question has been answered in part by the foregoing discussions. Although both direct-acting vasodilators and ACE inhibitors relax vascular smooth muscle, they do so in very different ways. The direct vasodilators are generally nonspecific, whereas ACE inhibitors dilate vessels that have been constricted by the neurohormonal systems they interdict. These systems may supply particularly important vascular beds. Indeed, the direct vasodilators may reflexly activate the same neurohormonal systems that the ACE inhibitors inhibit, with resulting tachycardia and sodium and fluid retention.[42,43] It is also now recognized that some vascular receptors and response mechanisms down regulate, leading to tolerance with agents such as the nitrates and prazosin.[42] Tolerance is only rarely, if ever, a problem with ACE inhibitors.

In addition to having more sustained and focused hemodynamic effects, the ACE inhibitors have other unique actions, such as mitigating diuretic-induced electrolyte changes. Furthermore, inhibition of the renin-angiotensin system and down regulation of the sympathetic nervous system may be cardioprotective.

However, the major reason to favor ACE inhibitors over direct vasodilators is the greater strength of the data supporting efficacy with the former. Among major trials, only the V-HeFT study has demonstrated a beneficial action of direct vasodilators—hydralazine and nitrates improved survival.[28] However, this regimen had little effect on exercise capacity,[29] and smaller controlled studies with hydralazine have been negative.[44] Studies with isosorbide dinitrate have been limited but do show favorable trends.[16,17] Studies with other predominantly arteriolar dilators, such as minoxidil and nifedipine, have shown no benefit.[45-47]

In contrast, numerous studies with several ACE inhibitors have yielded positive results, including improvements in symptoms, exercise tolerance, and survival.[18-27] Veterans Administration Cooperative Heart Failure Trial II (V-HeFT2) will provide a more definitive comparison of these approaches.

SUMMARY

From the discussion of these questions, several conclusions seem firm, whereas other issues await resolution. Patients with severe CHF should be treated with diuretics, digoxin, and an ACE inhibitor. In mild and moderate CHF, a diuretic should be combined with either digoxin or an ACE inhibitor—usually the latter. However, most of these patients would benefit from receiving all three drugs. Patients with asymptomatic left ventricular systolic dysfunction are at jeopardy for progressive deterioration. Angiotensin converting enzyme inhibitors and, possibly, direct vasodilators may prevent progression.

In initiating vasodilator therapy, ACE inhibitors usually should be the agent of choice. Exceptions may be patients with ongoing ischemia in whom nitrates are an appropriate alternative and those who are poor candidates because of hypotension, renal insufficiency, or hyperkalemia.

REFERENCES

1. Massie, BM: Exercise tolerance in congestive heart failure: Role of cardiac function, peripheral blood flow and muscle metabolism and effect of treatment. Am J Med 84 (Suppl 3A):75, 1988.

2. Massie, BM, Chatterjee, K, and Parmley, WW: Vasodilator therapy for acute and chronic heart failure. In Yu, PN and Goodwin, J: Progress in Cardiology, Vol 8. Lea & Febiger, Philadelphia, 1979.

3. Massie, B, Chatterjee, K, Werner, J, et al: Hemodynamic advantage of combined oral hydralazine and nonparenteral nitrates in the vasodilator therapy of chronic heart failure. Am J Cardiol 40:794, 1977.

4. Dzau, VJ, Hollenberg, NK, and Williams, GH: Neurohumoral mechanism in heart failure: Role of pathogenesis, therapy and drug tolerance. Fed Proc 42:3162, 1983.

5. Francis, GS, Goldsmith, SR, Levine, TB, et al: The neurohumoral axis in congestive heart failure. Ann Intern Med 101:370, 1984.

6. Zelis, R and Davis, D: The sympathetic nervous system in congestive heart failure. Heart Failure 2:21, 1986.

7. Clough, DP, Collis, MB, Conway, F, et al: Interaction of angiotensin-converting enzyme inhibitors with the function of the sympathetic nervous system. Am J Cardiol 49:1410, 1982.

8. Swartz, SL, Williams, GH, Hollenberg, NK, et al: Captopril-induced changes in prostaglandin production: Relationship to vascular responses in normal man. J Clin Invest 65:1257, 1980.

9. Zusman, RM: Renin and non-renin mediated antihypertensive action of converting enzyme inhibition. Kidney Int 25:976, 1984.

10. Chatterjee, K, Ports, TA, Massie, B, et al: Oral hydralazine in chronic heart failure: Sustained beneficial hemodynamic effects. Ann Intern Med 92:600, 1980.

11. Franciosa, JA and Cohn, JN: Sustained hemodynamic effects without tolerance during long-term isosorbide dinitrate treatment of chronic left ventricular failure. Am J Cardiol 45:648, 1980.

12. Dzau, VJ, Collucci, WS, and Williams, GH: Sustained effectiveness of converting-enzyme inhibition in patients with severe congestive heart failure. N Engl J Med 302:1373, 1980.

13. Massie, BM, Kramer, BL, and Topic, N: Long term captopril therapy on congestive heart failure. Am J Cardiol 53:1316, 1984.

14. Massie, B, Ports, T, Chatterjee, K, et al: Long term vasodilator therapy for heart failure: Clinical response and its relationship to hemodynamic measurements. Circulation 63:269, 1981.

15. The CONSENSUS Trial Study Group: Effects of enalapril on mortality in severe congestive heart failure. N Engl J Med 316:1429, 1987.

16. Franciosa, JA, Nordstrom, LA, and Cohn, JN: Nitrate therapy for congestive heart failure. Am J Cardiol 51:1346, 1983.

17. Leier, CV, Huss, P, Magorien, RD, et al: Improved exercise capacity and differing arterial and venous tolerance during chronic isosorbide dinitrate therapy for congestive heart failure. Circulation 67:817, 1983.

18. Kramer, BL, Massie, BM, and Topic, N: Controlled trial of captopril in chronic heart failure: A rest and exercise hemodynamic study. Circulation 67:807, 1983.

19. Captopril Multicenter Research Group: A placebo controlled trial of captopril in refractory chronic congestive heart failure. J Am Coll Cardiol 2:755, 1983.

20. Cleland, JGF, Dargie, JH, Hodsman, GP, et al: Captopril in heart failure: A double-blind controlled trial. Br Heart J 52:530, 1984.

21. Sharpe, DN, Murphy, J, Coxon, R, et al: Enalapril in patients with chronic heart failure: A placebo-controlled, randomized, double-blind study. Circulation 70:271, 1984.

22. Creager, MA, Massie, BM, Faxon, DP, et al: Acute and long-term effects of enalapril on the cardiovascular response to exercise and exercise tolerance in patients with congestive heart failure. J Am Coll Cardiol 6:163, 1985.

23. Franciosa, JA, Wilen, MM, and Jordan, R: Effects of enalapril, a new angiotensin-converting enzyme inhibitor, in a controlled trial in heart failure. J Am Coll Cardiol 5:101, 1985.

24. Cleland, JGF, Dargie, HJ, Bull, SG, et al: Effects of enalapril in heart failure: A double-blind study of the effects in exercise performance, renal function, hormone and metabolic state. Br Heart J 54:305, 1985.

25. The Captopril-Digitalis Multicenter Research Group: Comparative effects of captopril and digoxin in patients with mild-to-moderate heart failure. JAMA 259:539, 1988.

26. Newman, TJ, Maskin, CS, Dennick, LG, et al: Effects of captopril on survival in patients with heart failure. Am J Med 84(3A):140, 1988.

27. Kleber, FX: Influence of captopril on life-expectancy in chronic congestive heart failure. Herz 12 (Suppl 1):38, 1987.

28. Cohn, JN, Archibald, DG, Ziesche, S, et al: Effect of vasodilator therapy on mortality in chronic congestive heart failure: Results of a Veterans Administration Cooperative Study. N Engl J Med 314:1547, 1986.

29. Cohn, JN, Archibald, DG, and Johnson, G: Effects of vasodilator therapy on peak exercise oxygen consumption in heart failure (abstr). Circulation 76(Suppl IV):443, 1987.

30. Massie, BM and Conway, M: Survival of patients with congestive heart failure: Past, present, and future prospects. Circulation 75(Suppl IV):11, 1987.

31. Unverferth, DV, Magorien, RD, Lewis, RP, et al: The role of subendocardial ischemia in perpetuating myocardial failure in patients with non-ischemic congestive cardiomyopathy. Am Heart J 104:176, 1982.

32. Pfeffer, MA, Pfeffer, JM, and Braunwald, E: Influence of chronic captopril on the infarcted left ventricle of the rat. Circ Res 57:84, 1985.

33. Pfeffer, MA, Pfeffer, JM, Steinberg, CR, et al: Survival after an experimental myocardial infarction: Beneficial effects of long-term therapy with captopril. Circulation 72:406, 1985.

34. Sharpe, N, Murphy, J, Smith, H, et al: Treatment of patients with symptomless left ventricular dysfunction after myocardial infarction. Lancet 1:255, 1988.

35. Pfeffer, MA, Lamas, GA, Vaughan, DE, et al: Effect of captopril on progressive ventricular dilatation after anterior myocardial infarction. N Engl J Med 319:80, 1988.

36. Greenberg, B, Massie, BM, Bristow, JD, et al: Long-term vasodilator therapy of chronic aortic insufficiency: A randomized double-blinded, placebo controlled trial, Circulation 78:92, 1988.

37. Arnold, SB, Byrd, RC, Meister, W, et al: Long-term digitalis therapy improves left ventricular function in heart failure. N Engl J Med 303:1443, 1980.

38. Lee, DC-S, Johnson, RA, Bingham, JB, et al: Heart failure in outpatients: A randomized trial of digoxin versus placebo. N Engl J Med 306:699, 1982.

39. Guyatt, GH, Sullivan, MJJ, Fallen, EL, et al: A controlled trial of digoxin in congestive heart failure. Am J Cardiol 61:371, 1988.

40. DiBianco, R, Shabetai, R, Kostuk, W, et al: A comparison of oral milrinone, digoxin and their combination in the treatment of patients with chronic heart failure. N Engl J Med 320:677, 1989.

41. Fleg, JL, Gottlieb, SH, and Lakatta, EG: Is digoxin really important in treatment of uncomplicated heart failure? Am J Med 73:244, 1982.

42. Colucci, WS, Williams, GH, and Alexander, RW: Mechanisms and implications of vasodilator tolerance in the treatment of congestive heart failure. Am J Med 71:89, 1981.

43. Bayliss, J, Norell, MS, Canepa-Anson, R, et al: Clinical importance of the renin-angiotensin system in chronic heart failure: Double-blind comparison of captopril and prazosin. Br Med J 290:1861, 1985.

44. Franciosa, JA, Weber, KT, Levine, TB, et al: Hydralazine in the long term treatment of chronic heart failure: Lack of differences from placebo. Am Heart J 104:587, 1982.

45. Franciosa, JA, Jordan, RA, Wilen, MM, et al: Minoxidil in patients with chronic heart failure: Contrasting hemodynamic and clinical effects in a controlled trial. Circulation 70:63, 1984.

46. Agostini, PG, de Cesare, N, Doria, E, et al: Afterload reduction: A comparison of captopril and nifedipine in dilated cardiomyopathy. Br Heart J 55:391, 1986.

47. Elkayam, U, Weber, L, McKay, C, et al: Spectrum of acute hemodynamic effects of nifedipine in severe congestive heart failure. Am J Cardiol 45:560, 1985.

Commentary

By Melvin D. Cheitlin, M.D.

The treatment of congestive heart failure has three goals: (1) elimination of symptoms and the improvement of exercise tolerance; (2) prevention of progression of ventricular dysfunction; and (3) prolongation of life. The approach to the treatment of congestive heart failure has changed since we have better delineated the pathophysiology. Although the basic instigating problem in congestive heart failure due to systolic dysfunction is the decrease in myocardial contractility, the majority of the patient's symptoms and signs result from the excessive compensatory responses of sodium and water retention and activation of the sympathetic and renin-angiotensin systems. Although these responses lead to support of the stroke volume and cardiac output, they also result in excessive venous and arteriolar constriction. This effect increases impedance to ejection and initiates the downward spiral of decreasing stroke volume and tachycardia. The reduced arterial pressure combined with the elevated left ventricular filling pressure lead to decreased subendocardial perfusion, which can further compromise diastolic and systolic ventricular functions.

The three classes of drugs used to treat congestive heart failure address each of these pathophysiologic defects. Vasodilators and diuretics decrease preload, direct and indirect arteriolar vasodilators reduce afterload, and inotropes such as digitalis increase contractility.

There is abundant evidence that vasodilators improve mortality in dilated cardiomyopathy from a variety of etiologies. Within the classes of vasodilators, the converting enzyme inhibitors have the added advantage of combating the effects of the activated sympathetic nervous and renin-angiotensin systems. This may have additional cardioprotective effects. The CONSENSUS trial[1] showed that there is benefit in prolonging survival using converting enzyme inhibitors over and above that achieved by direct vasodilators.

There are several caveats. In all trials, patients have been on digoxin and diuretics as well as vasodilators. No trial has compared the response of patients on vasodilators alone with that of patients on digoxin and diuretics. Furthermore, digoxin has been shown to increase ejection fraction, whereas in the Captopril-Digoxin Study[2] captopril did not. Secondly, the Captopril-Digoxin Multicenter Study[2] showed the advantage of the use of both of these drugs with diuretics over diuretics alone. Because diuretics stimulate the renin-angiotensin system, there is considerable doubt whether diuretics should ever be used as a sole agent.

Following myocardial infarction, the most potent predictor of prognosis is the status of left ventricular function.[3] Although ejection fraction is usually employed

263

as an indicator of left ventricular function, ejection fraction is dependent on afterload as well as preload and, therefore, reflects contractility only indirectly. Theoretically the end-systolic pressure-volume relationship is a better reflection of contractility and is less dependent upon loading conditions. White and colleagues[4] have shown by following patients after acute myocardial infarction that end-systolic volume is the best predictor of prognosis, and even end-diastolic volume is better than ejection fraction. Pfeffer and colleagues[5] and Sharpe and associates[6] have shown that after acute myocardial infarction captopril is capable of preventing left ventricular dilatation and therefore of limiting the increase in left ventricular end-diastolic and end-systolic volumes. The hope here is that the remodeling that occurs after the loss of contracting myocardium may be prevented by a converting enzyme inhibitor, and therefore these drugs truly would be a preventive treatment for congestive heart failure.

For these reasons Dr. Massie's conclusions are quite appropriate, that is, that patients with symptomatic heart failure should be treated with agents from all three drug groups. In patients with less symptomatic congestive heart failure, two agents—probably a vasodilator (preferably a converting enzyme inhibitor) and a diuretic—should be used; although if the predominant symptom is fatigue rather than dyspnea, I would use digoxin with converting enzyme inhibitor. In patients with dilated cardiomyopathy and systolic dysfunction who are not yet symptomatic, an argument could be generated for the use of no drug treatment, because all of these drugs have side effects. Furthermore, neither digoxin nor diuretics have been shown to be of benefit in the asymptomatic patient. There is, however, preliminary evidence that ventricular dilatation might be inhibited by converting enzyme inhibitors, and, if there are no contraindications, it is recommended that these agents be started.

Finally, what has been said is true only for dilated cardiomyopathy with systolic dysfunction. The syndrome of congestive heart failure can be caused by the pathophysiologic mechanism of diastolic dysfunction, as is encountered in hypertrophic cardiomyopathy and in patients with hypertension or other reasons for left ventricular hypertrophy. If diastolic dysfunction is the cause of congestive heart failure, then diuretics and vasodilators sometimes may make the patient more symptomatic. For this reason, when evaluating a patient with heart failure, both the etiology and the pathophysiologic mechanism of the failure must be determined first, frequently using echocardiographic or echo-Doppler techniques, before a logical plan of therapy can be initiated.

REFERENCES

1. The CONSENSUS Trial Study Group: Effects of enalapril on mortality in severe congestive heart failure. N Engl J Med 316:1429, 1987.
2. The Captopril-Digitalis Multicenter Research Group: Comparative effects of captopril and digoxin in patients with mild-to-moderate heart failure. JAMA 259:539, 1988.
3. Taylor, GJ, Humphries, JO, Mellits, ED, et al: Predictors of clinical course, coronary anatomy and left ventricular function after recovery from acute myocardial infarction. Circulation 62:960, 1980.
4. White, HD, Norris, RM, Brown, MA, et al: Left ventricular end-systolic volume as the major determinant of survival after recovery from myocardial infarction. Circulation 76:44, 1987.
5. Pfeffer, MA, Lamas, GA, Vaughan, DE, et al: Effect of captopril on progressive ventricular dilatation after anterior myocardial infarction. N Engl J Med 319:80, 1988.
6. Sharpe, N, Murphy, J, Smith, H, et al: Treatment of patients with symptomless left ventricular dysfunction after myocardial infarction. Lancet 1:255, 1988.

CHAPTER 15

Should Patients with Pulmonary Hypertension and Increased Pulmonary Resistance be Treated with Vasodilators?

Stuart Rich, M.D.

THE ACTIONS OF VASODILATORS ON THE PULMONARY VASCULAR BED IN PULMONARY HYPERTENSION

The medical literature suggests that most systemic vasodilator drugs also will dilate the pulmonary vascular bed, presumably by direct vasodilator effects on the pulmonary arterioles. The basis for this vasodilator effect assumes pulmonary vascular vasoconstriction as an underlying etiologic mechanism of pulmonary hypertension. However, evidence that vasodilation occurs in the normal pulmonary vascular bed suggests the presence of substantial vascular tone in the resting state.[1] Chronic pulmonary hypertension appears to promote structural changes in the pulmonary vasculature, which includes medial hypertrophy, intimal proliferation, and intimal fibrosis.[2] In the face of advanced intimal changes, one would not expect much vascular responsiveness to vasodilators. In fact, the structural changes that occur in the pulmonary vascular bed appear to be related to the level of the pulmonary artery pressure, and it has been postulated that pulmonary hypertension promotes further intimal proliferation and fibrosis of the arterioles, which sustains the pulmonary hypertension. A reduction in pulmonary arterial pressure with a vasodilator might end this vicious cycle and possibly even promote regression of the pulmonary vascular changes that have already occurred.

It is becoming apparent that many pulmonary hypertensive states probably arise from damage to the pulmonary endothelium, which leads to increased pulmonary resistance. Two mechanisms for this damage are becoming defined. Plexogenic pulmonary arteriopathy—encountered most commonly in congenital heart disease, aminorex-induced pulmonary hypertension, and primary pulmonary hypertension—can be explained on the basis of increased pulmonary vascular tone, which could be attributed to the loss of endothelial inhibitors of smooth muscle.[3-5]

265

The effectiveness of a vasodilator would depend, in part, on its mechanism of action. A drug that appears to work via endothelial mediators, such as nitroglycerin, might not be effective if endothelial damage was widespread; whereas the effects of a direct smooth muscle vasodilator, such as hydralazine, would depend on the degree of smooth muscle hypertrophy.

Thrombotic pulmonary arteriopathy, most often found in congenital heart disease or primary pulmonary hypertension, also can be explained on the basis of endothelial cell damage.[3,4] There is now considerable evidence indicating that perturbations of the pulmonary vascular endothelium can lead to a procoagulant environment that could promote *in situ* thrombosis.[6,7] The effects on the pulmonary vasculature would depend on the degree of intimal proliferation and the extent of thrombosis, both of which could elevate the pulmonary vascular resistance. In this setting, the effectiveness of a vasodilator might depend on the extent of secondary medial hypertrophy. If the pulmonary vascular bed is maximally vasodilated via autoregulation in an attempt to normalize the pulmonary artery pressure, vasodilators may have no effect.

The vasodilators now in clinical use have been developed because of their ability to dilate systemic vascular beds. It is an expected effect of these drugs, when administered to patients with pulmonary hypertension, to achieve a reduction in systemic blood pressure and systemic vascular resistance. The physiologic mechanism for the drug effect depends largely upon the class of agent being used. Consequently, drugs that are considered direct smooth muscle vasodilators, such as hydralazine and minoxidil, will have direct effects on systemic and pulmonary vascular smooth muscle, whereas alpha-blocking agents reduce vascular resistance by a reduction in alpha-adrenergic vascular tone, and calcium blockers via limiting calcium influx and reducing increased vascular tone. This becomes an important consideration when selecting a vasodilator for clinical use. Severe pulmonary hypertension is often associated with systemic hypotension due to the low cardiac output that results. Patients often will have marked systemic vasoconstriction, as a compensatory mechanism, to maintain an adequate blood pressure. A vasodilator that does not exert a preferential pulmonary effect may result in hypotension and subsequent right ventricular ischemia and failure.

Vasodilator drugs commonly cause an increase in cardiac output when administered to patients with cor pulmonale. Because both the left and right ventricles are influenced by changes in afterload, it is expected that a reduction in afterload will be associated with a concomitant increase in stroke volume and cardiac output. In pulmonary hypertension, however, it appears that in the majority of the cases the increase in cardiac output that occurs is related to the reduction in systemic vascular resistance rather than pulmonary vascular resistance.[8] Because of the complexity of the interaction between the two ventricles, it is extremely difficult for one to sort out the basis for an increased cardiac output that might be observed following the administration of a vasodilator to any patient with pulmonary hypertension.

It is also an assumption that a fall in calculated pulmonary resistance represents a real reduction in the pulmonary vascular resistance. However, the relationship between pulmonary blood flow and pulmonary pressure, which is a reflection of the inherent pulmonary vascular resistance, is a complex one. In the normal lung, the curve is nonlinear and skewed to the pressure axis at lower flow rates and to the flow axis at higher flow rates.[9] Consequently, as flow increases, the calculated vascular resistance will decrease. This makes it difficult to assess the effect of a drug on the pressure/flow curve of a diseased lung on the basis of one point on a curve before and another during treatment. Accurate measurements of pulmonary outflow pressure are also required to calculate pulmonary vascular resistance, which is problematic.[10,11] Typically the pulmonary wedge pressure is assumed to be the downstream resistance pressure, but wedge pressure, left atrial pressure, and pulmonary diastolic pressures may not be similar in patients with pulmonary hypertension.[11] Calculations also need to take into account the fact that in the normal lung, left atrial pressure appears to be linearly related to the pulmonary arterial pressure at high pressures only if flow remains constant. For these reasons, the meaning of a fall in pulmonary resistance in the absence of a fall in pulmonary pressure is somewhat uncertain.

Finally, the clinician should be sensitive to the fact that there is considerable difficulty in establishing reproducible baseline hemodynamic measurements in patients with pulmonary hypertension. A previous study showed that spontaneous hemodynamic changes may account for changes in pulmonary artery pressure of 22 percent, and pulmonary vascular resistance of 36 percent, in the normal resting state.[12] Thus any conclusions made from small changes in pulmonary pressure and resistance must be made with caution. The mechanism for this biologic variability appears related to impaired feedback control mechanisms, as occurs in most disease states. Patients who are normotensive have relatively stable blood pressures, for example, whereas those who are hypertensive have not only high systemic pressures but also greater swings in their systemic blood pressure over time. The same has been shown to occur with respect to blood glucose in patients who are diabetic, and to systemic arterial oxygen saturation in patients with chronic lung disease. Impaired biofeedback appears to be a biologic manifestation of disease, with the degree of impairment in biofeedback control proportional to the severity of the disease itself. Patients with the highest levels of pulmonary vascular resistance appear to have the greatest variability as well. The experience with antiarrhythmic therapy in patients with ventricular extrasystolic beats has shown that reductions in frequency of at least 80 percent on a 24-hour Holter monitor may be required in order to establish a true drug effect.[13] These same caveats apply to the treatment of pulmonary hypertension with vasodilator drugs.

DEFINING BENEFICIAL EFFECTS FROM VASODILATORS IN PULMONARY HYPERTENSION

The chronic hemodynamic changes in patients with primary pulmonary hypertension who underwent serial catheterization studies have been described.[14] It appears that early in the onset of the disease pulmonary arterial pressure rises, while stroke volume remains normal and right ventricular systolic wall stress increases.[15] This leads to the development of right ventricular hypertrophy and eventually an impairment of right ventricular performance, which is ultimately manifest by a progressive reduction in cardiac output. Most patients who die with chronic pulmonary hypertension die from right ventricular failure. Consequently, a beneficial drug effect in these patients would be one in which pulmonary arterial pressure is reduced, thus reducing right ventricular systolic wall stress, while cardiac output is maintained. Owing to the afterload-dependent nature of the right ventricle, one is likely to observe an increase in cardiac output if a real reduction in right ventricular afterload occurs. Thus, a reduction in pulmonary artery pressure and calculated pulmonary vascular resistance, associated with a normalization of cardiac output, should be the goal of vasodilator therapy.

One also can characterize benefit from vasodilators by an increase in systemic oxygen transport. The low cardiac output and high systemic vascular resistance that occur in these patients can lead to systemic hypoperfusion. Any treatment that would increase the systemic oxygen transport, either by an improvement in pulmonary blood flow or by a reduction in perfusion/ventilation mismatch, also might be considered beneficial as long as no other adverse consequences of the drug therapy were manifest.

Inasmuch as patients with pulmonary hypertension are often in chronic low cardiac output states, one might argue that any intervention that results in an improvement in cardiac output, as long as it does not increase pulmonary artery pressure, is potentially beneficial to the patient. There are faults with this argument, however, when we realize that increasing cardiac output will result in an increase in venous return and volume of the right ventricle. If a concomitant reduction in pulmonary pressure is not realized, stroke work of the right ventricle will increase and might not be well tolerated.

DEFINING ADVERSE EFFECTS OF VASODILATORS IN PULMONARY HYPERTENSION

It is well-documented also that vasodilator therapy in patients with pulmonary hypertension can produce adverse effects, with an adverse clinical outcome and even death.[16] As previously stated, increasing the stroke work of the right ventricle might contribute to progressive right heart failure unless a *real* reduction in right ventricular afterload is realized. In addition, there may be inherent properties of vasodilator drugs that also contribute to worsening right ventricular performance. For example, the calcium blocker drugs possess negative inotropic properties.[17] Although the negative inotropic influence of these drugs in healthy patients is hard to detect clinically, it can become important in patients who already have underlying cardiac dysfunction. In the patient with pulmonary hypertension, calcium blockers may induce right ventricular failure if there is not substantial concomitant reduction in afterload.[18] During calcium blocker administration, one should pay close attention to right ventricular end-diastolic pressure (RVEDP) (or right atrial pressure) and cardiac output. A fall in calculated pulmonary resistance that occurs via a fall in cardiac output should be considered factitious. Likewise, an increase in cardiac output that is associated with an increase in right atrial pressure suggests impending right ventricular failure and usually predicts an adverse chronic response.

It should be appreciated also that vasodilators can promote right ventricular ischemia via a reduction in systemic blood pressure. There is considerable evidence to suggest that patients with pulmonary hypertension have some degree of chronic right ventricular ischemia owing to the loss of the aortic-right ventricular pressure gradient in systole.[19] The right ventricular coronary vasculature, which is relatively limited in anatomic supply, becomes diastolic-flow dependent in pulmonary hypertension, similar to the left ventricular system. A reduction in the systolic flow gradient will be exacerbated by any intervention that further reduces systemic blood pressure.

Lastly, vasodilator drugs can worsen ventilation-perfusion mismatching, especially in patients with underlying chronic lung disease.[20] Although the mechanism remains to be defined, it has been speculated to be related to vasodilatation of blood vessels in areas that have undergone compensatory vasoconstriction because of reduced alveolar ventilation.[21] Thus, it is not uncommon to encounter systemic arterial oxygen saturation fall with vasodilator administration, particularly in patients who have baseline hypoxemia. If one believes that enhancing systemic oxygen transport is an important goal of therapy, this would be considered an adverse outcome.

DOCUMENTATION OF CLINICAL BENEFITS OF VASODILATORS IN PULMONARY HYPERTENSION

PRIMARY PULMONARY HYPERTENSION

There have been many published studies on the acute effectiveness of vasodilators given to patients with primary pulmonary hypertension (PPH). Most of these studies have shown a substantial reduction in calculated pulmonary vascular resistance, with little influence on pulmonary arterial pressure. When one reviews the published experience with tolazoline, acetylcholine, isoproterenol, alpha-adrenergic blockers, diazoxide, nitroprusside, hydralazine, converting enzyme inhibitors, and calcium blockers, it is apparent that the literature remains equivocal as to the effectiveness of these drugs over the long term.[22] Given the common current practice to administer vasodilator drugs empirically to patients when the diagnosis of PPH is made, there is a surprising paucity of information to suggest that any of these agents alters the clinical course of the disease. In occasional case reports, substantial reductions in pulmonary arterial pressure and pulmonary vascular resistance in patients with PPH have been noted by investigators using a variety of different vasodilators, including the calcium channel blockers.[23,24] In these instances the patients responded to conventional doses of the drugs used, suggesting perhaps that their disease was less advanced. Rich and coworkers[25] evaluated the chronic treatment of 18 patients with PPH who responded acutely to conventional doses of hydralazine and/or nifedipine, with a reduction in pulmonary vascular resistance of 20 percent or greater that was not associated with a significant fall in pulmonary artery pressure. Half of the patients opted to be treated with a vasodilator, with the other nine declining. Both groups were followed prospectively over a 2-year period. Patients who were unable to achieve an acute reduction in pulmonary resistance of 20 percent or greater had a poor prognosis, with four of the five dead within six months. However, of the patients who did have an acute 20 percent or greater fall in pulmonary vascular resistance, there was no difference observed between their clinical course or mortality over the 2-year period. For the reasons mentioned, one has to wonder if acute reductions in pulmonary vascular resistance alone will be of long-term benefit to these patients.

It should be noted that most studies assessing the effectiveness of vasodilator agents in PPH have generally utilized conventional doses of drugs. It is understandable for one to expect that the dose of a drug that works effectively for one condition might work similarly for another. However, for the very reason that no drug has been shown to be specific for the pulmonary vascular bed, it should not be surprising that there might be a different dose-responsiveness for pulmonary vascular diseases. Rich and Brundage[26] reported their preliminary experience using a new regimen of high doses of calcium blockers as therapy for PPH. Under the premise that conventional doses of these agents may not be adequate for patients with PPH, a drug protocol was developed in which patients were challenged initially with conventional doses of nifedipine or diltiazem and then given consecutive hourly doses until a 50 percent fall in pulmonary vascular resistance and a 33 percent fall in pulmonary artery pressure were achieved, or until untoward side effects became manifest. The initial drug challenges produced only marginal reductions in pulmonary artery pressure and pulmonary vascular resistance, similar to previous published experiences. However, of the 13 patients initially tested, 8 responded to continued hourly doses, with a mean reduction in pulmonary pressure of 48 percent and of pulmonary vascular resistance of 60 percent. These patients were discharged on the high doses of nifedipine (up to 240 mg per day) or diltiazem (up to 720 mg per day) as chronic therapy and followed as outpatients. Each of the patients returned for restudy after one year. In seven of the eight patients, the reduction in pulmonary artery pressure and pulmonary vascular resistance was sustained over the year and associated with regression of right ventricular hypertrophy, as evidenced by changes on the electrocardiagram and echocardiogram and verified hemodynamically at catheterization. The five patients who failed to respond to the high-dose drug challenge did not appear to differ from the responders by their age, duration of symptoms, or level of pulmonary hypertension. Thus, they were unable to predict who would respond to this regimen. Surprisingly, although adverse effects of these drugs in high doses were anticipated, no patient who was placed on chronic therapy had the drug discontinued because of systemic hypotension or other intolerable side effects.

The reason for the apparent selective pulmonary effects of the high doses of calcium blockers observed in these patients is not known. It is possible, however, that rather than being selective for a specific arterial bed, calcium channel blockers work preferentially on vascular smooth muscle that has heightened tone and is vasoconstricted, leaving the other vascular beds largely unaffected. The large doses of calcium blockers required in patients with PPH suggest that there is a different sensitivity of either vascular beds or disease states to the effects of calcium channel blockers.

In the more recent experience, it has been observed that not all of the patients who tolerate the high doses of calcium blockers will have large reductions in pulmonary artery pressure. In some, there is a substantial fall in pulmonary vascular resistance without a fall in pulmonary artery pressure. Some patients also manifest responsiveness to intermediate-level doses of calcium blockers. The number of hourly doses of drug providing the greatest reduction in pulmonary vascular resistance can be highly variable and may range from one to eight. In some patients the fall in pulmonary vascular resistance is greater at low doses than at high doses. Inasmuch as the fall in pulmonary vascular resistance in these latter patients closely parallels an increase in cardiac output, this response may be a reflection of the negative inotropic effects of the calcium blockers which, in the absence of a fall in pulmonary artery pressure, limit cardiac output by affecting right ventricular function at high doses.

Recently there has been interest in prostacyclin as a pulmonary vasodilator. Rubin and colleagues[27] published their initial observations on the acute effects of intravenous prostacyclin in seven patients with PPH. They observed that prostacyclin reduced pulmonary vascular resistance in a dose-dependent manner, which suggested that it may be a useful agent in the initial evaluation of vasodilator therapy, and perhaps in the short-term management of seriously ill patients. Prostacyclin is particularly attractive as a test drug because it is known to be a potent pulmonary vasodilator, has a short duration of action, and has platelet inhibitory activity that might decrease the likelihood of thrombotic or embolic complications of the procedure, which require the use of indwelling catheters.

In studies comparing the effects of prostacyclin acutely with chronic calcium blockers, Groves and associates[28] made the observation that the best responders to diltiazem have been predicted by the acute response to intravenous prostacyclin. A similar experience has been reported by Barst,[29] using prostacyclin in children with PPH. In her series she noted a good correlation between the acute pulmonary vasodilator response to increasing doses of prostacyclin and increasing doses of nifedipine in nine patients. Similar reductions in pulmonary artery pressure occurred with both agents in the five respondents. The four patients who were nonrespondents to prostacyclin also failed to respond to nifedipine.

The published experience with chronic prostacyclin infusions in PPH is quite limited. In one study, patients with advanced PPH were maintained on prostacyclin until a heart-lung transplant could be performed.[30] Although substantial reductions in pulmonary artery pressure did not occur, it was noted that many patients were made clinically stable and symptomatically improved by the infusions.

SECONDARY PULMONARY HYPERTENSION

In spite of the renewed enthusiasm about the potential role of vasodilator drugs in patients with primary pulmonary hypertension, to date there is not one published experience documenting long-term benefits to patients with secondary pulmonary hypertension. It is likely that this relates to the basic etiology of the pulmonary hypertensive state. Patients who have pulmonary hypertension due to increased filling of the left ventricle, often labeled as passive pulmonary hypertension, seem to have little benefit from vasodilator administration. The only long-term benefits with respect to therapy in this group of patients are those that are directed at lowering left ventricular filling pressures (such as mitral valve replacement in mitral stenosis or relief of ischemia in patients with coronary heart disease). Likewise, vasodilators appear to have minimal effect in patients with pulmonary hypertension from Eisenmenger's physiology, and in fact they might be quite dangerous. The presence of a communication between the pulmonary and systemic bed will allow for shunting of blood toward the circulation with the lowest resistance. In the face of vasodilator therapy, if the drug lowers systemic resistance without having impact on pulmonary vascular resistance, there might be a marked increase in right-to-left shunting with severe hypoxemia. On the other hand, the effect of lowering pulmonary vascular resistance in these patients might be negated by increasing left-to-right shunting.

Some patients who have congenital heart disease with pulmonary hypertension will experience a progressive worsening of their pulmonary hypertension postoperatively, even though the shunt is closed. Inasmuch as these cases are very uncommon, it is understandable that there is no large experience on the use of vasodilators postoperatively. However, it would be reasonable to test these patients with vasodilators postoperatively inasmuch as the concerns about a communication between the systemic and pulmonary beds become negated. An open lung biopsy performed at the time of surgery would be helpful also in assessing the type of pulmonary vascular changes that have occurred.

Vasodilators have been administered to many patients with chronic obstructive pulmonary disease and cor pulmonale. The results in these patients are equivocal as well, inasmuch as there have been no studies documenting long-term effectiveness and reversal of cor pulmonale. As highlighted earlier, it can be quite hazardous to administer vasodilators to patients who have resting arterial hypoxemia because these drugs tend to worsen ventilation/perfusion mismatching. To date, the only agent that has been shown to be effective in reducing mortality when administered chronically to patients with chronic obstructive pulmonary disease (COPD) has been oxygen.[30]

Finally, collagen vascular disease also may manifest as pulmonary hypertension, with or without hypoxemia. Once pulmonary hypertension develops in these patients, it usually leads to their rapid demise. They have been particularly resistant to vasodilator challenge, inasmuch as there is not a single case report showing a substantial reduction in pulmonary artery pressure from vasodilator therapy. It is very possible that, owing to the structural changes that occur in the pulmonary vasculature as a result of the disease process in these patients, vasodilator therapy will be unsuccessful in any case.

CONCLUSION

It is clear from the published literature that vasodilators have the potential to improve acute and chronic pulmonary hypertension in selected patients. The long-term experience with high doses of calcium blockers in patients with primary pulmonary hypertension, now documented for periods in excess of 3½ years, offers promise that a subset of patients who are responsive to this therapy may have a remarkable prolongation in life as well as improvement in life-style. We define a beneficial effect of vasodilators in pulmonary hypertension as one that results in a reduction in pulmonary artery pressure and pulmonary vascular resistance, associated with a normalization in cardiac output and maintenance of systemic blood pressure. Patients who have a reduction in pulmonary vascular resistance without a substantial change in pulmonary artery pressure represent an unknown group. Only a randomized, clinical trial will be able to address whether this type of treatment is beneficial, or even potentially harmful, to these patients.

It should be recognized also that vasodilator treatment of patients with pulmonary hypertension has real potential for harm. Systemic hypotension, exacerbation of pulmonary hypertension, worsening of right ventricular function, and systemic arterial oxygen desaturation are all documented adverse effects of treatment and need to be closely guarded against. For these reasons we strongly advocate that testing of vasodilator drugs in patients with pulmonary hypertension be done acutely, with hemodynamic monitoring, and that all chronic follow-up should be closely monitored. Those patients who have a true beneficial influence of the drug should have consistent clinical improvements in noninvasive measures of pulmonary hypertension, such as a reduction in cardiac size on chest x-ray examination, a reduction in right ventricular size on echocardiogram, and a reduction in right ventricular voltage on the ECG. It is our bias not to treat patients chronically with vasodilator drugs empirically, or if an equivocal reduction in pulmonary vascular resistance was obtained.

Finally, it needs to be reemphasized that there has not been any series documenting long-term effectiveness of vasodilator drugs for patients who have any of the secondary forms of pulmonary hypertension. This is not to say that continued trials are not useful, but it should discourage against the empiric administration of vasodilator drugs in cor pulmonale.

REFERENCES

1. Bergofsky, E: Mechanisms underlying vasomotor regulation of regional pulmonary blood flow in normal and disease states. Am J Med 57:378, 1974.
2. Wagenvoort, CA and Wagenvoort, N: Primary pulmonary hypertension: A pathologic study of the lung vessels in 156 clinically diagnosed cases. Circulation 42:1163, 1970.
3. Bjornsson, J and Edwards, WD: Primary pulmonary hypertension: A histopathologic study of 80 cases. Mayo Clin Proc 60:16, 1985.
4. Rabinovitch, M, Bothwell, T, Hayakawa, BN, et al: Pulmonary artery endothelial abnormalities in patients with congenital heart defects and pulmonary hypertension. Lab Invest 55:632, 1986.
5. Gomez-Sanchez, MA, Mestre de Juan, MJ, Gomez-Pajuelo, C, et al: Pulmonary hypertension due to toxic oil syndrome: A clinicopathologic study. Chest 95:325, 1989.
6. Ryan, US: The endothelial surface and responses to injury. Fed Proc 45:101, 1986.
7. Rich, S, Levitsky, S, and Brundage, BH: Pulmonary hypertension from chronic pulmonary thromboembolism. Ann Intern Med 108:425, 1988.
8. Rich, S, Martinez, J, Lam, W, et al: A reassessment of the effects of vasodilator drugs in primary pulmonary hypertension: Guidelines for determining a pulmonary vasodilator response. Am Heart J 105:119, 1983.
9. Harris, P, Segel, N, and Bishop, JM: The relation between pressure and flow in the pulmonary circulation in normal subjects and patients with chronic bronchitis and mitral stenosis. Cardiovasc Res 2:73, 1968.
10. Versprille, A: Pulmonary vascular resistance: A meaningless variable. Intensive Care Med 10:51, 1984.
11. McGregor, M and Sniderman, A: On pulmonary vascular resistance: The need for a more precise definition. Am J Cardiol 55:217, 1985.
12. Rich, S, D'Alonzo, GE, Dantzker, DR, et al: Magnitude and implications of spontaneous hemodynamic variability in primary pulmonary hypertension. Am J Cardiol 55:159, 1985.
13. Winkle, RA: Antiarrhythmic drug effect mimicked by spontaneous variability of ventricular ectopy. Circulation 57:1116, 1978.
14. Rich, S and Levy, PS: Characteristics of surviving and nonsurviving patients with primary pulmonary hypertension. Am J Med 76:573, 1984.
15. Rich, S, Dantzker, DR, Ayres, S, et al: Primary pulmonary hypertension: A national prospective study. Ann Intern Med 107:216, 1987.
16. Packer, M: Vasodilator therapy for primary pulmonary hypertension: Limitations and hazards. Ann Intern Med 103:258, 1985.
17. Braunwald, E: Mechanism of action of calcium channel blocking agents. N Engl J Med 307:1618, 1982.
18. Packer, M, Medina, N, and Yushak, M: Adverse hemodynamic and clinical effects of calcium channel blockade in pulmonary hypertension secondary to obliterative pulmonary vascular disease. J Am Coll Cardiol 4:890, 1984.
19. Vlahakes, GJ, Turley, K, and Hoffman, JIE: The pathophysiology of failure in acute right ventricular hypertension: Hemodynamic and biochemical correlations. Circulation 63:87, 1981.
20. Melot, C, Hallemans, R, Naeije, R, et al: Deleterious effect of nifedipine on pulmonary gas exchange in chronic obstructive pulmonary disease. Am Rev Respir Dis 130:612, 1984.
21. Dantzker, DR and Bower, JS: Pulmonary vascular tone improves VA/Q matching in obliterative pulmonary hypertension. J Appl Physiol 51:607, 1981.
22. Rich, S: Primary pulmonary hypertension. Prog Cardiovasc Dis 31:205, 1988.
23. Saito, D, Haraoka, S, Yoshida, H, et al: Primary pulmonary hypertension improved by long-term oral administration of nifedipine. Am Heart J 105:1041, 1983.
24. Wise, JR: Nifedipine in the treatment of primary pulmonary hypertension. Am Heart J 105:693, 1983.

25. Rich, S, Brundage, BH, and Levy, PS: The effect of vasodilator therapy on the clinical outcome of patients with primary pulmonary hypertension. Circulation 71:1191, 1985.
26. Rich, S and Brundage, BH: High dose calcium blocking therapy for primary pulmonary hypertension: Evidence for long-term reduction in pulmonary arterial pressure and regression of right ventricular hypertrophy. Circulation 76:135, 1987.
27. Rubin, LJ, Groves, BM, Reeves, JT, et al: Prostacyclin-induced pulmonary vasodilation in primary pulmonary hypertension. Circulation 66:334, 1982.
28. Groves, BH, Rubin, LJ, Reeves, JT, et al: Comparable hemodynamic effects of prostacyclin and hydralazine in primary pulmonary hypertension. Circulation 64:IV297, 1980.
29. Barst, RJ: Pharmacologically induced pulmonary vasodilation in children and young adults with primary pulmonary hypertension. Chest 89:497, 1986.
30. Abraham, AS, Cole, RB, and Bishop, JB: Reversal of pulmonary hypertension by prolonged oxygen administration to patients with chronic bronchitis. Circ Res 23:147, 1968.

Commentary

By Melvin D. Cheitlin, M.D.

One of the unresolved problems in cardiology is the treatment of the patient with severe pulmonary hypertension who has increased pulmonary vascular resistance. In the past, occasionally patients with pulmonary hypertension of diverse etiologies have been reported to respond to vasodilators. Lately, a fascinating suggestion has been made that patients with primary pulmonary hypertension, a disease of increased pulmonary vascular resistance of unknown etiology, respond to calcium channel blocking agents, either nifedipine or diltiazem in very large doses.[1] The chronic dose is determined by increasing dosage every hour while monitoring pulmonary artery pressure and cardiac output and stopping at a dose at which there is a fall of 50 percent in pulmonary vascular resistance or 33 percent in pulmonary artery pressure without a substantial fall in systemic arterial pressure. Dr. Rich is the author of this report, and this approach was successful in 13 patients, eight of whom had a long-term reduction in right ventricular size and right ventricular hypertrophy by electrocardiogram. As far as I am aware, this is the first evidence of long-term successful therapy in such very sick patients.

In this chapter, Dr. Rich reviews the pathophysiologic basis for pulmonary hypertension and suggests reasons that even a drop in pulmonary vascular resistance and a rise in cardiac output without a drop in pulmonary artery pressure might be harmful. Also, the possibility of reducing both pulmonary vascular resistance and systemic vascular resistance without increasing output sufficiently to maintain blood pressure would result in a drop in systemic arterial blood pressure. At the very least, this could result in right ventricular myocardial ischemia and further compromise of right ventricular function.

Pathogenesis of pulmonary vascular disease in these patients can differ depending on the underlying etiology, and this might affect the response of the diseased pulmonary vessels to vasodilators. For instance, Rabinovitch and colleagues[2] have shown that in congenital heart disease with ventricular septal defect and/or patent ductus arteriosis, the high flow-high pressure existing from birth causes intimal damage and proliferation, hypertrophy of medial smooth muscle with extension further out in the vascular tree than is normal, and a failure of the vascular tree to branch as does the bronchial tree as the lung grows, so that there are fewer vessels in the periphery of the lung. How these patients could benefit by vasodilators is difficult to imagine, and there is little evidence in these patients that there has been such benefit. Similarly, with pulmonary vascular disease secondary to chronic lung disease there are several irreversible reasons for increased pulmo-

275

nary vascular resistance. Some increase in pulmonary vascular resistance is due to destruction of the lung and pulmonary vascular bed. There also may be medial smooth muscle hypertrophy. Additionally, damage to the intima can occur as well as thrombosis, and vessels affected in these ways probably will respond poorly to vasodilators. Those patients with chronic lung disease who have increased pulmonary vascular resistance due to hypoxia will respond to improvement of oxygenation with low-flow oxygen, and they do not need vasodilators. In patients with pulmonary disease, vasoconstriction secondary to poor aeration and hypoxia commonly occurs. With vasodilators, a marked increase in right-to-left shunting and a worsening of the hypoxemia can occur, which must be avoided, as must an increase in cardiac output without a drop in pulmonary artery pressure.

At the very least, if vasodilators are to be used, the patient with severe pulmonary hypertension should be hospitalized under conditions in which cardiac output, arterial oxygen saturation, and pulmonary artery pressure can be monitored. Vasodilators should be tried, although at present patients with increased pulmonary vascular resistance due to diseases other than primary pulmonary hypertension have not proved responsive. So far, apparently only patients with primary pulmonary hypertension have been shown to have long-term success.

REFERENCES

1. Rich, S and Brundage, BH: High-dose calcium blocking therapy for primary pulmonary hypertension: Evidence for long-term reduction in pulmonary arterial pressure and regression of right ventricular hypertrophy. Circulation 76:135, 1987.
2. Rabinovitch, M, Haworth, SG, Castenada, AR, et al: Lung biopsy in congenital heart disease: A morphometric approach to pulmonary vascular disease. Circulation 58:1107, 1978.

CHAPTER 16

Is Intermittent Dobutamine Infusion Useful in the Treatment of Patients with Refractory Congestive Heart Failure?

Peter Stecy, M.D.
Rolf M. Gunnar, M.D., F.A.C.P., F.R.C.P.

The management of congestive heart failure (CHF) has changed substantially over the past 20 years. Medical therapy has expanded to include such new pharmaceuticals as positive inotropic agents, vasodilators, beta-blocking drugs, and antiarrhythmics. Surgical treatment also has advanced dramatically with orthotopic heart transplantation and mechanical support devices.

The population in which to apply these modalities is vast and appears to be growing.[1] It is estimated that between two and three million persons have CHF in the United States, with an annual death rate of 10 percent per year.[2] The prognosis of patients in more severe heart failure—New York Heart Association (NYHA) functional classes III and IV—is poorer, with one-year mortalities between 34 and 58 percent.[3]

Despite the growing treatment choices for this condition, a sizable percentage of patients are refractory to medical management, and only a small number of them are able to undergo cardiac transplantation. For the remaining patients, novel approaches have been investigated, including intermittent therapy with the synthetic adrenergic receptor agonist, dobutamine. Although the clinical utility of dobutamine for the treatment of acutely decompensated CHF is well accepted, there is uncertainty regarding its value as intermittent chronic therapy.

To assess the possible role of intermittent dobutamine in a subset of patients with refractory CHF, several questions must be raised: Will the treatment improve such parameters as the patients' symptoms, exercise tolerance, and quality of life? Will the therapy effect sustained improvement in left ventricular function or peripheral hemodynamics? What is the optimal dose, duration, and frequency of administration of the drug? Finally, does dobutamine improve or worsen survival in this severely ill group of patients?

PHARMACOLOGY AND CLINICAL PROFILE OF
DOBUTAMINE

BASIC PHARMACOLOGY

In an effort to overcome some of the negative aspects of isoproteronol, Tuttle and Mills[4] systematically modified its chemical structure. The resulting molecule, dobutamine, was found to have less than one fourth the chronotropic effect of isoproteronol but had the same inotropic potency of epinephrine.

Dobutamine is a racemic mixture that stimulates $beta_1$-, $beta_2$-, and alpha-adrenergic receptors. Stimulation of the beta-receptors activates adenylate cyclase present in the cell membrane, which then encourages the conversion of adenosine triphosphate (ATP) to cyclic adenosine monophosphate (cAMP). In turn, cAMP stimulates a host of intracellular reactions leading to increased Ca^{++} transport by the sarcoplasmic reticulum. In the myocyte, these reactions enhance contractility.[5,6]

Increased left ventricular contractility is mainly effected via $beta_1$ receptor stimulation. In addition, dobutamine activates $beta_2$ receptors in the periphery and alpha receptors both in the myocardium and periphery. The two isoforms differ in their action. The L-isomer is a potent $alpha_1$ agonist, whereas the D-isomer is primarily a $beta_1$ and $beta_2$ agonist and a partial alpha receptor blocker.[7] The net sum of these effects is augmentation of cardiac contractility with little change in the systemic vascular bed. Unlike dopamine, dobutamine does not have a norepinephrine-releasing action and it does not stimulate the dopaminergic receptors in the renal and mesenteric vascular beds.[5,6]

CLINICAL EFFECTS

At intravenous doses of 2 to 15 mcg per kg per minute, dobutamine improves ventricular contractility, as evidenced by an increased stroke volume, cardiac output, ejection fraction, and maximum rate of rise of ventricular pressure (dP/dt). At the same time, it lowers systemic and pulmonary vascular resistance, probably as a result of reflex withdrawal of sympathetic tone. Consequently, left ventricular end-diastolic pressure (LVEDP) and pulmonary artery wedge pressure are usually reduced.[6,8,9] At low doses the improved hemodynamics generally occur without a significant effect in systemic blood pressure or heart rate (Fig. 16–1).[10] Although less arrhythmogenic than dopamine, dobutamine can be associated with increased ventricular ectopy.[11]

Renal parameters of urine output, urine sodium excretion, blood urea nitrogen, and serum creatinine are improved secondary to the enhanced cardiac output.[12–14]

Dobutamine increases coronary artery blood flow. Thus, although myocardial oxygen (O_2) demand usually rises with its use, the overall balance of O_2 supply and demand is little changed. The coronary arteriovenous (A-V) O_2 difference and myocardial O_2 extraction remain constant.[12,14] In heart failure, dobutamine even may improve myocardial O_2 balance by decreasing left ventricular size and wall stress.[12]

The pharmacologic effects of dobutamine are directly proportional to its serum level, which in turn is linearly related to its dose.[15] Its onset of activity occurs within minutes, and a steady state is achieved in 15 minutes. The half-life of the drug in patients with CHF averages 2.37 ± 0.70 minutes.[16] These pharmacokinetic properties make it an ideal drug to titrate rapidly in the acute heart failure setting.

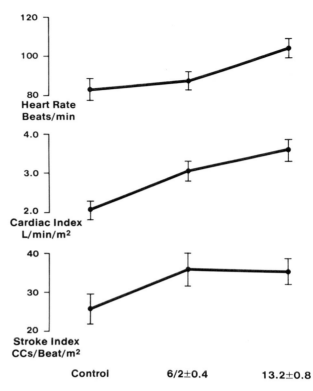

Figure 16-1. Mean value ($+/-$ SEM) for heart rate, cardiac index, and stroke index during the control period and during two different dobutamine infusion rates in 13 patients. (From Loeb, HS, et al,[10] with permission.)

TOLERANCE TO DOBUTAMINE

Tolerance to dobutamine's therapeutic effects may limit its use as chronic therapy. Unverferth and coworkers[17] administered dobutamine at a dose of 10 mcg per kg per minute to 14 patients over a period of 96 hours. Heart rate (HR), blood pressure (BP), cardiac output (CO), and systolic time intervals (STI) were measured at baseline, at two hours, and then at daily intervals. The benefit of the infusion began to decline slowly by 24 hours, reaching statistical significance at 72 hours when the CO fell to 66 percent of the two-hour value.

This clinical feature of tolerance is similar to other sympathomimetic agents that act via the beta receptor-adenylate cyclase- cAMP system. It has been explained by the term *receptor down-regulation.*[18]

EVIDENCE OF PROLONGED BENEFIT

UNCONTROLLED STUDIES

The possible efficacy of intermittent dobutamine in the treatment of chronic CHF is based on an assumption that the drug can induce sustained positive effects long after its 15 minute life span in the circulation. The first indication that this hypothesis might be true was found in a 1977 study by Leier and colleagues.[13] Their group studied 25 patients with severe CHF and placed them on 10 to 15 mcg per kg per minute of dobutamine for a 3-day period. Systolic time intervals, echocardiograms, and thermodilution CO (nine patients) were obtained at baseline and at approximately every 12 hours. As expected, the CO increased from 1.97 to 3.33 liters per minute, and the pre-ejection period/left ventricular ejection time (PEP/LVET) improved from 0.76 to 0.58. Unexpectedly, 30 minutes after the end of the infusion, the parameters of left ventricular (LV) function were still significantly above baseline values. In addition, 17 of 25 patients maintained functional class improvement for at least 1 week.

The same laboratory further investigated this fascinating finding. They reported an uncontrolled series of 38 patients suffering from nonischemic cardiomyopathy.[19] The patients were severely compromised with an average left ventricular ejection fraction (LVEF) of 25 percent and a NYHA functional class of 3.8. They were treated with dobutamine for 72 hours, titrated to maximize CO without the development of significant side effects. Functional class, PEP/LVET, and echocardiographic percent change in LV diameter (percent change D) were assessed at baseline and periodically up to 20 months after the initial infusion.

All of these parameters improved acutely, and some maintained improvement for months. At 4 weeks after infusion, the group's NYHA class was still improved above baseline (3.1 versus 3.8), and about one half the patients still showed enhanced LV function (percent change D, STI) at 3 months.

This study suffered from the lack of a control group, the use of a poorly reproducible end point (NYHA class),[20,21] and incomplete data collection. It did, however, suggest a possible long-term benefit of a 72-hour infusion of dobutamine.

In another uncontrolled series of 23 patients with nonischemic CHF,[14] a 72-hour infusion of dobutamine was administered and the patients were followed for 6 months. Approximately 50 percent of the patients had NYHA functional class improvement at 2 months, but only 13 percent showed sustained improvement at 6 months.

A RANDOMIZED, CONTROLLED TRIAL

The first randomized, blinded, placebo-controlled trial of a 72-hour infusion of dobutamine was reported in 1984.[22] Fifteen patients with stable, nonischemic CHF in functional classes III to IV were randomized to dobutamine or placebo. At 4-week follow-up, functional class, echocardiographic velocity of circumferential fiber shortening (Vcf), gated blood pool LVEF, and treadmill exercise time were all significantly improved in the dobutamine group but were unchanged in the placebo-treated patients. Although this study was small, its trial design and results lent weight to the data suggesting efficacy for intermittent dobutamine infusion.

MECHANISMS FOR SUSTAINED EFFECTS

MYOCARDIAL EFFECTS

The underlying mechanisms for the sustained action of dobutamine are uncertain, but data indicate that both myocardial and peripheral conditioning effects may occur.

A report in 1980 described changes in myocardial ultrastructure after a 72-hour dobutamine infusion.[23] Sixteen patients with nonischemic cardiomyopathy were treated with 2.5 to 15 mcg per kg per minute of dobutamine. Echocardiography, STI, and endomyocardial biopsies were performed immediately before and after treatment. The number of electron-dense particles seen on electronmicroscopy (EM), typically present in degenerating or ischemic myocytes, decreased by 20 percent ($P < 0.005$) after treatment. Also, the cristae-to-matrix ratio in the mitochondria (lower in failing cells) improved with dobutamine. The same laboratory also looked at ATP/creatine content in myocardial biopsy tissue and found an improvement after the 72-hour infusion.[14]

The investigators theorized that the enhanced coronary blood flow achieved with dobutamine, combined with unloading effects, could relieve subendomyocardial ischemia. Additional factors may play a role. Dobutamine-induced reduction in LV size and wall stress could allow the heart to function on a more efficient point on the Starling curve. Also, beta-receptor down-regulation induced by dobutamine possibly could be beneficial by protecting the heart from the effects of high levels of circulating catecholamines.

Conditioning Effects

Data indicating a conditioning effect, at least for *repetitive,* intermittent dobutamine have been emerging. A *single,* 72-hour dobutamine infusion, however, did not appear to have this result in a previously cited study by Liang and associates.[22] Fifteen subjects with nonischemic cardiomyopathy were randomized to placebo or dobutamine and underwent exercise testing before and after treatment. The data collection was elaborate with the measurement of CO; oxygen consumption (VO_2); gated blood pool LVEF; and serum lactate, pyruvate, and norepinephrine levels. They found none of the common changes induced by conditioning, such as a blunted exercise HR, delay in serum lactate rise, and an increase in $VO_{2\ max}$.

The effect of repetitive, intermittent dobutamine was examined by the same laboratory in a controlled experiment using a dog model.[24] Three groups of dogs were treated with either normal saline, dobutamine, or treadmill exercise for two hours per day, five days per week over a five-week period. Only the dobutamine and exercise groups had a decrease in the exercise HR, BP, lactate levels, and CO (for a given workload).

Sullivan and coworkers[25] studied the prevention of deconditioning of repetitive, intermittent dobutamine as compared with exercise in 24 normal, active males. The subjects were randomized into three groups, all of whom received monitored bedrest for three weeks to induce deconditioning. During this period, the groups were treated with either normal saline, moderate bicycle exercise, or dobutamine for two hours per day. The exercise and dobutamine therapies were adjusted to produce a HR of 20 percent of the maximal HR response over baseline for one hour. This level was increased to 40 percent for the next 45 minutes and to 60 percent for the final 15 minutes. To achieve this, the dobutamine doses were higher than the previous studies, averaging 17 to 34 mcg per kg per minute. Extensive pre- and post-treatment tests were performed, including bicycle ergometry, gated blood pool scans, and skeletal muscle biopsies for enzyme measurements.

Heart rate response, exercise capacity, CO, $VO_{2\ max}$, and delay in lactate production were maintained in the exercise and dobutamine groups. The aerobic enzyme activity (citrate synthetase, succinate dehydrogenase) remained constant or increased in the two active treatment groups.

This study on normal subjects showed that dobutamine in high doses can reproduce many of the physiologic responses of exercise, and deconditioning can be prevented. The effects may be mediated by changes in skeletal muscle enzymes and peripheral vascular responsiveness.[25]

Finally, the effects of exercise training alone were studied in a group of 12 patients with compensated, mild to moderate CHF.[26] After four to six months of aerobic training (one hour, three days per week), significant improvements were found. The average NYHA functional class decreased from 2.4 to 1.7, and the $VO_{2\ max}$ increased from 1.1 to 1.4 ml per kg per minute. The resting HR decreased, and the exercise time improved by 16 percent.

TRIALS OF UNMONITORED, AMBULATORY THERAPY

Encouraged by preliminary findings, several investigators expanded the use of dobutamine to weekly, 48-hour infusions given in an unmonitored, ambulatory setting. Case reports began emerging in 1982, involving patients with severe, refractory CHF.[27–29] Unlike those in previous studies, some of these patients had underlying ischemic heart disease. The five reported patients all received chronic, indwelling venous access systems, and dobutamine was administered via a portable infusion pump. In one case the pump was totally implanted and the infusate was driven by fluorocarbon vapor.[28] Improvement was reported in all patients in their functional class and in a reduction in their hospital admissions.

A larger, uncontrolled series was published in 1986 by Krell and associates.[30] They treated 13 patients in functional classes III to IV with 48-hour weekly dobutamine infusions over a 26-week period. Nine of the 13 patients had ischemic heart disease, but patients with angina, ventricular tachycardia, or a recent myocardial infarction were excluded. This was a severely compromised group with an average LVEF of 16 percent.

The mean dobutamine dose was 7.5 mcg per kg per minute, titrated in the hospital to obtain a maximum CO without side effects. With this initial dosing, the average CO rose from 1.6 to 3.2 liters per minute.

The long-term results were less than anticipated. Improvement in functional class was found in only seven (54 percent) patients, and only three patients survived the trial. Six of the patients died suddenly, although none demonstrated dobutamine-induced ectopy during initial monitoring.

An additional series of patients was reported in 1984.[31] Twenty-one subjects, approximately half with ischemic heart disease, were treated with intermittent dobutamine over a 4-year period. Dopamine was added to four treatment regimens for its renal and inotropic effects. The average functional class improved significantly from 3.8 to 2.8 after a mean follow-up of 7.8 months. Complications included drug tolerance (two patients), bacteremia (two patients), catheter exit-site infections (eight patients), and pump malfunction (two patients). Most significantly, 20 of the 21 patients died during the study period.

From this early information it became clear that intermittent dobutamine in an ambulatory setting provided symptomatic relief to some patients. It did not, however, dramatically improve survival and may have had a detrimental effect.

A randomized, placebo-controlled, double-blinded trial was conducted to further investigate this method of dobutamine therapy.[32] Sixty subjects with refractory CHF (mean LVEF 20 percent) were allocated randomly to either placebo or dobutamine treatment over a 24-week period. The average dobutamine dose was 8.1

mcg per kg per minute, given for 48 hours per week via a portable infusion pump. Seven control patients crossed over to the dobutamine group, and one dobutamine patient crossed over to placebo. These changes were made blindly when the patients were deemed treatment failures.

The study was prematurely halted when interim analysis revealed a disturbing trend for increased mortality in the dobutamine group. Overall, 20 of the 60 patients died: 5 originally assigned to placebo and 13 in the dobutamine group (P = 0.147). When analyzed on an actual treatment basis, 5 of 23 placebo-treated patients died, whereas 15 of 37 dobutamine-treated subjects died (P = 0.06). Nearly half of the deaths in the dobutamine group occurred suddenly during the actual infusions. It was discovered also that patients were more likely to die if initial monitoring revealed greater than four episodes of ventricular tachycardia per day. Despite this effect on mortality, dobutamine still significantly increased the patients' exercise time and tended to improve their symptoms.

This study raised an important question: Was chronic inotropic stimulation harmful to patients with refractory heart failure, or was simply the method of delivery at fault? The trial did support the fact that this mode of therapy can confer symptomatic improvement.

INTERMITTENT, MONITORED INFUSIONS

OHIO STATE UNIVERSITY EXPERIENCE

Another approach to intermittent dobutamine therapy is to administer the agent for short periods of time in a monitored, outpatient setting. This method was examined by Leier and colleagues[33] in 1982. They randomized 26 patients with nonischemic CHF to a four-hour weekly infusion of dobutamine given in an outpatient center or to routine treatment. Four additional patients entered the study but were not included in the analysis because they did not complete the 24-week trial period.

This group of patients was not as seriously compromised as patients in previous reports. Twenty-three subjects (88 percent) were in functional class III, and the mean cardiac index of the group was 2.06 liters per minute/M^2 as measured by the ^{131}I serum albumin radioisotope technique (RISA). The study design was single blinded, randomized, and employed a nonplacebo control group. The control group was evaluated every 2 weeks whereas the dobutamine group was seen weekly during the study period.

Dobutamine was titrated to a dose that increased the resting HR up to 40 percent or to a maximum dose of 10 mcg per kg per minute. Functional class, exercise testing, echocardiography, STI, and RISA cardiac output were assessed at baseline and at 2- to 8-week intervals. One of the infusions resulted in sustained ventricular tachycardia requiring cardioversion and hospitalization.

Parameters of LV function (percent change D, Vcf) improved only slightly in the dobutamine group while the STI and CO remained unchanged. There was, however, a significant improvement in both exercise duration and in functional class. Exercise time on a Bruce protocol treadmill test improved by nearly 2 minutes in the dobutamine group, but there was no improvement in the control subjects. Twelve of 15 dobutamine-treated patients improved at least one functional class, compared with only 2 of 11 control patients.

These results appeared more consistent with a conditioning effect than with a direct myocardial action. It is possible also that the improvement was due to the extra attention that the dobutamine patients received.

LOYOLA UNIVERSITY EXPERIENCE

Loyola University Medical Center has an active interest in end-stage CHF. It has a large population of patients awaiting heart transplantation and many refractory patients not eligible for such treatment. It adopted a therapeutic approach utilizing four-hour dobutamine infusions in an attempt to modify the downward spiral of this subset of patients.

Treatment Protocol

The dobutamine was administered in the ambulatory care facility adjacent to Loyola University Hospital. All patients were continuously attended by a nurse and had constant electrocardiographic monitoring. A cardiologist was in the immediate vicinity at all times. The dose of dobutamine ranged between 2.5 and 10 mcg per kg per minute and was adjusted to the highest level that did not elicit side effects. The average infusion rate was 5 mcg per kg per minute for 4 hours, one time per week.

Results

Thirty-seven patients were treated over a period of 2.5 years beginning on July 1, 1986. The data were obtained and analyzed retrospectively. All of the patients had been in NYHA class IV during their recent pretreatment course, and most remained in this class at the initiation of dobutamine treatment. The patients had all demonstrated clinical improvement with dobutamine during previous hospitalizations.

The group's baseline characteristics are shown in Table 16-1. They were predominantly male (78 percent) and middle-aged, and ischemic heart disease was the most frequent underlying etiology of their CHF. Sixteen patients were eligible for, and were awaiting, cardiac transplantation. The remaining patients were ineligible, most commonly because of age. The patients' indices of cardiac function were markedly diminished, with an averge LVEF of 19 percent.

Table 16-1. Patient Characteristics

Age (yr)	59 ± 13	(range 21–75)
Sex (M/F)	29/8	
Patients awaiting transplant	16 (43%)	
Diagnosis		
ischemic	18 (49%)	
idiopathic	12 (32%)	
valvular	5 (14%)	
miscellaneous	2 (6%)	
LVEF (n = 35)	19% ± 7	(range 10–41%)
RVEF (n = 29)	27% ± 12	(range 11–51%)
CI (n = 26)	2.1 ± 0.5 (liters/min/M²)	(range 1.2–3.1)

LVEF = left ventricular ejection fraction, RVEF = right ventricular ejection fraction, CI = cardiac index.

Table 16–2. Patients'
Medications (n = 36)

Furosemide (mg/d)	137 ± 58
Additional diuretics	25 (69%)
ACE inhibitors	23 (64%)
Other unloaders	23 (64%)
Antiarrhythmics	16 (44%)

ACE = angiotensin converting enzyme;
unloaders = nitrates, hydralazine, prazosin.

The patients' medications, as shown in Table 16–2, reflect the refractory nature of their heart failure. Large doses of furosemide were required, and 64 percent of the group were on angiotensin converting enzyme (ACE) inhibitors for afterload reduction. Additional diuretics and antiarrhythmics were commonly needed.

The treatment results are shown in Table 16–3. There was a wide range of treatment durations, with death being the most common reason for termination of the protocol. Seven patients received an orthotopic heart transplant. Four of them did not survive beyond 2 months after the procedure, and the remaining three patients are alive and well. The average survival time of the entire group was 40 weeks. Cumulative survival is shown in Figure 16–2. The 1-year survival rate was 35 percent. Three of the four patients that survived over 20 months were successful transplant recipients.

There were two serious complications of the dobutamine treatments. A 63-year-old patient with an idiopathic dilated cardiomyopathy developed ventricular fibrillation during the infusion. The arrhythmia was converted rapidly to sinus rhythm, and after a complicated 3.5-month hospitalization he underwent successful cardiac transplantation. The second complication occurred in a 43-year-old male, also with an idiopathic dilated cardiomyopathy. He developed ventricular tachycardia during the infusion and required cardioversion. He was hospitalized but died 4 days later in cardiogenic shock.

Discussion

The survival rate of the group was quite poor. It compares unfavorably with some studies of severe, refractory CHF patients that showed 1-year survival rates

Table 16–3. Treatment Data

Duration of R_x (mo)	4.7 ± 5.6 (range = 0.25–22)
Current patients	7
Reasons for Rx	
Death	16 (53%)
Transplant	7 (23%)
Transfer	2 (7%)
Side effects	3 (10%)
Other	2 (7%)
Mean survival after Rx in wk (n = 36)	40.2

R_x = treatment

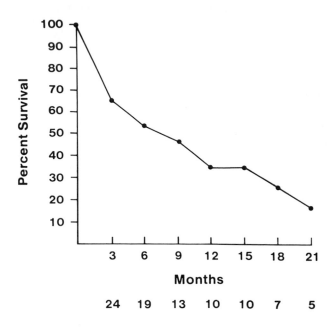

Figure 16-2. The probability of survival after beginning dobutamine therapy; numbers below months equal patients at risk.

of 50 to 70 percent.[34–37] It is, however, difficult to match the group with historical controls accurately. There are many factors related to prognosis, including age, etiology, functional class, and recent clinical deterioration.[3] This last factor was present in the vast majority of the Loyola group. When Massie and associates[34] examined patients in this category, they found only a 30 to 40 percent one-year survival. Despite the lack of matched controls, it is doubtful that intermittent dobutamine improved outcome in the group, and, indeed, it may have diminished survival.

There were anecdotal data from some individual patients and their physicians indicating that symptomatic relief and reduced hospitalizations occurred during the course of the dobutamine infusions. Whether this occurred *because of* or *in spite of* the dobutamine is unknown. The patients also received intensified outpatient monitoring with weekly histories, physical examinations and blood drawing, and additional diuretics and potassium as needed. It is possible that any improvement was due to this more aggressive standard treatment.

POTENTIAL ADVERSE EFFECTS

There has been a growing concern that chronic inotropic stimulation may not be beneficial in CHF and may even adversely affect survival. As opposed to recent data on vasodilator therapy,[38,39] studies proving a mortality benefit in CHF with inotropic agents are lacking.

Preliminary data support two different methods that could lead to adverse outcomes. The first questions whether chronic inotropic therapy may accelerate the underlying disease process. There is accumulating evidence that the myocytes of a failing heart are relatively energy depleted. Anversa and coworkers,[40] using quantitative electron microscopic techniques, examined cardiac myocyte composition in a pressure-overloaded rat ventricle. The ratio of the energy-producing mitochondria to the energy-consuming myofibrils was decreased in the rat heart. Earlier studies[41] have shown a decrease in high-energy phosphate compounds in a pressure-overloaded heart model.

As proposed by Katz,[42,43] depression of cardiac contractility may be a protective mechanism of the failing heart. Further depletion of the myocardial energy stores by inotropes may accelerate cell death. Also, dobutamine acts by increasing the intracellular level of cAMP, which can become a cardiotoxin at high concentrations. There is no clinical proof, however, for this potential myocyte-damaging effect. The actual energy cost of an inotrope is variable and is dependent not only on contractility but also on the cardiac loading conditions.

The second area of concern is the ability of dobutamine and other inotropic agents to precipitate ventricular arrhythmias. Ventricular ectopy is quite common in both ischemic and nonischemic causes of severe CHF. As discussed by Massie and Conway,[3] greater than 91 percent of heart failure patients have premature ventricular depolarizations. Complex arrhythmias, Lown grade 3 or greater, are found in 36 to 95 percent of the patients.

In general, this ectopy correlates with more severe symptoms and poorer LV function. Thus, it has been difficult to determine whether ventricular arrhythmias have an independant effect on mortality.

If dobutamine worsened these already common arrhythmias, then a negative effect on survival might be encountered. All of the positive inotropic agents have the potential to elicit ventricular ectopy. Cyclic AMP, the messenger of dobutamine's inotropic action, has been demonstrated to be arrhythmogenic.[44] In addition, the elevated cytoplasmic Ca^{++} that results from cAMP stimulation theoretically may lead to delayed afterdepolarizations and ventricular ectopy.[42]

There is one brief report on outpatient dobutamine and its potential to induce such arrhythmias.[11] Two class IV heart failure patients were treated with placebo and then 2 to 4 mcg per kg per minute of dobutamine for 4 hours every other day. Ambulatory electrocardiography quantified the ventricular ectopy over a 4-week period. The placebo treatment was associated with 487 premature ventricular complexes (PVCs) and 4 episodes of ventricular tachycardia over 23 hours. During a 4 mcg per kg per minute infusion the ectopy increased to 15,858 PVCs and 360 episodes of ventricular tachycardia. When this information is added to the problems with sudden death in the report by Dies and associates,[32] the danger of unmonitored dobutamine treatment appears to be a justified concern.

CONCLUSIONS

1. Intermittent dobutamine, especially when given in a repetitive fashion, may cause prolonged improvement in the symptoms, functional class, and exercise capacity of patients with severe heart failure. There are no data to indicate that it improves survival, and dobutamine may actually increase mortality when used as chronic therapy.
2. Current studies show an adverse effect on mortality when dobutamine is given in an unmonitored setting, particularly with sudden death occurring during infusions. This form of administration cannot be recommended.
4. Intermittent dobutamine given in a monitored environment may improve symptoms in refractory CHF patients. This treatment's effect on mortality is unknown and must await further study.
5. In the subset of patients refractory to more conventional therapy or awaiting cardiac transplantation, intermittent dobutamine therapy may be justified in an attempt to provide symptomatic relief. The best-studied proto-

cols are brief infusions given in a monitored, outpatient setting and longer— 48-to 72-hour—treatments given in the hospital.

REFERENCES

1. Gorlin, R: Incidence, etiology and prognosis of heart failure. Cardiovasc Rev Rep 4:765, 1983.
2. Leier, CV and Unverferth, DV: Medical therapy of end-stage congestive and ischemic cardiomyopathy. In Shaver, JA (ed): Cardiomyopathies: Clinical Presentation, Differential Diagnosis, and Management. FA Davis, Philadelphia, 1988, pp 243–251.
3. Massie, BM and Conway, M: Survival of patients with congestive heart failure: Past, present, and future prospects. Circulation (75 (Suppl IV):11, 1987.
4. Tuttle, RR and Mills, J: Dobutamine: Development of a new catecholamine to selectively increase cardiac contractility. Circ Res 36:185, 1975.
5. Braunwald, E, Sonnenblick, EH, and Ross, J: Mechanisms of cardiac contraction and relaxation. In Braunwald, E (ed): Heart Disease. WB Saunders, Philadelphia, 1988, pp 383–425.
6. Leier, CV and Unverferth, DV: Diagnosis and treatment, drugs five years later—Dobutamine. Ann Intern Med 99:490, 1983.
7. Ruffolo, RR, Spradlin, TA, Pollock, GD, et al: Alpha and beta adrenergic effects of the stereoisomers of dobutamine. J Pharmacol Exp Ther 219:447, 1981.
8. Loeb, HS, Bredakis, J, and Gunnar, RM: Superiority of dobutamine over dopamine for augmentation of cardiac output in patients with chronic low output cardiac failure. Circulation 55:375, 1977.
9. Berkowitz, C, McKeever, L, Croke, RP, et al: Comparative responses to dobutamine and nitroprusside in patients with chronic low output cardiac failure. Circulation 56:918, 1977.
10. Loeb, HS, Khan, M, Klodnycky, ML, et al: Hemodynamic effects of dobutamine in man. Circ Shock 2:29, 1975.
11. David, S and Zaks, JM: Arrhythmias associated with intermittent outpatient dobutamine infusion. Angiology 37:86, 1986.
12. Magorien, RD, Unverferth, DV, Brown, GP, et al: Dobutamine and hydralazine: Comparative influences of positive inotropy and vasodilation on coronary blood flow and myocardial energetics in non-ischemic congestive heart failure. J Am Coll Cardiol 1:499, 1983.
13. Leier, CV, Webel, J, and Bush, CA: The cardiovascular effects of the continuous infusion of dobutamine in patients with severe cardiac failure.Circulation 56:468, 1977.
14. Unverferth, DV, Magorien, RD, Altschuld, R, et al: The hemodynamic and metabolic advantages gained by a three-day infusion of dobutamine in patients with congestive cardiomyopathy. Am Heart J 106:29, 1983.
15. Leier, CV, Unverferth, DV, and Kates, RE: The relationship between plasma dobutamine concentrations and cardiovascular responses in cardiac failure. Am J Med 66:238, 1979.
16. Kates, RE and Leier, CV: Dobutamine pharmacokinetics in severe heart failure. Clin Pharmacol Ther 24:537, 1978.
17. Unverferth, DV, Blanford, M, and Kates, RE: Tolerance to dobutamine after a 72-hour continuous infusion. Am J Med 69:262, 1980.
18. Lefkowitz, RJ, Caron, MG, and Stiles, GL: Mechanisms of membrane-receptor regulation. N Engl J Med 310:1570, 1984.
19. Unverferth, DV, Magorien, RD, Lewis, RP, et al.: Long-term benefit of dobutamine in patients with congestive cardiomyopathy. Am Heart J 100:622, 1980.
20. Goldman, L, Hashimoto, B, Cook, EF, et al: Comparative reproducibility and validity of systems for assessing cardiovascular functional class: Advantages of a new specific activity scale. Circulation 64:1227, 1981.
21. Goldman, L, Cook, EF, Mitchell, N, et al: Pitfalls in the serial assessment of cardiac functional status. J Chron Dis 35:763, 1982.
22. Liang, C, Sherman, LG, Doherty, JU, et al: Sustained improvement of cardiac function in patients with congestive heart failure after short-term infusion of dobutamine. Circulation 69:113, 1984.
23. Unverferth, DV, Leier, CV, Magorien, RD, et al: Improvement of human myocardial mitochondria after dobutamine: A quantitative ultrastructural study. J Pharmacol Exp Ther 215:527, 1980.
24. Liang, C, Tuttle, RR, Hood, WB, et al: Conditioning effects of chronic infusions of dobutamine— Comparison with exercise training. J Clin Invest 64:613, 1979.

25. Sullivan, MJ, Binkley, PF, Unverferth, DV, et al: Prevention of bedrest-induced physical deconditioning by daily dobutamine infusions: Implications for drug-induced physical conditioning. J Clin Invest 76:1632, 1985.

26. Sullivan, MJ, Higginbotham, MB, and Cobb, FR: Exercise training in patients with severe left ventricular dysfunction: Hemodynamic and metabolic effects. Circulation 78:506, 1988.

27. Applefeld, MM, Newman, KA, Grove, WR, et al: Intermittent, continuous outpatient dobutamine infusion in the management of congestive heart failure. Am J Cardiol 51:455, 1983.

28. Berger, M and McSherry, CK: Outpatient dobutamine infusion using a totally implantable infusion pump for refractory congestive heart failure. Chest 88:295, 1985.

29. Hodgson, JM, Aja, M, and Sorkin, RP: Intermittent ambulatory dobutamine infusions for patients awaiting cardiac transplantation. Am J Cardiol 53:375, 1984.

30. Krell, MJ, Kline, EM, Bates, ER, et al: Intermittent, ambulatory dobutamine infusions in patients with severe congestive heart failure. Am Heart J 112:787, 1986.

31. Applefeld, MM, Newman, KA, Sutton, FJ, et al: Outpatient dobutamine and dopamine infusions in the management of chronic heart failure: Clinical experience in 21 patients. Am Heart J 114:589, 1987.

32. Dies, F, Krell, MJ, Whitlow, P, et al: Intermittent dobutamine in ambulatory outpatients with chronic cardiac failure. Circulation 74 (Suppl II):38, 1986.

33. Leier, CV, Huss, P, Lewis, RP, et al: Drug-induced conditioning in congestive heart failure. Circulation 65:1382, 1982.

34. Massie, B, Ports, T, Chatterjee, K, et al: Long-term vasodilator therapy for heart failure: Clinical Response and its relationship to hemodynamic measurements. Circulation 63:269, 1981.

35. Franciosa, JA, Wilen, M, Ziesche, S, et al: Survival in men with severe chronic left ventricular failure due to either coronary heart disease or idiopathic dilated cardiomyopathy. Am J Cardiol 51:831, 1983.

36. Wilson, JR, Schwartz, JS, St. John Stutton, M, et al: Prognosis in severe heart failure: Relation to hemodynamic measurements and ventricular ectopic activity. J Am Coll Cardiol 2:403, 1983.

37. Cohn, JN, Levine, TB, Olivari, MT, et al: Plasma norepinephrine as a guide to prognosis in patients with chronic congestive heart failure. N Engl J Med 311:819, 1984.

38. Cohn, JN, Archibald, DG, Ziesche, S, et al: Effect of vasodilator therapy on mortality in chronic congestive heart failure: Results of a Veterans Administration cooperative study (V-HeFT). N Engl J Med 314:1547, 1986.

39. The Consensus Trial Study Group: Effects of enalapril on mortality in severe congestive heart failure: Results of the Cooperative North Scandinavian Enalapril Survival Study. N Engl J Med 316:1429, 1987.

40. Anversa, P, Olivetti, G, Melissari, M, et al: Stereological measurement of cellular and subcellular hypertrophy and hyperplasia in the papillary muscle of adult rat. J Mol Cell Cardiol 12:781, 1980.

41. Pool, PE, Spann, JF, Buccino, RA, et al: Myocardial high energy phosphate stores in cardiac hypertrophy and heart failure. Circ Res 21:365, 1967.

42. Katz, AM: Potential deleterious effects of inotropic agents in the therapy of chronic heart failure. Circulation 73 (Suppl III):184, 1986.

43. Katz, AM: Cellular mechanisms in congestive heart failure. Am J Cardiol 62:3A, 1988.

44. Podzuweit, T, Lubbe, WF, and Opie, LH: Cyclic adenosine monophosphate, ventricular fibrillation and antiarrhythmic drugs. Lancet 1:341, 1976.

Commentary

By Melvin D. Cheitlin, M.D.

In the last half century the treatment of the patient with congestive heart failure has progressed from bedrest, digitalis, and a salt-free diet as our only courses of treatment, to a multiplicity of drugs and surgical approaches including cardiac transplantation. These new therapeutic modalities have markedly improved and extended life. The road ends now in sudden death or refractory heart failure, and it is at these termini, short of transplantation, that we still look for medications to extend life—even a little. The observation that dobutamine, a sympathetic adrenergic receptor agonist, not only could improve cardiac function in patients with refractory heart failure while being given acutely but also might have an extended effect long after the five half-life elimination period of 15 to 20 minutes has stimulated a great deal of interest in intermittent dobutamine infusions.

Many uncontrolled studies have indicated improvement in symptoms and even fewer hospitalizations for heart failure than before the intermittent infusions were given; however, when objective data for continued, sustained improvement in ventricular function are sought, there is little evidence that this symptomatic improvement can be explained by the dobutamine effect on ventricular function. A better explanation is either the *peripheral conditioning effect* of dobutamine, acting like exercise and physical conditioning, or else the improved conventional management secondary to more frequent visits and closer observation.

The few randomized, placebo-controlled, blinded studies of intermittent dobutamine infusion in congestive heart failure that have been done suggest little benefit except for mild symptomatic improvement and increased exercise time. The largest study, by Dies and colleagues,[1] was prematurely stopped when a disturbing trend emerged for increased mortality in the dobutamine group compared with the placebo group. In this chapter Stecy and Gunnar review the Loyola clinical experience with intermittent dobutamine infusion in outpatients. In individual patients, marked symptomatic improvement has been found, but whether this was due to the dobutamine infusion or the closer monitoring and conventional drug treatment or to other factors is not clear. The survival in this group in the first year was 35 percent, so no benefit in mortality is shown; and again the question is raised as to whether mortality has been increased.

Over a decade ago Leier and associates[2] reported the prolonged benefit of an infusion of dobutamine in patients with severe congestive heart failure. The evidence at present is that if intermittent dobutamine infusion is used, it should be employed only in a monitored setting with resuscitation capabilities immediately available, and only limited and short-lived symptomatic improvement can be hoped for. Its most useful application may be in temporarily improving the patient with severe refractory congestive heart failure who is awaiting transplantation.

REFERENCES

1. Dies, F, Krell, MJ, Whitlow, P, et al: Intermittent dobutamine in the ambulatory outpatient with chronic cardiac failure. Circulation 74 (Suppl II):38, 1986.
2. Leier, CV, Webel, J, and Bush, CA: The cardiovascular effects of a continuous infusion of dobutamine in patients with severe cardiac failure. Circulation 56:468, 1977.

CHAPTER 17

Should the Patient with Suspected Acute Dissection of the Aorta Have MRI, CAT Scan, or Aortography as the Definitive Study?

Mark W. Anderson, M.D.
Charles B. Higgins, M.D.

Acute aortic dissection is a potentially lethal condition that requires prompt and accurate diagnosis for optimal therapeutic results. If untreated, it has a mortality of approximately 36 to 72 percent at 48 hours and 90 percent at one year.[1]

Aortic dissection is thought to be related to a structural defect in or degeneration of the aortic media.[2] Hemorrhage of the vasa vasorum into the aortic media without intimal rupture has been described and may represent a precursor to dissection.[3] Thus the disease can exist without a direct luminal component.

Classically, an intimal tear allows dissection of blood through the media, ultimately resulting in the development in two channels that are separated by an intimal flap. The dissecting blood may then reenter the lumen, come to a halt, or rupture into the pericardium or periaortic tissues. Conditions associated with aortic dissection include hypertension, atherosclerosis, connective tissue diseases such as Marfan's syndrome, congenital heart disease (bicuspid aortic valve, coarctation of the aorta), pregnancy, or previous coronary artery bypass surgery.[1-4]

CLINICAL FEATURES

Clinical assessment can be difficult. The condition is encountered most frequently in males between the ages of 50 and 60 years. Females are more often affected over the age of 60.[1] Although the vast majority of patients will present with severe chest pain, the classic pattern of pain beginning in the chest and spreading down the back into the abdomen or extremities is uncommon.[5] The differentiation of acute aortic dissection from acute myocardial infarction can be challenging. Similarly, the pain may be localized primarily within the abdomen, leading to a primary consideration of an acute intra-abdominal process.[5]

293

Approximately 90 percent of patients will be hypertensive at presentation or will have a history of hypertension.[5] Physical signs such as precordial murmurs, differential blood pressures in the upper extremities, or neurologic findings in the setting of severe chest pain are helpful, especially when the electrocardiogram (ECG) shows no signs of acute myocardial infarction.[5] However, these signs are not invariably present.

In addition to diagnosing the presence of a dissection, accurate localization of the segment of aorta that is involved is crucial because both prognosis and treatment are related to the location of the dissection. Stanford type A lesions (DeBakey I and II) involve the ascending aorta and are generally treated surgically, whereas Stanford type B lesions (DeBakey III) which propagate distally from the ligamentum arteriosum, are usually treated medically.[2]

IMAGING

PLAIN FILM

The plain chest film is of limited use in evaluating a patient with a suspected dissection[6] and may in fact be normal in this setting. Although widening of the mediastinal contour is sometimes present, absence of this sign does not rule out the diagnosis inasmuch as this finding is absent in 40 to 50 percent of cases.[5] Other signs such as inward displacement of intimal calcifications, tracheal shift, or pleural effusion are even less specific.

ANGIOGRAPHY

Traditionally, angiography has provided the "gold standard" in the diagnosis of aortic dissection. Although visualization of the intimal flap between true and false lumens is the hallmark of dissection, other angiographic signs include narrowing of the true lumen by the nonopacified false channel, differential opacification of the two channels, or failure to opacify branch vessels.[7] Angiography also can define the extent of dissection, involvement of branch vessels, and the presence of aortic regurgitation. However, angiography is not without significant drawbacks, such as the need for catheterization of the already abnormal aorta and the use of contrast media in these patients who often have borderline renal function.[8] Other factors can lead to difficulties in interpreting the study. Failure to opacify the false lumen, simultaneous opacification of both channels (simulating a normal aorta), and failure to detect the intimal flap separating the two channels may lead to false-negative studies[9] (Fig. 17–1). False-positive studies also have been reported. With the advent of newer noninvasive imaging modalities such as computed axial tomography (CAT), transesophageal echocardiography (TEC), and magnetic resonance imaging (MRI), the role of angiography, especially as a screening examination, has been declining.

COMPUTED AXIAL TOMOGRAPHY

Computed axial tomography (CAT) provides a very useful, noninvasive means for evaluating the thoracic aorta and has been shown to be at least as accurate as angiography in the diagnosis of aortic dissection.[10–14] Several investigators have documented type A dissections diagnosed by CAT that were not detected on aor-

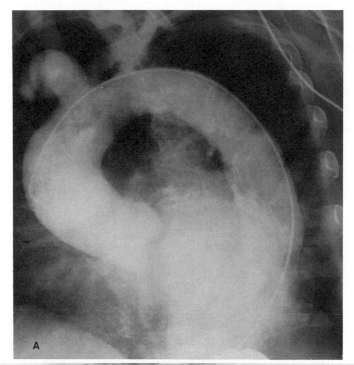

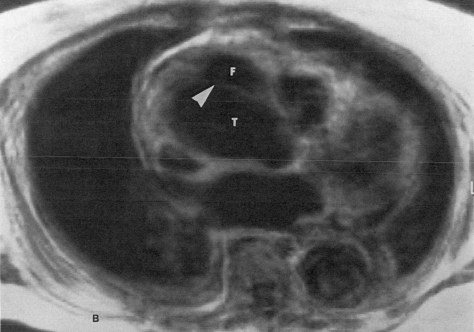

Figure 17–1. Female (age 79) with chest pain. (*A*) Aortogram (LAO projection) demonstrates aneurysmal dilation of the ascending aorta, but no evidence of intimal flap or extravasation. (*B*) ECG gated, T1 weighted transaxial MR scan at a level just above the aortic valve displays the intimal flap *(arrowhead)* separating true (T) or false (F) channels within the dilated ascending aorta. The dissecting aneurysm of the ascending aorta was confirmed at surgery.

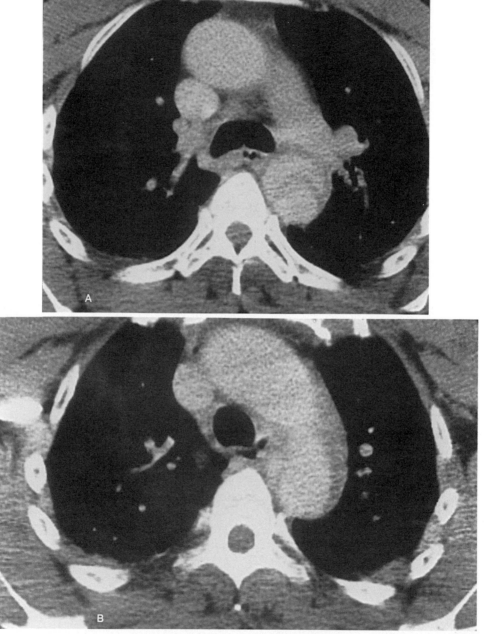

Figure 17–2. Male (age 40) presenting with chest pain and significant hypertension. (*A*) Contrast enhanced CT defines the intimal flap in the descending aorta; however, the exact point of origin of the dissection cannot be determined at the level of the arch (*B*).

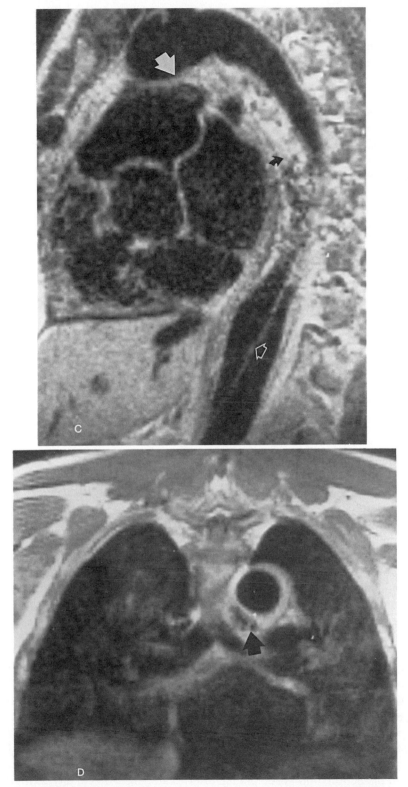

Figure 17–2. *Continued.* Sagittal (*C*) and coronal (*D*) ECG gated, T1 weighted MRI images reveal that the dissection begins at the floor of the aortic arch *(straight arrows),* well away from the brachiocephalic vessels. Note the flow artifact in false channel, *(curved arrow)* and intimal flap in distal thoracic aorta *(open arrow).*

tography.[12,15] Because of its superb contrast resolution, mediastinal structures are clearly defined, and with the use of intravenous contrast media, definition of the true and false channels, the intimal flap, and aortic wall thickness can be obtained. Differential opacification of the two channels, related to differences in flow, may also be helpful in diagnosis. Inward displacement of intimal calcifications, widening of the aorta, or fluid in the pericardial or pleural spaces are supportive but less specific signs. Computed axial tomography also has proven to be extremely useful in the follow-up of chronic dissections and in patients who have undergone previous surgical repair.[15-17] Patency or thrombosis of the false channel, extension of the dissection, and progressive dilation of the aorta have all been documented.

Potential weaknesses of CAT include its limitation to the transaxial plane as well as its reliance on an adequate bolus of intravenous contrast material (Fig. 17-2). Although detection of the intimal flap on noncontrast-enhanced scans has been reported,[18] contrast media are routinely required with their inherent risks of allergic reaction or impairment of renal function in this population of patients, who often have borderline renal function due to chronic hypertension. Interpretive pitfalls can occur secondary to streak artifacts[13] or extra-aortic structures that may resemble a false channel such as the superior pericardial recess, the left superior intercostal vein, or the left pulmonary vein.[19] Also, the distinction between a fusiform aneurysm of the aorta and a dissection with thrombus in the false channel can be very difficult.[20]

ECHOCARDIOGRAPHY

Two-dimensional echocardiography has been advocated as a useful adjunct in the noninvasive evaluation of aortic dissection.[21-23] It is relatively inexpensive, noninvasive, and does not require contrast media. The ascending aorta can be evaluated using a left parasternal approach or through the second right intercostal space. By imaging through the suprasternal notch, the aortic arch can be visualized, and evaluation of the descending aorta is performed via the left parasternal or subcostal approach.[2] Two-dimensional echocardiography has been shown to be reliable in demonstrating involvement of the ascending aorta, and aortic regurgitation or pericardial effusion also can be detected with this modality.[22] Color-flow Doppler echocardiography may provide some information about the flow dynamics of the true and false channels.[24]

Drawbacks of echocardiography include a limited field of view, lack of visualization of branch vessels, and the need for optimal technical performance of the scan, which is not possible in some patients. False-positive and false-negative results do occur.

Transesophageal echocardiography has been advocated recently in this setting to provide a more detailed look at the aorta.[25] However, this is technically more difficult to perform and requires a greater degree of patient cooperation, which may not be feasible in the acute setting. Moreover, it has an even more limited field of view than standard echocardiography. Because large segments of the aorta are involved with dissection, and aortic branch arteries are jeopardized, any technique with such a limited field of view is not optimal for the comprehensive evaluation of aortic dissection.

MAGNETIC RESONANCE IMAGING

Magnetic resonance imaging (MRI) has proven to be very accurate in the evaluation of thoracic aortic disease and in particular in the diagnosis of acute aortic dissection.[26-31] Exquisite depiction of both intraluminal and extraluminal aortic anatomy is possible without the use of contrast material. The protons within rapidly flowing blood exit the imaging plane prior to giving off any signal, resulting in a black *flow void* within the vessel when the spin echo technique is used (Fig. 17–3). The intimal flap, the hallmark of dissection, is seen as a thin linear structure of medium signal intensity separating the true and false channels (Fig. 17–4). Because slowly flowing blood (as within a false channel) will give off some signal, information regarding differential flow velocities is also provided (Fig. 17–5). Slowly flowing blood sometimes may be differentiated from intraluminal thrombus by its characteristic increase in signal intensity on second echo images.[8] Other techniques, such as phase images[32] or rotating gated studies,[8] can be helpful in this differentiation (Fig. 17–6 A and B). Images can be obtained directly in virtually any plane—a feature that may better define any branch vessel involvement.

A complete scan can be obtained in 30 to 45 minutes. Electrocardiogram gating is utilized to eliminate phase-encoding artifacts from cardiac motion. Motion artifacts from breathing also can be suppressed through reordering of the phase-encoding gradients.[33]

In a recent study of 54 patients with suspected aortic dissections, the sensitivity of MRI ranged from 96 to 100 percent at specificity levels of 90 and 95 percent, respectively.[8] In the vast majority of dissections, the intimal flap was well seen and the diagnosis was made with certainty.

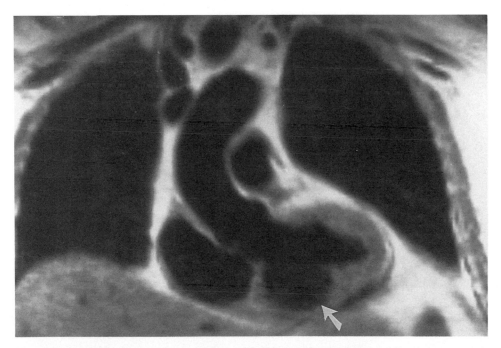

Figure 17–3. Rapidly flowing blood results in a dark *flow void* within the ascending aorta, and main pulmonary artery. A left ventricular aneurysm is also demonstrated *(arrow).*

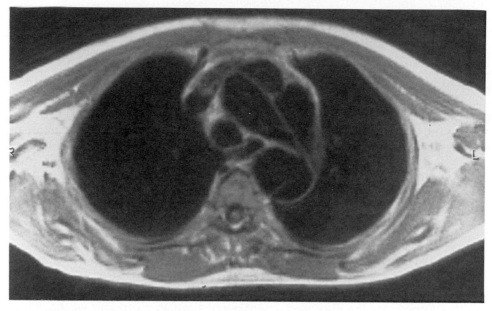

Figure 17–4. Stanford type A aortic dissection with a complex intimal flap involving both ascending and descending aorta.

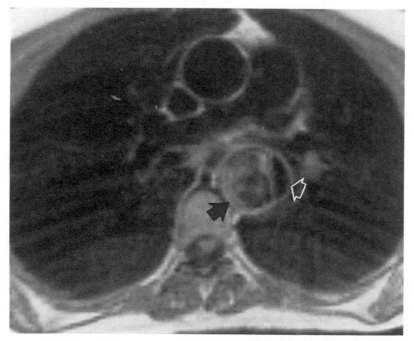

Figure 17–5. Increased signal due to slow flow within the false lumen *(arrow)* of a Stanford type B dissection *(open arrow* = true lumen).

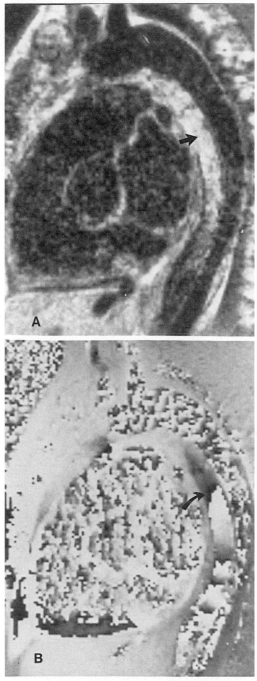

Figure 17–6. Type B dissection with increased signal in false channel *(A straight arrow)* shown to be due to slow flow rather than thrombus on subsequent phase image. *(B curved arrow).* (Same patient as in Fig. 17–2.)

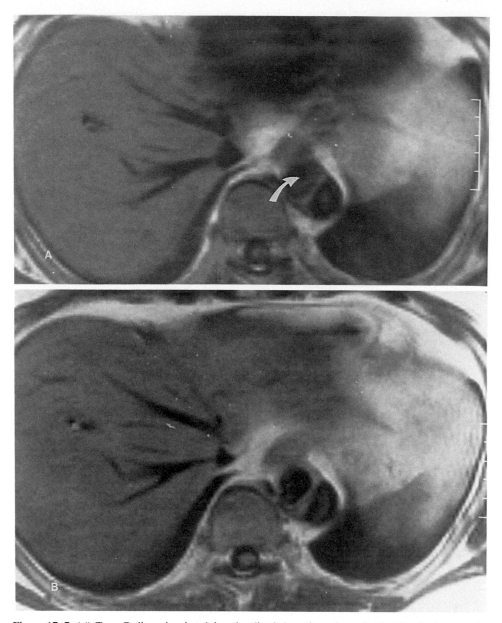

Figure 17–7. (*A*) Type B dissection involving the distal thoracic and proximal abdominal aorta with thrombus and central flow (*curved arrow*) in false channel. (*B*) Follow-up study seven months later reveals no change in the appearance of the false channel.

Both MRI and CAT also have been shown to be of value in detecting intramural hemorrhage without an associated intimal tear—the so-called aortic dissection without intimal rupture.[3] This is thought to be related to hemorrhage of the vasa vasorum within the wall of the aorta and may be a precursor of true dissection. Hematoma has a characteristic signal intensity in MRI; it causes high signal intensity on T1 weighted images. Thus, the early stage of aortic dissection can be detected by MRI; however, because there is no luminal component to this stage of the disease, angiography is useless.

Magnetic resonance imaging has also been shown to be an accurate, noninvasive method for follow-up of chronic aortic dissections[34] (Fig. 17-7). No contrast medium is needed, thus providing a clear advantage over CAT in this setting.

A potential weakness of the technique is that the status of the aortic valve cannot be determined with conventional MRI. However, this can usually be evaluated intraoperatively without compromising the surgical result.[35] Also, some patients cannot be studied with MRI. Pacemakers, intracranial aneurysm clips, and retained intraocular metallic fragments are clear contraindications. Random patient motion can degrade the images, and if a patient is unable to cooperate, the study most likely will be of suboptimal quality.

There is a common fallacy that patients requiring monitoring or with multiple intravenous lines cannot be studied by MRI. In general, we have not found this to be a significant problem. With any critical or sedated patient, we require that a physician or nurse remain in the room during scanning. Mechanical infusion pumps can usually be used or the drip can be set to a *to keep open* rate or monitored visually for the duration of the scan. Pulse rate and oxygenation can be monitored via a pulse oximeter, which will suffice during scanning in most cases. Oxygen is available from a wall port if required.

CONCLUSION

Whereas the three noninvasive modalities discussed have a somewhat complimentary relationship, each with certain strengths and weaknesses, MRI appears to provide the maximum diagnostic information with the minimum risk to the patient when ruling out an acute aortic dissection. Its wide field of view, multiplanar capability, and exquisite tissue contrast and precise definition of intravascular anatomy without the need of a contrast agent make it an ideal modality for evaluating this clinical dilemma. The ability to accomplish MRI rapidly in a period of 30 minutes or less may be critical. Moreover, the potential nephrotoxicity of contrast media must be a consideration in patients with hemodynamic stresses (acute dissection and imminent cardiopulmonary bypass) superimposed upon reduced renal reserve. One may find the use of contrast media in this setting to be indefensible when a completely noninvasive diagnostic modality is available. Therefore, MRI should be the examination of choice in this setting, with angiography and the other noninvasive tests assuming a secondary, problem-solving role.

REFERENCES

1. Anagnostopoulos, C, Prabhakar, M, and Kittle, C: Aortic dissection and dissecting aneurysms. Am J Cardiol 30:263, 1972.
2. Wechsler, R, Kotler, M, and Steiner, R: Multimodality approach to thoracic aortic dissection. Cardiovasc Clin 17:385, 1986.
3. Yamada, T, Tada, S, and Harada, J: Aortic dissection without intimal rupture: Diagnosis with MR imaging and CT. Radiology 168:347, 1988.
4. Thorsen, M, Goodman, L, Sagel, S, et al: Ascending aorta complications of cardiac surgery: CT evaluation. J Comput Assist Tomagr 10:219, 1986.
5. Wheat, M: Acute dissection of the aorta. Cardiovasc Clin 17:241, 1987.
6. Jagannath, A, Sos, T, and Lockhart, S: Aortic dissection: A statistical analysis of the usefulness of plain chest radiographic findings. AJR 147:1123, 1986.
8. Kersting-Sommerhoff, B, Higgins, CB, White, R, et al: Aortic dissection: Sensitivity and specificity of MR imaging. Radiology 166:651, 1988.

9. Shuford, W, Sybers, R, and Weens, H: Problems in the aortographic diagnosis of dissecting aneurysms of the aorta. N Engl J Med 280:225, 1969.

10. Thorsen, M, Lawson, T, and Foley, W: CT of aortic dissections. CRC Crt Rev Diagn Imaging 26:291, 1986.

11. Thorsen, M, San Dretto, M, Lawson, T, et al: Dissecting aortic aneurysms: Accuracy of computed tomographic diagnosis. Radiology 148:773, 1983.

12. Oudkerk, M, Overbosch, E, and Dee, P: CT recognition of acute aortic dissection. AJR 141:671, 1983.

13. Vasile, N. Mathieu, D, Keita, K. et al: Computed tomography of thoracic aortic dissection: Accuracy and pitfalls. J Comput Assist Tomogr 10:211, 1986.

14. White, R, Lipton, M, Higgins, CB, et al: Noninvasive evaluation of suspected thoracic aortic diseases by contrast enhanced computed tomography. Am J Cardiol 57:282, 1986.

15. Godwin, J, Turley, K, Herfkens, R, et al: Computed tomography for follow-up of chronic aortic dissections. Radiology 139:655, 1981.

16. Mathieu, D, Keita, K, Loisanc, D: Postoperative CT follow up of aortic dissection. J Comput Assist Tomogr 10:216, 1986.

17. Yamaguchi, T, Naito, K, Loisance, D, et al: False lumens in type III aortic dissections: Progress CT study. Radiology 156:757, 1985.

18. Demos, T, Posniak H, and Churchill R: Detection of the intimal flap of aortic dissection on unenhanced CT images. AJR 146:601, 1986.

19. Chiles, C, Baker, M, and Silverman, P: Superior pericardial recess simulating aortic dissection on computed tomography. J Comput Assist Tomogr 10:421, 1986.

20. Heiberg, E. Wolverson, M, Sundaram, M. et al: CT characteristics of atherosclerotic aneurysm versus aortic dissection. J Comput Assist Tomogr 9:78, 1985.

21. De Maria, A, Bommer, W, Neuman, A, et al: Identification of aneurysms of the ascending aorta by cross-sectional echocardiography. Circulation 59:755, 1979.

22. Victor, M, Mintz, G, Kotler, M, et al: Two dimensional echocardiographic diagnosis of aortic dissection. Am J Cardiol 48:1155, 1981.

23. Goldman, A, Kotler, M, Scanlon,M, et al: Magnetic resonance imaging and two dimensional echocardiography: Alternative approach to aortography in diagnosis of aortic dissecting aneurysm. Am J Med 80:1225, 1986.

24. Ileceto, S, Nanda, W, Rizzon, P, et al: Color Doppler evaluation of aortic dissection. Circulation 75:748, 1987.

25. Mohr-Kahaly, S, Erbel, R, Steller, D, et al: Aortic dissection detected by transesophageal echocardiography. Int J Card Imaging 2: 31, 1986–87.

26. Amparo, E, Higgins, CB, Hoddick, E, et al: Magnetic resonance imaging of aortic disease: Preliminary results. AJR 143:1203, 1984.

27. Amparo, E, Higgins, CB, Hricak,H, et al: Aortic dissection: Magnetic resonance imaging. Radiology 155:399, 1985.

28. Geisinger, M, Risius, B, O'Donnell, J, et al: Thoracic aortic dissections: Magnetic resonance imaging. Radiology 155:40-7, 1985.

29. Glazer, H, Gutierrez, F. Levitt, R, et al: The thoracic aorta studied by MR imaging. Radiology 157:149, 1985.

30. Dinsmore, RE, Liberthson, RR, Wismer, GL, et al: Magnetic resonance imaging of thoracic aortic aneurysms: Comparisons with other imaging methods. AJR 146:309, 1986.

31. Kersting-Sommerhoff, B, Sechtem, U, Schiller, N, et al: MR imaging of the thoracic aorta in Marfan patients. J Comput Assist Tomogr 11:633, 1987.

32. Dinsmore, R, Wedeen, V, Miller, S, et al: MRI of dissection of the aorta: Recognition of the intimal tear and differential flow velocities. AJR 146:1286, 1986.

33. Bailes, D, Gilderdale, D, Bydder, G, et al: Respiratory ordered phase encoding (ROPE): A method for reducing respiratory motion artifacts in MR imaging. J Comput Assist Tomogr 9:835, 1985.

34. Pernes,J, Grenier, P, Desbleds, M, et al: MR evaluation of chronic aortic dissection. J Comput Assist Tomogr 11:975, 1987.

35. Miller, D, Stinson, E, Oyer, P, et al: Operative treatment of aortic dissections: Experience with 125 patients over a sixteen year period. J Thorac Cardiovasc Surg 78:365, 1979.

Commentary

by Melvin D. Cheitlin, M.D.

Anderson and Higgins have described the qualities of magnetic resonance imaging (MRI) that theoretically make it the diagnostic modality of choice in acute aortic dissection. There is no question that, with the newest technology allowing rapid scans, MRI scanning in a hospital with appropriate facilities and technical support is as rapidly performed as any technique, including aortography. Magnetic resonance imaging also has the advantage over a computerized axial tomography (CAT) scan and aortography in that it needs no contrast material. This is most helpful in patients with compromised renal function. If a CAT scan was done first and the study was inconclusive, later cardiac catheterization and aortography are limited because of the amount of contrast agent that has already been used.

Because motion artifact is a problem in CAT scan and NMR scan and because patients with suspected aortic dissection are acutely ill patients in pain, not infrequently a less than good technical study is obtained. This obviously would be less of a problem in the patient with a chronic aortic dissection. Also, I would not lightly dismiss the isolation of the acutely ill patient in an MRI facility. Because of the strong magnetic field generated, these facilities are frequently in less accessible places in the hospital than usual, and with the patient in a magnetic coil and frequently not easily observed, it would be very difficult to run a code in an arrested patient in these circumstances.

The question of false-positive and false-negative studies is not well described. In the study done by Kersting-Sommerhoff and colleagues[1] at the University of California at San Francisco although the patients were suspected of having aortic dissections, many had suspected old dissections or had atherosclerotic aortic anuerysm. Most of the atherosclerotic aneurysms were not operated upon, and therefore the *true* diagnosis is not known with certainty. Because acute aortic dissections have thin intimal flaps and the false lumen may not be dilated, it is possible that some dissections could have been missed and the figures given may be incorrect.

Sensitivity is not 100 percent for any study, so one cannot be sure that acute dissection has really been ruled out. Even with specificity of 90 to 95 percent, there are 5 to 10 percent false-negative studies. Therefore, a negative MRI cannot rule out the possibility of acute dissection. Because this can also happen in aortography, these techniques are complementary, and one should be able and willing to perform another technique to avoid missing acute dissections if the clinical suspicion for dissection is high enough.

Certainly the large field that MRI, CAT scans, and aortography have over echo-Doppler is important when comparing these techniques for use in acute aortic dissection. With echo-Doppler only the proximal ascending aorta, and with trans-esophageal echo-Doppler a good length of the descending aorta, can be visualized. However, if the echo-Doppler clearly shows an intimal flap and if one can be certain the dissection involves the ascending aorta, then it is questionable what aortography could add. Certainly with aortography it is possible to identify involvement of the coronary arteries, the severity of aortic valve incompetence, and which aortic branches are involved. However, what the surgeon really needs to know is whether the ascending aorta is involved, because a midsternal thoracotomy is necessary if it is involved. It really appears that the technique done in an acute situation—aortography or MRI or CAT scan—depends upon the facility, the availability of technical assistance at any hour of the day or night, as well as on the surgeon's confidence that a diagnosis can be accurately made on the basis of a non-invasive study.

REFERENCES

1. Kersting-Sommerhott, B, Higgins, CB, White, R, et al: Aortic dissection: Sensitivity and specificity of MR imaging. Radiology 166:651, 1988.

Index

A page number in *italics* indicates a figure. A "t" following a page number indicates a table.